WORLD HEALTH ORGANIZATION

INTERNATIONAL AGENCY FOR RESEARCH ON CANCER

IARC MONOGRAPHS

ON THE

EVALUATION OF THE CARCINOGENIC RISK OF CHEMICALS TO HUMANS

Some Naturally Occurring and Synthetic Food Components, Furocoumarins and Ultraviolet Radiation

VOLUME 40

This publication represents the views and expert opinions
of an IARC Working Group on the
Evaluation of the Carcinogenic Risk of Chemicals to Humans
which met in Lyon,

15-22 October 1985

1986

IARC MONOGRAPHS

In 1969, the International Agency for Research on Cancer (IARC) initiated a programme on the evaluation of the carcinogenic risk of chemicals to humans involving the production of critically evaluated monographs on individual chemicals. In 1980, the programme was expanded to include the evaluation of the carcinogenic risk associated with exposures to complex mixtures.

The objective of the programme is to elaborate and publish in the form of monographs critical reviews of data on carcinogenicity for chemicals and complex mixtures to which humans are known to be exposed, and on specific occupational exposures, to evaluate these data in terms of human risk with the help of international working groups of experts in chemical carcinogenesis and related fields, and to indicate where additional research efforts are needed.

This project was supported by PHS Grant No. 2 UO1 CA33193-04 awarded by the US National Cancer Institute, Department of Health and Human Services.

CONTENTS

NOTE TO THE READER

The term 'carcinogenic risk' in the *IARC Monographs* series is taken to mean the probability that exposure to the chemical will lead to cancer in humans.

Inclusion of a chemical in the *Monographs* does not imply that it is a carcinogen, only that the published data have been examined. Equally, the fact that a chemical has not yet been evaluated in a monograph does not mean that it is not carcinogenic.

Anyone who is aware of published data that may alter the evaluation of the carcinogenic risk of a chemical to humans is encouraged to make this information available to the Unit of Carcinogen Identification and Evaluation, Division of Environmental Carcinogenesis, International Agency for Research on Cancer, 150 cours Albert Thomas, 69372 Lyon Cedex 08, France, in order that the chemical may be considered for re-evaluation by a future Working Group.

Although every effort is made to prepare the monographs as accurately as possible, mistakes may occur. Readers are requested to communicate any errors to the Unit of Carcinogen Identification and Evaluation, so that corrections can be reported in future volumes.

IARC WORKING GROUP ON THE EVALUATION OF THE CARCINOGENIC RISK OF CHEMICALS TO HUMANS: SOME NATURALLY OCCURRING AND SYNTHETIC FOOD COMPONENTS, FUROCOUMARINS AND ULTRAVIOLET RADIATION

Lyon, 15-22 October 1985

Members

C.F. Arlett, MRC Cell Mutation Unit, University of Sussex, Falmer, Brighton BN1 9RR, UK

B.K. Armstrong, NH & MRC Unit in Epidemiology and Preventive Medicine, University Department of Medicine, The Queen Elizabeth II Medical Centre, Nedlands, Western Australia 6009 (*Chairman*)

P.K.C. Austwick, Occupational Health Unit, The Robens Institute of Industrial and Environmental Health and Safety, University of Surrey, Guildford, Surrey GU2 5XH, UK

D. Averbeck, Section de Biologie, Institut Curie, 26 rue d'Ulm, 75231 Paris Cedex 05, France

R. Bass, Institut für Arzneimittel des Bundesgesundheitsamtes, Postfach 330013, 1000 Berlin (West) 33, Federal Republic of Germany

V. Beral, Epidemiological Monitoring Unit, London School of Hygiene and Tropical Medicine, Keppel Street, London WC1E 7HT, UK

F. Dall'Aqua, Department of Pharmaceutical Sciences, Padova University, via Marzolo 5, 35131 Padova, Italy

E.A. Emmett, Johns Hopkins University, Center for Occupational and Environmental Health, Building 6, 3100 Wyman Parks Drive, Baltimore, MD 21211, USA

J.W. Grisham, Chapel Hill Preclinical Educational Building 228H, University of North Carolina, Chapel Hill, NC 27514, USA

C.A. van der Heijden, Laboratory for Carcinogenesis and Mutagenesis, National Institute of Public Health, Antonie van Leeuwenhoeklaan 9, PO Box 1, 3720 BA Bilthoven, The Netherlands

J.E. Huff, National Toxicology Program, US Public Health Service, PO Box 12233, Research Triangle Park, NC 27709, USA

N. Ito, First Department of Pathology, Nagoya City University Medical School, Kawasumi Mizuhi-cho, Mizuho-ku, Nagoya 467, Japan

I. Knudsen, Institute of Toxicology, National Food Institute, 19 Mørkhøj Bygade, 2860 Søborg, Denmark

M. Nagao, National Cancer Center Research Institute, Tsukiji 5-chome, Chuo-ku, Tokyo 104, Japan

J. Rafter, Department of Medical Nutrition, Karolinska Institute, Huddinge University Hospital F69, 14186 Huddinge, Sweden

D.C.G. Skegg, University of Otago Medical School, PO Box 913, Dunedin, New Zealand

F. Stenbäck, Nordic Council for Arctic Medical Research, Aapistie 3, 90220 Oulu 22, Finland

G.M. Williams, Naylor Dana Institute for Disease Prevention, American Health Foundation, Valhalla, NY 10595, USA (*Vice-chairman*)

A.R. Young, Department of Photobiology, The Institute of Dermatology, Homerton Grove, London E9 6BX, UK

F. Zajdela, Unité de Physiologie Cellulaire, Institut National de la Santé et de la Recherche Médicale, Bâtiment 110 (Institut Curie), 91405 Orsay, France

G. Zetterberg, Department of Genetics, University of Uppsala, Box 7003, 75007 Uppsala, Sweden

Representative of the National Cancer Institute

S.S. Thorgeirsson, Laboratory of Experimental Carcinogenesis, Division of Cancer Etiology, National Cancer Institute, Building 37, Room 3B25, Bethesda, MD 20892, USA

Representative of Tracor Jitco, Inc.

S. Olin, Tracor Jitco, Inc., 1601 Research Boulevard, Rockville, MD 20850, USA

Representative of the International Programme on Chemical Safety

G. Vettorazzi, International Programme on Chemical Safety, Division of Environmental Carcinogenesis, World Health Organization, 1211 Geneva 27, Switzerland

Observers[1]

Representative of the Food and Drug Administration

R.J. Scheuplein, Center for Food Safety and Applied Nutrition, Food and Drug Administration, Washington DC 20204, USA

---

[1]Unable to attend: J.L. Emerson, External Technical Affairs Department, The Coca-Cola Company, PO Drawer 1734, Atlanta, GA 30301, USA

Representative of the National Institute of Hygienic Sciences

M. Hayashi, Department of Mutagenesis, Biological Safety Research Center, National Institute of Hygienic Sciences, 1-18-1 Kami-Yooga, Setagaya-ku, Tokyo 158, Japan

Secretariat

H. Bartsch, Division of Environmental Carcinogenesis

J.R.P. Cabral, Division of Environmental Carcinogenesis

B. Dodet, Division of Environmental Carcinogenesis

M. Friesen, Division of Environmental Carcinogenesis

L. Haroun, Division of Environmental Carcinogenesis (*Co-secretary*)

E. Heseltine, Editorial and Publications Services

J. Kaldor, Division of Epidemiology and Biostatistics

B. McKnight[1], Division of Epidemiology and Biostatistics

D. Mietton, Division of Environmental Carcinogenesis

R. Montesano, Division of Environmental Carcinogenesis

I. O'Neill, Division of Environmental Carcinogenesis

C. Partensky, Division of Environmental Carcinogenesis

I. Peterschmitt, Division of Environmental Carcinogenesis, Geneva, Switzerland

S. Poole, Birmingham, UK

R. Saracci, Division of Epidemiology and Biostatistics

L. Shuker, Division of Environmental Carcinogenesis

L. Simonato, Division of Epidemiology and Biostatistics

L. Tomatis, Director

A. Tossavainen, Division of Environmental Carcinogenesis

H. Vainio, Division of Environmental Carcinogenesis (*Head of the Programme*)

J.D. Wilbourn, Division of Environmental Carcinogenesis (*Co-secretary*)

H. Yamasaki, Division of Environmental Carcinogenesis

Secretarial assistance

J. Cazeaux

M.-J. Ghess

M. Lézère

A.-M. Maillol

M. Mainaud

S. Reynaud

---

[1]Present address: University of Washington, Department of Biostatistics SC-32, Seattle, WA 98195, USA

PREAMBLE

IARC MONOGRAPHS PROGRAMME ON THE EVALUATION OF THE CARCINOGENIC RISK OF CHEMICALS TO HUMANS[1]

PREAMBLE

1. BACKGROUND

In 1969, the International Agency for Research on Cancer (IARC) initiated a programme to evaluate the carcinogenic risk of chemicals to humans and to produce monographs on individual chemicals. Following the recommendations of an ad-hoc Working Group, which met in Lyon in 1979 to prepare criteria to select chemicals for *IARC Monographs*(1), the *Monographs* programme was expanded to include consideration of exposures to complex mixtures which may occur, for example, in many occupations or as a result of human habits.

The criteria established in 1971 to evaluate carcinogenic risk to humans were adopted by all the working groups whose deliberations resulted in the first 16 volumes of the *IARC Monographs* series. This preamble reflects subsequent re-evaluation of those criteria by working groups which met in 1977(2), 1978(3), 1982(4) and 1983(5).

2. OBJECTIVE AND SCOPE

The objective of the programme is to elaborate and publish in the form of monographs critical reviews of data on carcinogenicity for chemicals, groups of chemicals, industrial processes and other complex mixtures to which humans are known to be exposed, to evaluate the data in terms of human risk with the help of international working groups of experts, and to indicate where additional research efforts are needed. These evaluations are intended to assist national and international authorities in formulating decisions concerning preventive measures. No recommendation is given concerning legislation, since this depends on risk-benefit evaluations, which seem best made by individual governments and/or other international agencies.

---

[1]This project is supported by PHS Grant No. 2 U01 CA33193-04 awarded by the US National Cancer Institute, Department of Health and Human Services.

The *IARC Monographs* are recognized as an authoritative source of information on the carcinogenicity of environmental and other chemicals. A users' survey, made in 1984, indicated that the monographs are consulted by various agencies in 45 countries. As of June 1986, 40 volumes of the *Monographs* had been published or were in press. Five supplements have been published: two summaries of evaluations of chemicals associated with human cancer, an evaluation of screening assays for carcinogens, and two cross indexes of synonyms and trade names of chemicals evaluated in the series(6).

3. SELECTION OF CHEMICALS AND COMPLEX EXPOSURES FOR MONOGRAPHS

The chemicals (natural and synthetic including those which occur as mixtures and in manufacturing processes) and complex exposures are selected for evaluation on the basis of two main criteria: (a) there is evidence of human exposure, and (b) there is some experimental evidence of carcinogenicity and/or there is some evidence or suspicion of a risk to humans. In certain instances, chemical analogues are also considered. The scientific literature is surveyed for published data relevant to the *Monographs* programme; and the IARC *Survey of Chemicals Being Tested for Carcinogenicity*(7) often indicates those chemicals that may be scheduled for future meetings.

As new data on chemicals for which monographs have already been prepared become available, re-evaluations are made at subsequent meetings, and revised monographs are published.

4. WORKING PROCEDURES

Approximately one year in advance of a meeting of a working group, a list of the substances or complex exposures to be considered is prepared by IARC staff in consultation with other experts. Subsequently, all relevant biological data are collected by IARC; recognized sources of information on chemical carcinogenesis and on-line systems such as CANCERLINE, MEDLINE and TOXLINE are used in conjunction with US Public Health Service Publication No. 149(8). Bibliographical sources for data on mutagenicity and teratogenicity are the Environmental Mutagen Information Center and the Environmental Teratology Information Center, both located at the Oak Ridge National Laboratory, TN, USA.

The major collection of data and the preparation of first drafts for the sections on chemical and physical properties, on production and use, on occurrence, and on analysis are carried out by Tracor Jitco, Inc., and its subcontractor, Technical Resources, Inc., both in Rockville, MD, USA, under a separate contract with the US National Cancer Institute. Most of the data so obtained refer to the USA and Japan; IARC attempts to supplement this information with that from other sources in Europe. Representatives from industrial associations may assist in the preparation of sections describing industrial processes.

Six months before the meeting, articles containing relevant biological data are sent to an expert(s), or are used by IARC staff, to prepare first drafts of the sections on biological effects. The complete drafts are then compiled by IARC staff and sent, prior to the meeting, to all participants of the Working Group for their comments.

The Working Group meets in Lyon for seven to eight days to discuss and finalize the texts of the monographs and to formulate the evaluations. After the meeting, the master copy of each monograph is verified by consulting the original literature, edited by a professional editor and prepared for reproduction. The aim is to publish monographs within nine months of the Working Group meeting. Each volume of monographs is printed in 4000 copies for distribution to governments, regulatory agencies and interested scientists. The monographs are also available *via* the WHO Distribution and Sales Service.

These procedures are followed for the preparation of most volumes of monographs, which cover chemicals and groups of chemicals; however, they may vary when the subject matter is an industry or life-style factor.

5. DATA FOR EVALUATIONS

With regard to biological data, only reports that have been published or accepted for publication are reviewed by the working groups, although a few exceptions have been made: in certain instances, reports from government agencies that have undergone peer review and are widely available are considered. The monographs do not cite all of the literature on a particular chemical or complex exposure: only those data considered by the Working Group to be relevant to the evaluation of carcinogenic risk to humans are included.

Anyone who is aware of data that have been published or are in press which are relevant to the evaluations of the carcinogenic risk to humans of chemicals or complex exposures for which monographs have appeared is asked to make them available to the Unit of Carcinogen Identification and Evaluation, Division of Environmental Carcinogenesis, International Agency for Research on Cancer, Lyon, France.

6. THE WORKING GROUP

The tasks of the Working Group are five-fold: (a) to ascertain that all data have been collected; (b) to select the data relevant for evaluation; (c) to ensure that the summaries of the data enable the reader to follow the reasoning of the Working Group; (d) to judge the significance of the results of experimental and epidemiological studies; and (e) to make an evaluation of the carcinogenicity of the chemical or complex exposure.

Working Group participants who contributed to the consideration and evaluation of chemicals or complex exposures within a particular volume are listed, with their addresses, at the beginning of each publication. Each member serves as an individual scientist and not as a representative of any organization or government. In addition, observers are often invited from national and international agencies and industrial associations.

7. GENERAL PRINCIPLES APPLIED BY THE WORKING GROUP IN EVALUATING CARCINOGENIC RISK OF CHEMICALS OR COMPLEX MIXTURES

The widely accepted meaning of the term 'chemical carcinogenesis', and that used in these monographs, is the induction by chemicals (or complex mixtures of chemicals) of neoplasms that are not usually observed, the earlier induction of neoplasms that are commonly observed, and/or the induction of more neoplasms than are usually found —although fundamentally different mechanisms may be involved in these three situations. Etymologically, the term 'carcinogenesis' means the induction of cancer, that is, of malignant neoplasms; however, the commonly accepted meaning is the induction of various types of neoplasms or of a combination of malignant and benign tumours. In the monographs, the words 'tumour' and 'neoplasm' are used interchangeably. (In the scientific literature, the terms 'tumorigen', 'oncogen' and 'blastomogen' have all been used synonymously with 'carcinogen', although occasionally 'tumorigen' has been used specifically to denote a substance that induces benign tumours.)

(a) Experimental Evidence

(i)   *Evidence for carcinogenicity in experimental animals*

The Working Group considers various aspects of the experimental evidence reported in the literature and formulates an evaluation of that evidence.

Qualitative aspects: Both the interpretation and evaluation of a particular study as well as the overall assessment of the carcinogenic activity of a chemical (or complex mixture) involve several considerations of qualitative importance, including: (a) the experimental parameters under which the chemical was tested, including route of administration and exposure, species, strain, sex, age, etc.; (b) the consistency with which the chemical has been shown to be carcinogenic, e.g., in how many species and at which target organ(s); (c) the spectrum of neoplastic response, from benign neoplasm to multiple malignant tumours; (d) the stage of tumour formation in which a chemical may be involved: some chemicals act as complete carcinogens and have initiating and promoting activity, while others may have promoting activity only; and (e) the possible role of modifying factors.

There are problems not only of differential survival but of differential toxicity, which may be manifested by unequal growth and weight gain in treated and control animals. These complexities are also considered in the interpretation of data.

Many chemicals induce both benign and malignant tumours. Among chemicals that have been studied extensively, there are few instances in which the only neoplasms induced are benign. Benign tumours may represent a stage in the evolution of a malignant neoplasm or they may be 'end-points' that do not readily undergo transition to malignancy. If a substance is found to induce only benign tumours in experimental animals, it should nevertheless be suspected of being a carcinogen, and it requires further investigation.

Hormonal carcinogenesis: Hormonal carcinogenesis presents certain distinctive features: the chemicals involved occur both endogenously and exogenously; in many instances, long exposure is required; and tumours occur in the target tissue in association with a stimulation of non-neoplastic growth, although in some cases hormones promote the proliferation of tumour cells in a target organ. For hormones that occur in excessive amounts, for hormone-mimetic agents and for agents that cause hyperactivity or imbalance in the endocrine system, evaluative methods comparable with those used to identify chemical carcinogens may be required; particular emphasis must be laid on quantitative aspects and duration of exposure. Some chemical carcinogens have significant side effects on the endocrine system, which may also result in hormonal carcinogenesis. Synthetic hormones and anti-hormones can be expected to possess other pharmacological and toxicological actions in addition to those on the endocrine system, and in this respect they must be treated like any other chemical with regard to intrinsic carcinogenic potential.

Complex mixtures: There is an increasing amount of data from long-term carcinogenicity studies on complex mixtures and on crude materials obtained by sampling in occupational environments. The representativity of such samples must be considered carefully.

Quantitative aspects: Dose-response studies are important in the evaluation of carcinogenesis: the confidence with which a carcinogenic effect can be established is strengthened by the observation of an increasing incidence of neoplasms with increasing exposure.

The assessment of carcinogenicity in animals is frequently complicated by recognized differences among the test animals (species, strain, sex, age) and route and schedule of administration; often, the target organs at which a cancer occurs and its histological type may vary with these parameters. Nevertheless, indices of carcinogenic potency in particular experimental systems (for instance, the dose-rate required under continuous exposure to halve the probability of the animals remaining tumourless(9)) have been formulated in the hope that, at least among categories of fairly similar agents, such indices may be of some predictive value in other species, including humans.

Chemical carcinogens share many common biological properties, which include metabolism to reactive (electrophilic(10-11)) intermediates capable of interacting with DNA. However, they may differ widely in the dose required to produce a given level of tumour induction. The reason for this variation in dose-response is not understood, but it may be due to differences in metabolic activation and detoxification processes, in different DNA repair capacities among various organs and species or to the operation of qualitatively distinct mechanisms.

Statistical analysis of animal studies: It is possible that an animal may die prematurely from unrelated causes, so that tumours that would have arisen had the animal lived longer may not be observed; this possibility must be allowed for. Various analytical techniques have been developed which use the assumption of independence of competing risks to allow for the effects of intercurrent mortality on the final numbers of tumour-bearing animals in particular treatment groups.

For externally visible tumours and for neoplasms that cause death, methods such as Kaplan-Meier (i.e., 'life-table', 'product-limit' or 'actuarial') estimates(9), with associated significance tests(12), have been recommended. For internal neoplasms that are discovered 'incidentally'(12) at autopsy but that did not cause the death of the host, different estimates(13) and significance tests(12) may be necessary for the unbiased study of the numbers of tumour-bearing animals.

The design and statistical analysis of long-term carcinogenicity experiments were reviewed in Supplement 2 to the *Monographs* series(14). That review outlined the way in which the context of observation of a given tumour (fatal or incidental) could be included in an analysis yielding a single combined result. This method requires information on time to death for each animal and is therefore comparable to only a limited extent with analyses which include global proportions of tumour-bearing animals.

Evaluation of carcinogenicity studies in experimental animals: The evidence of carcinogenicity in experimental animals is assessed by the Working Group and judged to fall into one of four groups, defined as follows:

(1) *Sufficient evidence* of carcinogenicity is provided when there is an increased incidence of malignant tumours: (a) in multiple species or strains; or (b) in multiple experiments (preferably with different routes of administration or using different dose levels); or (c) to an unusual degree with regard to incidence, site or type of tumour, or age at onset. Additional evidence may be provided by data on dose-response effects.

(2) *Limited evidence* of carcinogenicity is available when the data suggest a carcinogenic effect but are limited because: (a) the studies involve a single species, strain or experiment; or (b) the experiments are restricted by inadequate dosage levels, inadequate duration of exposure to the agent, inadequate period of follow-up, poor survival, too few animals, or inadequate reporting; or (c) the neoplasms produced often occur spontaneously and, in the past, have been difficult to classify as malignant by histological criteria alone (e.g., lung adenomas and adenocarcinomas and liver tumours in certain strains of mice).

(3) *Inadequate evidence* of carcinogenicity is available when, because of major qualitative or quantitative limitations, the studies cannot be interpreted as showing either the presence or absence of a carcinogenic effect.

(4) *No evidence* of carcinogenicity applies when several adequate studies are available which show that, within the limits of the tests used, the chemical or complex mixture is not carcinogenic.

It should be noted that the categories *sufficient evidence* and *limited evidence* refer only to the strength of the experimental evidence that these chemicals or complex mixtures are carcinogenic and not to the extent of their carcinogenic activity nor to the mechanism involved. The classification of any chemical may change as new information becomes available.

(ii)   *Evidence for activity in short-term tests*[1]

Many short-term tests bearing on postulated mechanisms of carcinogenesis or on the properties of known carcinogens have been developed in recent years. The induction of cancer is thought to proceed by a series of steps, some of which have been distinguished experimentally (15-19). The first step — initiation — is thought to involve damage to DNA, resulting in heritable alterations in or rearrangements of genetic information. Most short-term tests in common use today are designed to evaluate the genetic activity of a substance.

---

[1]Based on the recommendations of a working group which met in 1983(5).

Data from these assays are useful for identifying potential carcinogenic hazards, in identifying active metabolites of known carcinogens in human or animal body fluids, and in helping to elucidate mechanisms of carcinogenesis. Short-term tests to detect agents with tumour-promoting activity are, at this time, insufficiently developed.

Because of the large number of short-term tests, it is difficult to establish rigid criteria for adequacy that would be applicable to all studies. General considerations relevant to all tests, however, include (a) that the test system be valid with respect to known animal carcinogens and noncarcinogens; (b) that the experimental parameters under which the chemical (or complex mixture) is tested include a sufficiently wide dose range and duration of exposure to the agent and an appropriate metabolic system; (c) that appropriate controls be used; and (d) that the purity of the compound or, in the case of complex mixtures, that the source and representativity of the sample being tested be specified. Confidence in positive results is increased if a dose-response relationship is demonstrated and if this effect has been reported in two or more independent studies.

Most established short-term tests employ as end-points well-defined genetic markers in prokaryotes and lower eukaryotes and in mammalian cell lines. The tests can be grouped according to the end-point detected:

Tests of *DNA damage*. These include tests for covalent binding to DNA, induction of DNA breakage or repair, induction of prophage in bacteria and differential survival of DNA repair-proficient/-deficient strains of bacteria.

Tests of *mutation* (measurement of heritable alterations in phenotype and/or genotype). These include tests for detection of the loss or alteration of a gene product, and change of function through forward or reverse mutation, recombination and gene conversion; they may involve the nuclear genome, the mitochondrial genome and resident viral or plasmid genomes.

Tests of *chromosomal effects*. These include tests for detection of changes in chromosome number (aneuploidy), structural chromosomal aberrations, sister chromatid exchanges, micronuclei and dominant-lethal events. This classification does not imply that some chromosomal effects are not mutational events.

Tests for *cell transformation*, which monitor the production of preneoplastic or neoplastic cells in culture, are also of importance because they attempt to simulate essential steps in cellular carcinogenesis. These assays are not grouped with those listed above since the mechanisms by which chemicals induce cell transformation may not necessarily be the result of genetic change.

The selection of specific tests and end-points for consideration remains flexible and should reflect the most advanced state of knowledge in this field.

The data from short-term tests are summarized by the Working Group and the test results tabulated according to the end-points detected and the biological complexities of the test systems. The format of the table used is shown below. In these tables, a '+' indicates that the compound was judged by the Working Group to be significantly positive in one or more assays for the specific end-point and level of biological complexity; '-' indicates that it was judged to be negative in one or more assays; and '?' indicates that there were contradictory results from different laboratories or in different biological systems, or that the result was judged to be equivocal. These judgements reflect the assessment by the Working Group of the quality of the data (including such factors as the purity of the test compound, problems of metabolic activation and appropriateness of the test system) and the relative significance of the component tests.

Overall assessment of data from short-term tests

	Genetic activity			Cell transformation
	DNA damage	Mutation	Chromosomal effects	
Prokaryotes				
Fungi/ Green plants				
Insects				
Mammalian cells (*in vitro*)				
Mammals (*in vivo*)				
Humans (*in vivo*)				

An overall assessment of the evidence for *genetic activity* is then made on the basis of the entries in the table, and the evidence is judged to fall into one of four categories, defined as follows:

(1) *Sufficient evidence* is provided by at least three positive entries, one of which must involve mammalian cells *in vitro* or *in vivo* and which must include at least two of three end-points — DNA damage, mutation and chromosomal effects.

(2) *Limited evidence* is provided by at least two positive entries.

(3) *Inadequate evidence* is available when there is only one positive entry or when there are too few data to permit an evaluation of an absence of genetic activity or when there are unexplained, inconsistent findings in different test systems.

(4) *No evidence* applies when there are only negative entries; these must include entries for at least two end-points and two levels of biological complexity, one of which must involve mammalian cells *in vitro* or *in vivo*.

It is emphasized that the above definitions are operational, and that the assignment of a chemical or complex mixture into one of these categories is thus arbitrary.

In general, emphasis is placed on positive results; however, in view of the limitations of current knowledge about mechanisms of carcinogenesis, certain cautions should be respected: (i) At present, short-term tests should not be used by themselves to conclude whether or not an agent is carcinogenic nor can they predict reliably the relative potencies of compounds as carcinogens in intact animals. (ii) Since the currently available tests do not detect all classes of agents that are active in the carcinogenic process (e.g., hormones), one must be cautious in utilizing these tests as the sole criterion for setting priorities in carcinogenesis research and in selecting compounds for animal bioassays. (iii) Negative results from short-term tests cannot be considered as evidence to rule out carcinogenicity, nor does lack of demonstrable genetic activity attribute an epigenetic or any other property to a substance (5).

(b) Evaluation of Carcinogenicity in Humans

Evidence of carcinogenicity can be derived from case reports, descriptive epidemiological studies and analytical epidemiological studies.

An analytical study that shows a positive association between an exposure and a cancer may be interpreted as implying causality to a greater or lesser extent, on the basis of the following criteria: (a) There is no identifiable positive bias. (By 'positive bias' is meant the operation of factors in study design or execution that lead erroneously to a more strongly positive association between an exposure and disease than in fact exists. Examples of positive bias include, in case-control studies, better documentation of the exposure for cases than for controls, and, in cohort studies, the use of better means of detecting cancer in exposed individuals than in individuals not exposed.) (b) The possibility of positive confounding has been considered. (By 'positive confounding' is meant a situation in which the relationship between an exposure and a disease is rendered more strongly positive than it truly is as a result of an association between that exposure and another exposure which either causes or prevents the disease. An example of positive confounding is the association between coffee consumption and lung cancer, which results from their joint association with cigarette smoking.) (c) The association is unlikely to be due to chance alone. (d) The association is strong. (e) There is a dose-response relationship.

In some instances, a single epidemiological study may be strongly indicative of a cause-effect relationship; however, the most convincing evidence of causality comes when several independent studies done under different circumstances result in 'positive' findings.

Analytical epidemiological studies that show no association between an exposure and a cancer ('negative' studies) should be interpreted according to criteria analogous to those listed above: (a) there is no identifiable negative bias; (b) the possibility of negative confounding has been considered; and (c) the possible effects of misclassification of exposure or outcome have been weighed. In addition, it must be recognized that the probability that a given study can detect a certain effect is limited by its size. This can be perceived from the confidence limits around the estimate of association or relative risk. In a study regarded as 'negative', the upper confidence limit may indicate a relative risk substantially greater than unity; in that case, the study excludes only relative risks that are above the upper limit. This usually means that a 'negative' study must be large to be convincing. Confidence in a 'negative' result is increased when several independent studies carried out under different circumstances are in agreement. Finally, a 'negative' study may be considered to be relevant only to dose levels within or below the range of those observed in the study and is pertinent only if sufficient time has elapsed since first human exposure to the agent. Experience with human cancers of known etiology suggests that the period from first exposure to a chemical carcinogen to development of clinically observed cancer is usually measured in decades and may be in excess of 30 years.

The evidence for carcinogenicity from studies in humans is assessed by the Working Group and judged to fall into one of four groups, defined as follows:

(1) *Sufficient evidence* of carcinogenicity indicates that there is a causal relationship between the exposure and human cancer.

(2) *Limited evidence* of carcinogenicity indicates that a causal interpretation is credible, but that alternative explanations, such as chance, bias or confounding, could not adequately be excluded.

(3) *Inadequate evidence* of carcinogenicity, which applies to both positive and negative evidence, indicates that one of two conditions prevailed: (a) there are few pertinent data; or (b) the available studies, while showing evidence of association, do not exclude chance, bias or confounding.

(4) *No evidence* of carcinogenicity applies when several adequate studies are available which do not show evidence of carcinogenicity.

(c) Relevance of Experimental Data to the Evaluation of Carcinogenic Risk to Humans

Information compiled from the first 40 volumes of the *IARC Monographs* shows that, of the chemicals or groups of chemicals now generally accepted to cause or probably to cause cancer in humans, all of those that have been tested appropriately produce cancer in at least one animal species. For several of the chemicals (e.g., aflatoxins, 4-aminobiphenyl, diethylstilboestrol, melphalan, mustard gas and vinyl chloride), evidence of carcinogenicity in experimental animals preceded evidence obtained from epidemiological studies or case reports.

For many of the chemicals (or complex mixtures) evaluated in the *IARC Monographs* for which there is *sufficient evidence* of carcinogenicity in animals, data relating to carcinogenicity for humans are either insufficient or nonexistent. **In the absence of adequate data on humans, it is reasonable, for practical purposes, to regard chemicals or exposures for which there is sufficient evidence of carcinogenicity in animals as if they presented a carcinogenic risk to humans.** The use of the expressions 'for practical purposes' and 'as if they presented a carcinogenic risk' indicates that, at the present time, a correlation between carcinogenicity in animals and possible human risk cannot be made on a purely scientific basis, but only pragmatically. Such a pragmatic correlation may be useful to regulatory agencies in making decisions related to the primary prevention of cancer.

In the present state of knowledge, it would be difficult to define a predictable relationship between the dose (mg/kg bw per day) of a particular chemical required to produce cancer in test animals and the dose that would produce a similar incidence of cancer in humans. Some data, however, suggest that such a relationship may exist(20,21), at least for certain classes of carcinogenic chemicals, although no acceptable method is currently available for quantifying the possible errors that may be involved in such an extrapolation procedure.

8. EXPLANATORY NOTES ON THE CONTENTS OF MONOGRAPHS ON CHEMICALS AND COMPLEX MIXTURES

These notes apply to the format of most monographs, except for those that address industries or life-style factors. Thus, sections 1 and 2, as described below, are applicable in monographs on chemicals or groups of chemicals; in other monographs, they may be replaced by sections on the history of an industry or habit, a description of a process and other relevant information.

(a) Chemical and Physical Data (Section 1)

The Chemical Abstracts Services Registry Number, the Chemical Abstracts Primary Name (Ninth Collective Index)(22) and the IUPAC Systematic Name(23) are recorded in section 1. Other synonyms and trade names are given, but the list is not necessarily comprehensive. Some of the trade names may be those of mixtures in which the compound being evaluated is only one of the ingredients.

The structural and molecular formulae, molecular weight and chemical and physical properties are given. The properties listed refer to the pure substance, unless otherwise specified, and include, in particular, data that might be relevant to identification, environmental fate and human exposure, and biological effects, including carcinogenicity.

A separate description of the composition of technical products includes available information on impurities and formulated products.

(b) Production, Use, Occurrence and Analysis (Section 2)

The purpose of section 2 is to provide indications of the extent of past and present human exposure to the chemical.

Monographs on occupational exposures to complex mixtures or exposures to complex mixtures resulting from human habits include sections on: historical perspectives; description of the industry or habit; manufacturing processes and use patterns; exposures in the workplace; chemistry of the complex mixture.

(i) *Synthesis*

Since cancer is a delayed toxic effect, the dates of first synthesis and of first commercial production of the chemical are provided. This information allows a reasonable estimate to be made of the date before which no human exposure could have occurred. In addition, methods of synthesis used in past and present commercial production are described.

(ii) *Production*

Since Europe, Japan and the USA are reasonably representative industrialized areas of the world, most data on production, foreign trade and uses are obtained from those regions. It should not, however, be inferred that those areas or nations are the sole or even necessarily the major sources or users of any individual chemical.

Production and foreign trade data are obtained from both governmental and trade publications. In some cases, separate production data on organic chemicals manufactured in the USA are not available because their publication could disclose confidential information. In such cases, an indication of the minimum quantity produced can be inferred from the number of companies reporting commercial production. Each company is required to report on individual chemicals if the annual sales value or production volume exceeds a specified minimum level. These levels vary for chemicals classified for different uses, e.g., medicinals and plastics; in fact, the minimal reportable level for annual sales value ranges from $1000-$50 000, and the minimal reportable level for annual production volume ranges from 450-22 700 kg for different classes of use. Data on production are also obtained by means of general questionnaires sent to companies thought to produce the compounds being evaluated. Information from the completed questionnaires is compiled, by country, and the resulting estimates of production are included in the individual monographs.

(iii) *Use*

Information on uses is usually obtained from published sources but is often complemented by direct contact with manufacturers. Some uses identified may not be current or major applications, and the coverage is not necessarily comprehensive. In the case of drugs, mention of their therapeutic uses does not necessarily represent current practice nor does it imply judgement as to their clinical efficacy.

Statements concerning regulations, standards and guidelines (e.g., pesticide registrations, maximum levels permitted in foods, occupational standards and allowable limits) in specific countries may not reflect the most recent situation, since such standards are continuously reviewed and modified. The absence of information on regulatory status for a country should not be taken to imply that that country does not have regulations with regard to the chemical.

(iv) *Occurrence*

Information on the occurrence of a chemical in the environment is obtained from published data, including that derived from the monitoring and surveillance of levels of the chemical in occupational environments, air, water, soil, foods and tissues of animals and humans. When no published data are available to the Working Group, unpublished reports, deemed appropriate, may be considered. When available, data on the generation, persistence and bioaccumulation of a chemical are also included.

(v)   *Analysis*

The purpose of the section on analysis is to give the reader an overview, rather than a complete list, of current methods cited in the literature. No critical evaluation or recommendation of any of the methods is meant or implied.

(c)   Biological Data Relevant to the Evaluation of Carcinogenic Risk to Humans (Section 3)

In general, the data recorded in section 3 are summarized as given by the author; however, comments made by the Working Group on certain shortcomings of reporting, of statistical analysis or of experimental design are given in square brackets. The nature and extent of impurities/contaminants in the chemicals being tested are given when available.

(i)   *Carcinogenicity studies in animals*

The monographs are not intended to cover all reported studies. A few studies are purposely omitted because they are inadequate (e.g., too short a duration, too few animals, poor survival) or because they are judged irrelevant for the purpose of the evaluation. In certain cases, however, such studies are mentioned briefly, particularly when the information is considered to be a useful supplement to other reports or when it is the only data available. Their inclusion does not, however, imply acceptance of the adequacy of their experimental design or of the analysis and interpretation of their results.

Mention is made of all routes of administration by which the test material has been adequately tested and of all species in which relevant tests have been done(24). In most cases, animal strains are given. Quantitative data are given to indicate the order of magnitude of the effective carcinogenic doses. In general, the doses and schedules are indicated as they appear in the original report; sometimes units have been converted for easier comparison. Experiments in which the compound was administered in conjunction with known carcinogens and experiments on factors that modify the carcinogenic effect are also reported. Experiments on the carcinogenicity of known metabolites and derivatives are also included.

(ii)   *Other relevant biological data*

LD_{50} data are given when available, and other data on toxicity are included when considered relevant.

Data on effects on reproduction, on teratogenicity and embryo- and fetotoxicity and on placental transfer, from studies in experimental animals and from observations in humans, are included when considered relevant.

Information is given on absorption, distribution and excretion. Data on metabolism are usually restricted to studies that show the metabolic fate of the chemical in experimental animals and humans, and comparisons of data from animals and humans are made when possible.

Data from short-term tests are also included. In addition to the tests for genetic activity and cell transformation described previously (see pages 18-19), data from studies of related effects, but for which the relevance to the carcinogenic process is less well established, may also be mentioned.

The criteria used for considering short-term tests and for evaluating their results have been described (see pages 19-21). In general, the authors' results are given as reported. An assessment of the data by the Working Group which differs from that of the authors, and comments concerning aspects of the study that might affect its interpretation are given in square brackets. Reports of studies in which few or no experimental details are given, or in which the data on which a reported positive or negative result is based are not available for examination, are cited, but are identified as 'abstract' or 'details not given' and are not considered in the summary tables or in making the overall assessment of genetic activity.

For several recent reviews on short-term tests, see IARC(24), Montesano et al.(25), de Serres and Ashby(26), Sugimura et al.(27), Bartsch et al.(28) and Hollstein et al.(29).

(iii) *Case reports and epidemiological studies of carcinogenicity to humans*

Observations in humans are summarized in this section. These include case reports, descriptive epidemiological studies (which correlate cancer incidence in space or time to an exposure) and analytical epidemiological studies of the case-control or cohort type. In principle, a comprehensive coverage is made of observations in humans; however, reports are excluded when judged to be clearly not pertinent. This applies in particular to case reports, in which either the clinico-pathological description of the tumours or the exposure history, or both, are poorly described; and to published routine statistics, for example, of cancer mortality by occupational category, when the categories are so broadly defined as to contribute virtually no specific information on the possible relation between cancer occurrence and a given exposure. Results of studies are assessed on the basis of the data and analyses that are presented in the published papers. Some additional analyses of the published data may be performed by the Working Group to gain better insight into the relation between cancer occurrence and the exposure under consideration. The Working Group may use these analyses in its assessment of the evidence or may actually include them in the text to summarize a study; in such cases, the results of the supplementary analyses are given in square brackets. Any comments by the Working Group are also reported in square brackets; however, these are kept to a minimum, being restricted to those instances in which it is felt that an important aspect of a study, directly impinging on its interpretation, should be brought to the attention of the reader.

(d) Summary of Data Reported and Evaluation (Section 4)

Section 4 summarizes the relevant data from animals and humans and gives the critical views of the Working Group on those data.

(i) *Exposures*

Human exposure to the chemical or complex mixture is summarized on the basis of data on production, use and occurrence.

(ii) *Experimental data*

Data relevant to the evaluation of the carcinogenicity of the test material in animals are summarized in this section. The animal species mentioned are those in which the carcinogenicity of the substance was clearly demonstrated. Tumour sites are also indicated. If the substance has produced tumours after prenatal exposure or in single-dose experiments, this is indicated. Dose-response data are given when available.

Significant findings on effects on reproduction and prenatal toxicity, and results from short-term tests for genetic activity and cell transformation assays are summarized, and the latter are presented in tables. An overall assessment is made of the degree of evidence for genetic activity in short-term tests.

(iii) *Human data*

Case reports and epidemiological studies that are considered to be pertinent to an assessment of human carcinogenicity are described. Other biological data that are considered to be relevant are also mentioned.

(iv) *Evaluation*

This section comprises evaluations by the Working Group of the degrees of evidence for carcinogenicity of the exposure to experimental animals and to humans. An overall evaluation is then made of the carcinogenic risk of the chemical or complex mixture to humans. This section should be read in conjunction with pages 18 and 22 of this Preamble for definitions of degrees of evidence.

When no data are available from epidemiological studies but there is *sufficient evidence* that the exposure is carcinogenic to animals, a footnote is included, reading: 'In the absence of adequate data on humans, it is reasonable, for practical purposes, to regard chemicals or exposures for which there is *sufficient evidence* of carcinogenicity in animals as if they presented a carcinogenic risk to humans' (see pp. 22-23 of this Preamble).

References

1. IARC (1979) Criteria to select chemicals for *IARC Monographs. IARC intern. tech. Rep. No. 79/003*

2. IARC (1977) IARC Monographs Programme on the Evaluation of the Carcinogenic Risk of Chemicals to Humans. Preamble. *IARC intern. tech. Rep. No. 77/002*

3. IARC (1978) Chemicals with *sufficient evidence* of carcinogenicity in experimental animals — *IARC Monographs* volumes 1-17. *IARC intern. tech. Rep. No. 78/003*

4. IARC (1982) *IARC Monographs on the Evaluation of the Carcinogenic Risk of Chemicals to Humans*, Supplement 4, *Chemicals, Industrial Processes and Industries Associated with Cancer in Humans* (IARC Monographs Volumes 1 to 29)

5. IARC (1983) Approaches to classifying chemical carcinogens according to mechanism of action. *IARC intern. tech. Rep. No. 83/001*

6. IARC (1972-1986) *IARC Monographs on the Evaluation of the Carcinogenic Risk of Chemicals to Humans*, Volumes 1-41, Lyon, France

    Volume 1 (1972) Some Inorganic Substances, Chlorinated Hydrocarbons, Aromatic Amines, N-Nitroso Compounds and Natural Products (19 monographs), 184 pages

    Volume 2 (1973) Some Inorganic and Organometallic Compounds (7 monographs), 181 pages

    Volume 3 (1973) Certain Polycyclic Aromatic Hydrocarbons and Heterocyclic Compounds (17 monographs), 271 pages

    Volume 4 (1974) Some Aromatic Amines, Hydrazine and Related Substances, N-Nitroso Compounds and Miscellaneous Alkylating Agents (28 monographs), 286 pages

    Volume 5 (1974) Some Organochlorine Pesticides (12 monographs), 241 pages

    Volume 6 (1974) Sex Hormones (15 monographs), 243 pages

    Volume 7 (1974) Some Anti-thyroid and Related Substances, Nitrofurans and Industrial Chemicals (23 monographs), 326 pages

    Volume 8 (1975) Some Aromatic Azo Compounds (32 monographs), 357 pages

    Volume 9 (1975) Some Aziridines, N-, S- and O-Mustards and Selenium (24 monographs), 268 pages

    Volume 10 (1976) Some Naturally Occurring Substances (22 monographs), 353 pages

    Volume 11 (1976) Cadmium, Nickel, Some Epoxides, Miscellaneous Industrial Chemicals and General Considerations on Volatile Anaesthetics (24 monographs), 306 pages

    Volume 12 (1976) Some Carbamates, Thiocarbamates and Carbazides (24 monographs), 282 pages

    Volume 13 (1977) Some Miscellaneous Pharmaceutical Substances (17 monographs), 255 pages

    Volume 14 (1977) Asbestos (1 monograph), 106 pages

    Volume 15 (1977) Some Fumigants, the Herbicides, 2,4-D and 2,4,5-T, Chlorinated Dibenzodioxins and Miscellaneous Industrial Chemicals (18 monographs), 354 pages

    Volume 16 (1978) Some Aromatic Amines and Related Nitro Compounds — Hair Dyes, Colouring Agents, and Miscellaneous Industrial Chemicals (32 monographs), 400 pages

    Volume 17 (1978) Some N-Nitroso Compounds (17 monographs), 365 pages

    Volume 18 (1978) Polychlorinated Biphenyls and Polybrominated Biphenyls (2 monographs), 140 pages

Volume 19 (1979) Some Monomers, Plastics and Synthetic Elastomers, and Acrolein (17 monographs), 513 pages

Volume 20 (1979) Some Halogenated Hydrocarbons (25 monographs), 609 pages

Volume 21 (1979) Sex Hormones (II) (22 monographs), 583 pages

Volume 22 (1980) Some Non-nutritive Sweetening Agents (2 monographs), 208 pages

Volume 23 (1980) Some Metals and Metallic Compounds (4 monographs), 438 pages

Volume 24 (1980) Some Pharmaceutical Drugs (16 monographs), 337 pages

Volume 25 (1981) Wood, Leather and Some Associated Industries (7 monographs), 412 pages

Volume 26 (1981) Some Antineoplastic and Immunosuppressive Agents (18 monographs), 411 pages

Volume 27 (1981) Some Aromatic Amines, Anthraquinones and Nitroso Compounds, and Inorganic Fluorides Used in Drinking-Water and Dental Preparations (18 monographs), 344 pages

Volume 28 (1982) The Rubber Industry (1 monograph), 486 pages

Volume 29 (1982) Some Industrial Chemicals and Dyestuffs (18 monographs), 416 pages

Volume 30 (1982) Miscellaneous Pesticides (18 monographs), 424 pages

Volume 31 (1983) Some Food Additives, Feed Additives and Naturally Occurring Substances (21 monographs), 314 pages

Volume 32 (1983) Polynuclear Aromatic Compounds, Part 1, Chemical, Environmental and Experimental Data (42 monographs), 477 pages

Volume 33 (1984) Polynuclear Aromatic Compounds, Part 2, Carbon Blacks, Mineral Oils and Some Nitroarenes (8 monographs), 245 pages

Volume 34 (1984) Polynuclear Aromatic Compounds, Part 3, Industrial Exposures in Aluminium Production, Coal Gasification, Coke Production, and Iron and Steel Founding (4 monographs), 219 pages

Volume 35 (1984) Polynuclear Aromatic Compounds, Part 4, Bitumens, Coal-Tars and Derived Products, Shale-Oils and Soots (4 monographs), 271 pages

Volume 36 (1985) Allyl Compounds, Aldehydes, Epoxides and Peroxides (15 monographs), 369 pages

Volume 37 (1985) Tobacco Habits other than Smoking; Betel-quid and Areca-nut Chewing; and Some Nitroso Compounds (8 monographs), 291 pages

Volume 38 (1986) Tobacco Smoking (1 monograph), 421 pages

Volume 39 (1986) Some Chemicals Used in Plastics and Elastomers (19 monographs), 403 pages

Volume 40 (1986) Some Naturally Occurring and Synthetic Food Components, Furocoumarins and Ultraviolet Radiation (20 monographs), 444 pages

Supplement No. 1 (1979) Chemicals and Industrial Processes Associated with Cancer in Humans (IARC Monographs, Volumes 1 to 20), 71 pages

Supplement No. 2 (1980) Long-term and Short-term Screening Assays for Carcinogens: A Critical Appraisal, 426 pages

Supplement No. 3 (1982) Cross Index of Synonyms and Trade Names in Volumes 1 to 26, 199 pages

Supplement No. 4 (1982) Chemicals, Industrial Processes and Industries Associated with Cancer in Humans (IARC Monographs, Volumes 1 to 29), 292 pages

Supplement No. 5 (1985) Cross Index of Synonyms and Trade Names in Volumes 1 to 36, 259 pages

7. IARC (1973-1986) *Information Bulletin on the Survey of Chemicals Being Tested for Carcinogenicity*, Numbers 1-11, Lyon, France

    Number 1 (1973) 52 pages
    Number 2 (1973) 77 pages
    Number 3 (1974) 67 pages
    Number 4 (1974) 97 pages
    Number 5 (1975) 88 pages
    Number 6 (1976) 360 pages
    Number 7 (1978) 460 pages
    Number 8 (1979) 604 pages
    Number 9 (1981) 294 pages
    Number 10 (1983) 326 pages
    Number 11 (1984) 370 pages
    Number 12 (1986) 389 pages

8. PHS 149 (1951-1983) Public Health Service Publication No. 149, *Survey of Compounds which have been Tested for Carcinogenic Activity*, Washington DC, US Government Printing Office

    1951 Hartwell, J.L., 2nd ed., Literature up to 1947 on 1329 compounds, 583 pages

    1957 Shubik, P. & Hartwell, J.L., Supplement 1, Literature for the years 1948-1953 on 981 compounds, 388 pages

    1969 Shubik, P. & Hartwell, J.L., edited by Peters, J.A., Supplement 2, Literature for the years 1954-1960 on 1048 compounds, 655 pages

    1971 National Cancer Institute, Literature for the years 1968-1969 on 882 compounds, 653 pages

    1973 National Cancer Institute, Literature for the years 1961-1967 on 1632 compounds, 2343 pages

    1974 National Cancer Institute, Literature for the years 1970-1971 on 750 compounds, 1667 pages

    1976 National Cancer Institute, Literature for the years 1972-1973 on 966 compounds, 1638 pages

    1980 National Cancer Institute, Literature for the year 1978 on 664 compounds, 1331 pages

1983 National Cancer Institute, Literature for years 1974-1975 on 575 compounds, 1043 pages

9. Pike, M.C. & Roe, F.J.C. (1963) An actuarial method of analysis of an experiment in two-stage carcinogenesis. *Br. J. Cancer*, *17*, 605-610

10. Miller, E.C. (1978) Some current perspectives on chemical carcinogenesis in humans and experimental animals: Presidential address. *Cancer Res.*, *38*, 1479-1496

11. Miller, E.C. & Miller, J.A. (1981) Searches for ultimate chemical carcinogens and their reactions with cellular macromolecules. *Cancer*, *47*, 2327-2345

12. Peto, R. (1974) Guidelines on the analysis of tumour rates and death rates in experimental animals. *Br. J. Cancer*, *29*, 101-105

13. Hoel, D.G. & Walburg, H.E., Jr (1972) Statistical analysis of survival experiments. *J. natl Cancer Inst.*, *49*, 361-372

14. Peto, R., Pike, M.C., Day, N.E., Gray, R.G., Lee, P.N., Parish, S., Peto, J., Richards, S. & Wahrendorf, J. (1980) *Guidelines for simple sensitive significance tests for carcinogenic effects in long-term animal experiments*. In: *IARC Monographs on the Evaluation of the Carcinogenic Risk of Chemicals to Humans, Supplement 2, Long-term and Short-term Screening Assays for Carcinogens: A Critical Appraisal*, Lyon, pp. 311-426

15. Berenblum, I. (1975) *Sequential aspects of chemical carcinogenesis: Skin*. In: Becker, F.F., ed., *Cancer. A Comprehensive Treatise*, Vol. 1, New York, Plenum Press, pp. 323-344

16. Foulds, L. (1969) *Neoplastic Development*, Vol. 2, London, Academic Press

17. Farber, E. & Cameron, R. (1980) The sequential analysis of cancer development. *Adv. Cancer Res.*, *31*, 125-126

18. Weinstein, I.B. (1981) The scientific basis for carcinogen detection and primary cancer prevention. *Cancer*, *47*, 1133-1141

19. Slaga, T.J., Sivak, A. & Boutwell, R.K., eds (1978) *Mechanisms of Tumor Promotion and Cocarcinogenesis*, Vol. 2, New York, Raven Press

20. Rall, D.P. (1977) *Species differences in carcinogenesis testing*. In: Hiatt, H.H., Watson, J.D. & Winsten, J.A., eds, *Origins of Human Cancer*, Book C, Cold Spring Harbor, NY, Cold Spring Harbor Laboratory, pp. 1383-1390

21. National Academy of Sciences (NAS) (1975) *Contemporary Pest Control Practices and Prospects: The Report of the Executive Committee*, Washington DC

22. Chemical Abstracts Services (1978) *Chemical Abstracts Ninth Collective Index (9CI), 1972-1976*, Vols 76-85, Columbus, OH

23. International Union of Pure & Applied Chemistry (1965) *Nomenclature of Organic Chemistry*, Section C, London, Butterworths

24. IARC (1980) *IARC Monographs on the Evaluation of the Carcinogenic Risk of Chemicals to Humans*, Supplement 2, *Long-term and Short-term Screening Assays for Carcinogens: A Critical Appraisal*, Lyon

25. Montesano, R., Bartsch, H. & Tomatis, L., eds (1980) *Molecular and Cellular Aspects of Carcinogen Screening Tests (IARC Scientific Publications No. 27)*, Lyon

26. de Serres, F.J. & Ashby, J., eds (1981) *Evaluation of Short-Term Tests for Carcinogens. Report of the International Collaborative Program*, Amsterdam, Elsevier/North-Holland Biomedical Press

27. Sugimura, T., Sato, S., Nagao, M., Yahagi, T., Matsushima, T., Seino, Y., Takeuchi, M. & Kawachi, T. (1976) *Overlapping of carcinogens and mutagens*. In: Magee, P.N., Takayama, S., Sugimura, T. & Matsushima, T., eds, *Fundamentals in Cancer Prevention*, Tokyo/Baltimore, University of Tokyo/University Park Press, pp. 191-215

28. Bartsch, H., Tomatis, L. & Malaveille, C. (1982) *Qualitative and quantitative comparison between mutagenic and carcinogenic activities of chemicals*. In: Heddle, J.A., ed., *Mutagenicity: New Horizons in Genetic Toxicology*, New York, Academic Press, pp. 35-72

29. Hollstein, M., McCann, J., Angelosanto, F.A. & Nichols, W.W. (1979) Short-term tests for carcinogens and mutagens. *Mutat. Res., 65*, 133-226

GENERAL REMARKS

This fortieth volume of *IARC Monographs* comprises 20 monographs on foods and food components and naturally occurring and synthesized compounds that have been investigated for use in therapy of dermatological conditions in conjunction with ultraviolet light.

Diet has been investigated in many recent studies as one of the factors that may be involved in human cancer. Most of the substances considered here that occur in food may be found in the diets of large numbers of people. The food additives and contaminants considered fall into three broad classes, resulting in different human exposures: (1) naturally occurring components of food and compounds formed by fungal contamination; (2) deliberate additions to food; and (3) mutagenic heterocyclic compounds that may be formed during cooking of food. The food additives and contaminants considered in previous *IARC Monographs* are listed in Table 1. Exposure to naturally occurring components and contaminants and to pyrolysis products may be presumed to be worldwide, the levels being modified by local climatic and cooking practices. Occupational exposures may occur during the production of food additives.

Of the naturally occurring products, bracken fern is the most abundant, being found throughout the temperate zones of the world. It is harvested for a wide variety of uses and is eaten as a delicacy in some countries. Bracken 'poisoning' in grazing animals has been recognized for many decades. Humans may also be exposed to bracken constituents in milk and other food products derived from animals that have eaten bracken. In view of the long and common use of bracken fern in certain populations and knowledge about its toxicity, the paucity of clear epidemiological studies on humans exposed to this plant is unfortunate.

Three compounds occurring naturally in food were considered: citrinin, rugulosin and patulin are fungal metabolites that may contaminate various fruits, vegetables and cereal grains intended for human consumption. Patulin was evaluated previously, in Volume 10 of the *IARC Monographs* (IARC, 1976); new data on this compound were summarized and taken into consideration in the present evaluation. The known activity and widespread occurrence of these mycotoxins would appear to warrant their evaluation for carcinogenicity, but their involvement in human disease has not yet emerged.

The four food additives considered are benzyl acetate, butylated hydroxyanisole, butylated hydroxytoluene and potassium bromate. Benzyl acetate is a common flavouring and fragrance addition in food, beverages and cosmetics and is also a natural constituent of several essential oils and plant extracts. Potassium bromate is used primarily as a maturing agent in flour and as a dough conditioner in bread-making. It is also used in some other food and consumer products.

Table 1. Food additives, food contaminants and naturally occurring substances found in food that were evaluated in previous *IARC Monographs*

Compound	Evaluation[a]		IARC Monographs			Supplement 4	
	Humans	Animals	Vol.	Page	Year	Page	Classification[b]
FOOD ADDITIVES							
AF$_2$ [2-(2-Furyl)-3-(5-nitro-2-furyl)acrylamide]	ND	S	*31*	47	1983		
Allyl isothiocyanate	ND	L	*36*	55	1985		
Allyl isovalerate	ND	L	*36*	69	1985		
Amaranth	ND	I	*8*	41	1975		
Benzoyl peroxide	I	I	*36*	267	1985		
Benzyl violet 4B*	ND	S	*16*	153	1978		
Blue VRS*	ND	L	*16*	163	1978		
Brilliant blue FCF, disodium salt	ND	L	*16*	171	1978		
Carmoisine*	ND	I	*8*	83	1975		
Carrageenan	ND		*31*	79	1983		
native		N					
degraded	ND	S					
Cinnamyl anthranilate	ND	L	*31*	133	1983		
Citrus Red 2[c]	ND	S	*8*	101	1975		
Cyclamates	I	L	*22*	55	1980	97	3
Dulcin*	ND	I	*12*	97	1976		
Ethylene oxide	I	S	*36*	189	1985	126	2B
Eugenol	ND	L	*36*	75	1985		
Fast green FCF	ND	L	*16*	187	1978		
Guinea green B*	ND	L	*16*	199	1978		
Hydrogen peroxide	ND	L	*36*	285	1985		
Light green SF*	ND	L	*16*	209	1978		

Table 1 (contd)

Compound	Evaluation[a]		IARC Monographs			Supplement 4	
	Humans	Animals	Vol.	Page	Year	Page	Classification[b]
FOOD ADDITIVES (contd)							
Oil orange SS*	ND	S	8	165	1975		
Orange I*	ND	L	8	173	1975		
Orange G*	ND	I	8	181	1975		
Ponceau MX*	ND	S	8	189	1975		
Ponceau 3R*	ND	S	8	199	1975		
Ponceau SX*	ND	I	8	207	1975		
Saccharin	I	L	22	111	1980	224	3
Scarlet red*	ND	I	8	217	1975		
Sudan I*	ND	L	8	225	1975		
Sudan II*	ND	L	8	233	1975		
Sudan III*	ND	I	8	241	1975		
Sunset yellow FCF	ND	I	8	257	1975		
Yellow AB*	ND	I	8	279	1975		
Yellow OB*	ND	L	8	287	1975		
FOOD CONTAMINANTS							
Aflatoxins	L	S	10	51	1976	31	2A
Cyclochlorotine	ND	L	10	139	1976		
Ochratoxin A	ND	L	31	191	1983		
Quercetin	ND	L	31	213	1983		
Sterigmatocystin	ND	S	10	245	1976		
Trp-P-1 (3-Amino-1,4-dimethyl-5H-pyrido-[4,3-b]indole)	ND	S	31	247	1983		
Trp-P-2 (3-Amino-1-methyl-5H-pyrido[4,3-b]-indole)	ND	S	31	255	1983		
T_2-trichothecene	ND	I	31	265	1983		

Table 1 (contd)

Compound	Evaluation[a] Humans	Evaluation[a] Animals	IARC Monographs Vol.	IARC Monographs Page	IARC Monographs Year	Supplement 4 Page	Supplement 4 Classification[b]
NATURALLY OCCURRING SUBSTANCES							
Agaritine (L-Glutamic acid, 5-[2-(4-hydroxymethyl)phenylhydrazide])	ND	I	*31*	63	1983		
Cholesterol	I / L (breast, colo-rectal cancer)	I	*31*	95	1983		
Cycasin	ND	S	*10*	121	1976		
cis-9,10-Epoxystearic acid	ND	I	*11*	153	1976		
Fusarenon-X	ND	I	*31*	153	1983		
Gyromitrin (Acetaldehyde formylmethyl-hydrazone)	ND	S	*31*	163	1983		
Isosafrole	ND	L	*10*	232	1976		
Kaempferol	ND	I	*31*	171	1983		
Lasiocarpine	ND	S	*10*	281	1976		
Luteoskyrin	ND	L	*10*	163	1976		
Malonaldehyde	ND	I	*36*	163	1985		
Methylazoxymethanol and its acetate (*see also* Cycasin)	ND	S	*10*	121,131	1976		
Monocrotaline	ND	S	*10*	291	1976		
Parasorbic acid	ND	L	*10*	199	1976		
Penicillic acid	ND	L	*10*	211	1976		
Petasitenine	ND	L	*31*	207	1983		
Retrorsine	ND	L	*10*	303	1976		
Riddelliine	ND	I	*10*	313	1976		
Seneciphylline	ND	I	*10*	319	1976		

Table 1 (contd)

Compound	Evaluation[a]		IARC Monographs			Supplement 4	
	Humans	Animals	Vol.	Page	Year	Page	Classification[b]
NATURALLY OCCURRING SUBSTANCES (contd)							
Senkirkine	ND	L	*31*	231	1983		
Symphytine	ND	I	*31*	239	1983		
Tannic acid, tannins	ND	L	*10*	253	1976		
Zearalenone	ND	L	*31*	279	1983		

*Past use; no longer permitted in some countries

[a]Abbreviations: ND, no data; S, sufficient evidence; L, limited evidence; I, inadequate evidence; N, no evidence; for definitions of these terms, see Preamble, pp. 18 and 22.

[b]Group 2, The chemical, group of chemicals, industrial process or occupational exposure is probably carcinogenic to humans. This category includes exposures for which, at one extreme, the evidence of human carcinogenicity is almost *sufficient*, as well as exposures for which, at the other extreme, it is *inadequate*. To reflect this range, the category was divided into higher (*Group A*) and lower (*Group B*) degrees of evidence. Usually, category 2A was reserved for exposures for which there was at least *limited evidence* of carcinogenicity to humans. The data from studies in experimental animals played an important role in assigning studies to category 2, and particularly those in Group B; thus, the combination of *sufficient evidence* in animals and inadequate data in humans usually resulted in a classification of 2B.
Group 3, The chemical, group of chemicals, industrial process or occupational exposure cannot be classified as to its carcinogenicity to humans.

[c]For use on citrus fruits only

Butylated hydroxyanisole (BHA) and butylated hydroxytoluene (BHT) are the most commonly used synthetic antioxidants for preserving food and feed. They are also used in cosmetics, pharmaceuticals and food-packaging materials. By tonnage, the largest uses of BHT are as an additive to motor oils, in plastics and in rubber products; therefore, occupational exposure occurs.

Since BHA and BHT are antioxidizing agents and effective radical scavengers, it had been postulated that they could modify the effects of those carcinogens and mutagens that act by virtue of their oxidizing or radical-producing properties. Thus, many studies have been carried out on the modulating effects of these two compounds on the action of known carcinogens and mutagens. The experiments involved either administration of BHA or BHT for a relatively long time after administration of a known carcinogen, or administration of BHA or BHT for a short period (a few days or weeks) prior to or concurrently with a known carcinogen. The former type of experiment, which resulted in most instances in an increased carcinogenic response, provides some information about the carcinogenicity of BHA and BHT and about their mechanisms of action. The second type of experiment resulted in many instances, but not all, in a reduction in the carcinogenic effect of various carcinogens. In these experiments, the temporal relationship between exposure to BHA or BHT and to the carcinogen (i.e., whether before, with or following the carcinogen) appeared to be critical. In most of these experiments, only a single target organ was examined, which makes it impossible to assess the carcinogenicity of these compounds to other organs. In a study in which various organs were examined in an experiment with BHT and 2-acetyl-aminofluorene, an observed reduction in the carcinogenicity of 2-acetylaminofluorene to the liver of rats was parallelled by an increased incidence of bladder cancer (see also individual monographs).

No simplistic generalization can be made concerning any 'protective' effect that these agents may have on cancer development in humans. Although no attempt is made to reach a conclusion about the mechanisms involved or to evaluate the significance of combined exposures of humans to BHA or BHT and carcinogens and mutagens, the Working Group considered it valuable to summarize data from experiments on the modulating effects of BHA and BHT.

BHA and BHT also enhance a variety of enzymes in different tissues, and particularly in the liver. The enzyme induction is associated with a change in the generation of reactive metabolites of activation-dependent toxic chemicals and a reduction in the toxicity of such chemicals. Studies of these effects have made it possible to draw a number of conclusions concerning the mechanisms of the modulating effects of BHA and BHT. Most of the numerous reports of the results of short-term tests, in which a variety of endpoints and chemicals were used, were designed to study the effects of BHA and BHT on the metabolism of known carcinogens and mutagens. In the monographs, only selected data were used to evaluate the genetic activity and related effects of BHA and BHT, and these are summarized in tabular form.

With regard to evaluating the carcinogenicity of BHA, the Working Group experienced particular difficulty. In view of the extensive use of this compound, the Group thought it prudent to take into consideration whether the production (on present evidence) only of tumours of the rodent forestomach (an organ not possessed by humans) has the same significance to humans as would evidence of carcinogenesis in other organs.

The third group of compounds considered in this volume of *IARC Monographs* comprises seven heterocyclic amines in foods; two pyrolysis products of tryptophan were evaluated in Volume 31 of the *IARC Monographs* (IARC, 1983). Mutagenic compounds are formed from proteins heated to temperatures that may be reached during the grilling of food, and several mutagens have been isolated from cooked foods. These N-heterocyclic primary amines fall into two classes: derivatives of either carbolines or imidazoquinoline. For each of two amino acid pyrolysis products (A-α-C and MeA-α-C) reviewed in this volume, only one long-term study in experimental animals had been reported, but in each of these studies a very high incidence of tumours was observed in treated animals. In addition, these two compounds are closely related chemically to Glu-P-1 and Glu-P-2, which induced cancer in two species of animals; all four compounds gave positive results in short-term tests, with endpoints relevant to carcinogenesis. A-α-C and MeA-α-C were also shown, in separate studies, to produce certain lesions of the liver that are considered by some investigators to be preneoplastic. While these factors are not essential elements for the evaluations made, they support the conclusions of the Working Group.

It is surprising that several of the compounds reviewed here to which there is extensive human exposure — for example BHA, BHT, benzyl acetate and bracken fern — have been studied inadequately, if at all, in humans. While it would be desirable to obtain more human data, the Working Group did not underestimate the difficulties of carrying out epidemiological studies on some of the compounds, such as BHA and BHT, to which human exposure is ubiquitous.

The final group of compounds considered includes a number of furocoumarins (psoralens and angelicins). Some of these compounds are used clinically in conjunction with ultraviolet A radiation (UVA) in the treatment of several skin diseases, including psoriasis, vitiligo and the T-cell lymphoma mycosis fungoides. Humans may thus be exposed to psoralens for therapeutic purposes, but also by exposure to or consumption of plant material containing these compounds. Citrus oils such as bergamot oil, containing psoralens, are used not only in food and beverages but also in suntanning products, fragrances and other cosmetics.

Most psoralens have limited biological activity in the dark, but may have potent effects when activated by the absorption of UVA. In principle, furocoumarins can act under two distinct conditions: (1) in the absence of UVA, when the molecule is in the ground state; and (2) in the presence of UVA, when the molecule is in the excited state. Under the latter condition, the molecule provokes significant biological modifications (photosensitizing effects), which are dependent on the dose of UVA. In the monograph, therefore, both biological effects obtained in the dark — toxic, mutagenic and carcinogenic effects — and those dependent on exposure to UVA, including phototoxic, photomutagenic and photocarcinogenic effects, are considered.

In the absence of UVA, furocoumarins have no significant therapeutic or genotoxic effect. The photochemotherapeutic effect of PUVA (psoralen plus UVA) is thought to be closely related to the antiproliferative effect (i.e., inhibition of DNA synthesis) of the psoralen derivatives used and to their capacity to bind to DNA in the presence of UVA. In the presence of UVA, the bifunctional furocoumarin 8-methoxypsoralen (methoxsalen), which can induce mono- and bi-adducts with DNA and an antiproliferative effect, is photochemotherapeutically active. Methoxsalen, which is used with UVA in the treatment of psoriasis and vitiligo, was evaluated in Volume 24 (IARC, 1980) and Supplement 4 (IARC, 1982) of the *IARC Monographs*. There is *sufficient evidence* for its carcinogenicity in the presence of UVA to humans. In view of the carcinogenicity of this compound, alternative furocoumarin compounds have been studied for their clinical efficacy with UVA and for their carcinogenic hazard in comparison with methoxsalen.

Furocoumarins bind to DNA in the presence of UVA. It has been suggested that monofunctional furocoumarins might be photochemotherapeutically active but less toxic, mutagenic and carcinogenic than the bifunctional furocoumarin methoxsalen. For this volume, monographs were prepared on two additional bifunctional furocoumarins, 4,5′,8-trimethylpsoralen and 5-methoxypsoralen, and on several photoreactive, monofunctional furocoumarins — angelicin and its methylated derivatives, 3-carbethoxypsoralen and two pyridopsoralens.

Thus, most of the studies on the furocoumarins considered in this volume were designed to evaluate carcinogenicity in combination with UVA and relative to that of methoxsalen with UVA. Because of the specific objective of these studies, their design was usually inadequate to evaluate the dermal or systemic carcinogenicity of the furocoumarin *per se*. In addition, the endpoints of such studies are different from those of chemical carcinogenesis tests; a frequently used endpoint in tests of psoralens is the time in weeks for 50% of animals to develop a skin tumour.

Since the clinical and suntanning uses of the furocoumarins considered depend on concomitant exposure to UVA and since human exposure to sunlight (which contains UVA as well as UVB) alone is ubiquitous and a well-known risk factor for human cancer, it was deemed useful to provide the reader with information on the carcinogenic effects of ultraviolet radiation alone. This is provided as an appendix, in which a very brief overview is given of the nomenclature and of situations in which humans are exposed to ultraviolet radiation, information on other toxic effects is reviewed briefly, and the genetic and related effects are summarized. Some studies of UVA, UVB and UVC radiation in animals are reviewed. The available case reports and epidemiological studies are analysed in more detail. It was noted that studies of the association between sunlight and nonmelanocytic skin cancer suffered from deficiencies of design and reporting, largely because they were conducted many years ago when the criteria for conducting valid epidemiological studies were less clear than they are now. Studies of adequate quality have not been performed since, probably because the relationship between sunlight and nonmelanocytic skin cancer was believed to be self-evident. It is hoped that this clear presentation of available data will stimulate the necessary additional studies.

References

IARC (1976) *IARC Monographs on the Evaluation of Carcinogenic Risk of Chemicals to Man*, Vol. 10, *Some Naturally Occurring Substances*, Lyon, pp. 205-210

IARC (1980) *IARC Monographs on the Evaluation of the Carcinogenic Risk of Chemicals to Humans*, Vol. 24, *Some Pharmaceutical Drugs*, Lyon, pp. 101-124

IARC (1982) *IARC Monographs on the Evaluation of the Carcinogenic Risk of Chemicals to Humans*, Suppl. 4, *Chemicals, Industrial Processes and Industries Associated with Cancer in Humans (IARC Monographs Volumes 1 to 29)*, Lyon, pp. 158-160

IARC (1983) *IARC Monographs on the Evaluation of the Carcinogenic Risk of Chemicals to Humans*, Vol. 31, *Some Feed Additives, Food Additives and Naturally Occurring Substances*, Lyon, pp. 247-254, 255-263

THE MONOGRAPHS

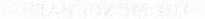

NATURALLY OCCURRING TOXINS

BRACKEN FERN (*Pteridium aquilinum*)
AND SOME OF ITS CONSTITUENTS

1. Historical Perspective

Bracken fern is a plant belonging to the Filicineae class, which comprises the ferns. They are one of the oldest plant forms and contributed to the formation of coal beds during the Carboniferous period (also known as the 'age of ferns'), beginning about 260 000 000 years ago. Since bracken fern grows rapidly in recently deforested areas, its abundance and impact have been attributed to the widespread clearance of forests which began about 5000 years ago (Page, 1976; Rymer, 1976). It has been harvested for centuries for a variety of uses, and is still eaten as a delicacy in some parts of the world (Rymer, 1976).

Bracken fern was first recognized as a potential health hazard to grazing animals less than 100 years ago (Evans, 1984). Syndromes such as 'cattle bracken poisoning', 'bracken staggers' and 'bright blindness' are now clearly associated with the ingestion of bracken fern by domestic animals (Roberts *et al.*, 1949; Evans *et al.*, 1954; Watson *et al.*, 1965; Taylor, 1980).

2. Occurrence, Use and Chemical Constituents

2.1 Occurrence

Bracken fern, a common pteridophyte, is found on every continent and in every climate, except the polar and desert regions, and is one of the most widespread of all vascular plants. Covering millions of acres of land from sea-level to 3000 m in altitude, this aggressive and resilient species thrives in pastures, deforested areas and abandoned farmlands (Page, 1976; Rymer, 1976; Taylor, 1980; Evans, 1984).

The large triangular fronds of bracken fern grow as high as 3-4 m. Reproduction and dispersal are by means of spores borne in spore cases (sori) beneath the fronds. The spores germinate to form prothalli bearing the sex organs and, after fertilization, the young sporophytes initiate the new colonies. Growth is slow, with the branching of the root-like rhizomes producing short shoots, each bearing a single frond, and long shoots which extend the colony peripherally. The rhizome endows the bracken fern with a hearty resilience to eradication programmes, such as cutting and burning, as it may grow many centimetres below the surface of the ground. Dead and decaying fronds which accumulate each winter also serve to protect the rhizome from freezing, covering the surrounding area with a thick fern litter. The growth of competing plants is inhibited through the leaching out of phytotoxins from bracken fern by rainfall. These phytotoxic compounds have not been identified or widely studied (Gliessman, 1976; Page, 1976; Watt, 1976).

Although the genus *Pteridium* has been considered monotypic (i.e., a sole species, *P. aquilinum*, occurs), data obtained experimentally on a particular geographic population of bracken may not necessarily be extrapolated to another. *P. aquilinum* has been divided into two subspecies geographically: *aquilinum* mainly in the northern hemisphere and Africa and *caudatum* principally in the southern hemisphere, and further into 12 different varieties, the distribution of which is as follows (Page, 1976):

Subspecies *aquilinum*

var. *aquilinum*	Europe and Africa
var. *wightianum*	South-east Asia (including India, China and the Malay Archipelago)
var. *pubescens*	western North America
var. *feei*	Central America
var. *decompositum*	Hawaiian Islands
var. *pseudocaudatum*	eastern North America
var. *latiusculum*	North America, northern Asia, Japan, northern Europe, USSR
var. *africanum*	south-west Africa

Subspecies *caudatum*

var. *caudatum*	Central America, Caribbean
var. *arachnoideum*	Central and South America, Caribbean
var. *esculentum*	Australia, New Zealand, Pacific Islands
var. *yarrabense*	Malay Archipelago, north-east India

Bracken is probably most abundant in parts of Europe, North America, Australia and New Zealand, and its spread has caused environmental problems in parts of the USSR, Romania, the UK, Brazil, Canada and the USA, including Hawaii (Taylor, 1980). Rapid deforestation, leading to loss of natural environmental control and subsequent abandonment of agricultural plots, is a major factor in this proliferation (Page, 1976; Rymer, 1976).

Bracken is one of the most important weeds in the UK, occurring in over 90% of all 10-km squares. In 1957, over 450 000 acres of farmland in Scotland were infested, a 2% increase over 1943; by 1970, it was estimated that 400 000 acres were invaded. In 1936, 3% of Wales was infested; by 1966, the percentage had increased to 5.7%. In New Zealand in 1923, over 35% of 11 million acres of former forest that had been converted to grassland was infested (Page, 1976; Rymer, 1976; Taylor, 1980; Evans, 1984).

2.2 Uses and human exposure

Bracken fern for human consumption is grown commercially in Japan, Canada, Siberia and north-eastern USA (Rymer, 1976; Bryan & Pamukcu, 1982).

In the UK, until the beginning of the 20th century, bracken fern was an important source of potash for glass, soap and bleaching manufacture. The plant has also been used for fuel, thatch, animal litter, floor covering, compost, dyestuffs, animal fodder and for medicinal purposes (Rymer, 1976).

Bracken rhizomes have been ground and used to make or augment bread flour by Maoris in New Zealand, and in Europe at times of severe food shortages. Bracken fern is used as a salad green; in Japan, bracken fronds are widely served as appetizers. Fresh bracken is prepared in two ways: either by immersion in plain boiling water or in boiling water containing wood ash or sodium bicarbonate, or by pickling in salt and immersion in boiling water before use. It has been reported that over 300 000 kg of young fronds are consumed every year in Tokyo alone (Rymer, 1976; Wang *et al.*, 1976; Mori *et al.*, 1977).

Bracken-derived toxins could potentially leach into and contaminate water supplies (Taylor, 1980), although no actual compound has been identified or isolated. Similarly, bracken toxins have been found to pass into the milk of cows feeding on the fern. In grazing areas where bracken infestation is prevalent, contamination of dairy products and subsequent human consumption is possible (Evans *et al.*, 1972; Pamukcu *et al.*, 1978; Evans, 1984).

2.3 Chemical constituents

Many compounds have been isolated from bracken fern in studies to identify the acutely toxic and carcinogenic principles. These include tannins and organic acids, such as chichoric acid (dicaffeyltartaric acid) and shikimic acid, at least five flavonoids, about 30 pterosin-sesquiterpenes, and also polysaccharides, glycosides, including cyanogenic glycosides, and ecdysones. Astragalin (kaempferol-3-glucoside) and isoquercitrin (quercetin-3-glucoside) have been isolated from the fronds; catecholamines and pteraquilin have been isolated from the rhizomes (Carlisle & Ellis, 1968; Cooper-Driver, 1976; Hikino *et al.*, 1976; Wang *et al.*, 1976; Fukuoka *et al.*, 1983; Jones, 1983; Evans, 1984). Some of these compounds may undergo seasonal and geographical variation in content (Cooper-Driver, 1976; Jones, 1983).

Recently, ptaquiloside (aquilide A), an unstable norsesquiterpene glucoside of the illudane type, has been isolated and characterized as a metabolic precursor of the pterosins (van der Hoeven *et al.*, 1983; Niwa *et al.*, 1983; Hirono *et al.*, 1984a,b).

Several components of bracken fern and the levels identified are given in Table 1.

Table 1. Levels of some major constituents of bracken fern

Compound	Chem. Abstr. Name [Chem. Abstr. Services Reg. No.]	IUPAC Systematic Name Synonyms	Structural and molecular formulae and molecular weight	Level found in bracken fern (mg/kg)[a]	References
Kaempferol	3,5,7-Trihydroxy-2-(4-hydroxyphenyl)-4H-1-benzopyran-4-one [520-18-3]	3,4',5,7-Tetrahydroxy-flavone; CI 75640; kempferol; nimbecetin; pelargidenolon 1497; populnetin; rhamnolutein; rhamnolutin; robigenin; swartziol; trifolitin; 5,7,4'-trihydroxyflavonol; 3,5,7-trihydroxy-2-(4-hydroxy-phenyl-4H-1-benzopyran-4-one)	$C_{15}H_{10}O_6$ Mol. wt: 286.24	1100	Pamukcu et al. (1980a)
Ptaquiloside	7a-(β-D-Glucopyranosyl-oxy)-1',3'a,4',7a-tetra-hydro-4'-hydroxy-2',4',6'-trimethylspiro[cyclo-propane-1,5'-(5H)-inden]-3'-(2'H)-one [87625-62-5]	Aquilide A	$C_{20}H_{30}O_8$ Mol. wt: 398.45	210-2400	van der Hoeven et al. (1983); Niwa et al. (1983)

Table 1 (contd)

Compound	Chem. Abstr. Name [Chem. Abstr. Services Reg. No.]	IUPAC Systematic Name Synonyms	Structural and molecular formulae and molecular weight	Level found in bracken fern (mg/kg)[a]	References
Quercetin	2-(3,4-Dihydroxyphenyl)-3,5,7-trihydroxy-4H-1-benzopyran-4-one [117-39-5]	3,3',4',5,7-Pentahydroxy-flavone; cyanidenolon 1522; meletin; NCI-C60106; 3,5,7,3',4'-pentahydroxyflavone; quercetine; quercetol; quercitin; quertine; sophoretin; 3',4',-5,7-tetrahydroxyflavan-3-ol; xanthaurine	$C_{15}H_{10}O_7$ Mol. wt: 302.24 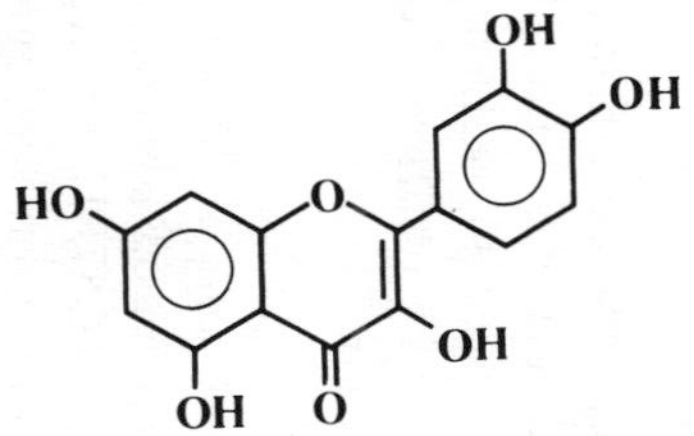	570	Pamukcu et al. (1980a)
Shikimic acid	3,4,5-Trihydroxy-1-cyclohexene-1-carboxylic acid [138-59-0]	3α,4α,5β-Trihydroxy-1-cyclohexene-1-carboxylic acid	$C_7H_{10}O_5$ Mol. wt: 174.15 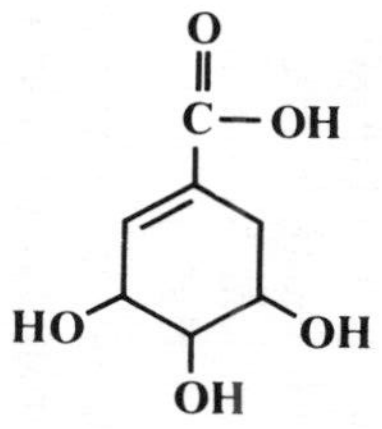	1440	Hirono et al. (1977)

[a] Dry weight

3. Biological Data Relevant to the Evaluation of
Carcinogenic Risk to Humans

Data on the carcinogenicity of bracken fern have been reviewed (Evans, 1984, 1987).

[The Working Group summarized the most relevant of the many reports on the carcinogenicity of bracken fern. They noted that many studies involved small numbers of animals and the results were incompletely reported.]

3.1 Carcinogenicity studies in animals

(a) Oral administration of bracken fern

Mouse: A group of 40 female Swiss mice, six weeks old, was fed a diet of dried bracken fern mixed with grain (1 part bracken fern:2 parts basal diet) [33%] every other week for a total of 60 weeks. All of the 33 mice that survived 30 weeks or more developed lymphatic leukaemia with multiple organ involvement; in addition, five mice developed multiple pulmonary tumours. No tumour was detected in 38 control mice that survived 30-60 weeks (Pamukcu *et al.*, 1972).

Groups of 34 male and female C57BL/6 and of 20 male and female dd mice [sex distribution unspecified], four weeks old, were fed 33% young bracken fern in basal diet for 17 weeks. Intestinal tumours developed in 11/34 C57BL/6 mice, and lung adenomas in 7/10 dd mice that survived more than 39 weeks. No tumour was reported in control mice fed the basal diet (Hirono *et al.*, 1975).

In a study described in a preliminary report, a group of 98 male and female TFI and Aber mice [age, sex and strain distribution unspecified] was administered bracken fern spores orally. Each animal received an aqueous suspension of a total of approximately 200 mg dried bracken fern spores that had been stored at room temperature for at least five months, or fresh spores, approximately one day old at the start of dosing (17 mice), in ten divided doses. A group of 49 mice served as controls. Survivors were killed at 87-117 weeks. Of the treated animals, 53/98 had tumours, 28 of which were leukaemias. Gastric tumours were reported in six mice, five of which had received the fresh spores. Two TFI females in the control group had mammary tumours; no tumour was observed in the Aber controls (Evans, 1987).

Rat: A group of 20 male and 20 female Glaxo rats, seven weeks of age, was fed a diet containing 34% dried bracken fern for 64 days and observed for 50 weeks. Animals also received three subcutaneous injections of thiamine[1] during treatment. A group of 40 rats served as controls. At the time of reporting, 20/20 males and 14/20 females in the treated group and no control rat had died. Multiple tumours that protruded into the lumen of the intestine were reported in treated animals; these occurred throughout the small intestines,

---

[1]In order to counteract the hypovitaminosis B induced by bracken fern

but predominantly in the ileal region. Most of the tumours were 5-18 mm in diameter, although ten animals developed a large tumour (2-4 cm in diameter) and other smaller widespread tumours. Some of the tumours were examined histologically and determined to be adenocarcinomas (Evans & Mason, 1965). [The Working Group noted the incomplete reporting of data on control animals.]

A group of 16 male and ten female ACI rats, four weeks old, was fed pelleted diets containing 33% dried bracken fern for 17 weeks. An untreated control group of six males and seven females was available. All treated animals died or were killed when moribund within 61 weeks. All of the 24 rats alive after 30 weeks developed tumours in the ileal region (16 adenomas, 18 adenocarcinomas and 12 sarcomas); six rats developed caecal adenomas and one, a caecal sarcoma. No such tumour was observed in the control group (Hirono et al., 1970, 1975).

A group of 12 male and 14 female albino rats [strain unspecified], 30-49 days of age, was fed 33% dried, powdered bracken fern in a grain diet; a second group of 38 males and 52 females received the same diet together with once-weekly subcutaneous injections of 2 mg thiamine hydrochloride[1]; and a third group of ten males and 12 females received the basal diet only and served as controls. Animals were observed for up to 52 weeks. All rats in the group receiving bracken fern alone that survived more than 26 weeks developed multiple intestinal adenomatous polyps or adenocarcinomas; 1/9 (11%) males and 1/13 (8%) females developed urinary-bladder carcinomas. Animals receiving bracken fern and thiamine also had a 100% incidence of multiple intestinal tumours, and 19/36 (53%) males and 35/51 (69%) females developed urinary-bladder carcinomas. No such tumour was observed in the control group (Pamukcu & Price, 1969; Pamukcu et al., 1970).

Groups of male and female ACI rats, four weeks of age, were administered pelleted diets containing 33% whole bracken frond, 33% bracken rhizomes or 33% starch made from rhizomes for 17 weeks and were observed for 70 weeks. Intestinal tumours were induced in 13/18 rats receiving whole bracken fern and in 13/13 rats receiving rhizomes; one animal in each of these groups developed bladder tumours. No tumour was reported in rats receiving the starch (Hirono et al., 1973).

A group of 15 male and 15 female Sprague-Dawley rats, six weeks old, was fed a diet containing 30% bracken fern fronds for 37 weeks. Eight females developed mammary adenocarcinomas, five developed anaplastic carcinomas of the mammary gland, and one, a squamous-cell carcinoma of the mammary gland. Ileal adenomas were observed in 14 males and nine females, and ileal adenocarcinomas in 13 males and 12 females. One male and one female had a spindle-cell fibrosarcoma of the ileum. Urinary-bladder carcinomas were observed in six males and six females; two females developed squamous-cell carcinomas of the Zymbal gland. No tumour was found in an untreated control group (Hirono et al., 1983).

Guinea-pig: A group of 13 guinea-pigs, six weeks old, was given a supplement of fresh bracken fern fronds in their diet [ratio unspecified] for 11 weeks. One guinea-pig died of an

---

[1]In order to counteract the hypovitaminosis B induced by bracken fern

adenocarcinoma of the jejunum after 100 weeks; urinary-bladder carcinomas were also observed in several animals. No tumour was reported in a control group (Evans, 1968). [The Working Group noted the incomplete reporting of the data.]

Cow: Thirty cows, aged 1.5 to four years, weighing 100-150 kg, were fed 400-1000 g fresh bracken fern or 300-600 g dried bracken fern per cow per day. A group of 14 cows served as untreated controls. Of the cows receiving the highest dose, six died within one year. Within 276-1920 days, 20 cows developed urinary-bladder tumours (macroscopically visible in 13, microscopically visible in seven); 18 of these tumours were either epithelial or epithelial and mesenchymal. Carcinomas occurred in ten cows and papillomas in eight. No bladder tumour was reported in the controls (Pamukcu *et al.*, 1976).

High incidences of alimentary-tract carcinomas (in association with papillomas) and of bladder tumours were reported in beef cattle in highland areas of the UK where bracken fern is common (Jarret, 1978; Jarret *et al.*, 1978).

Toad: A group of 98 toads (*Bufo regularis*), weighing 50 g, was fed 10 mg bracken fern per animal per week for five months. Seven animals developed ileal adenocarcinomas, and 16 developed hepatomas, six of which metastasized to the kidneys. No tumour developed in 100 control animals (El-Mofty *et al.*, 1980).

(b) Oral administration of processed bracken fern

Rat: A group of six male and six female ACI rats was fed a pelleted diet containing 33% bracken fern that had been immersed in boiled water for 5-10 min. A group of six male and seven female rats fed basal diet only served as controls. Animals were treated for 17 weeks and observed for approximately 70 weeks. In the treated group, nine animals developed intestinal tumours (seven adenomas and three adenocarcinomas); and three developed bladder carcinomas. The authors reported that the intestinal tumours occurred at a lower incidence and longer latent period [no data given] in this group of animals than in a group receiving untreated bracken fern [see above]. One urinary bladder papilloma was observed in the control group (Hirono *et al.*, 1970, 1975).

Groups of 10-14 male and female ACI rats, four to six weeks old, were fed diets containing 33% untreated bracken fern for 17 weeks (group A), 33% bracken fern immersed in boiled water plus wood ash for 17 weeks (group B), 33% bracken fern immersed in boiled water plus sodium bicarbonate for 17 weeks (group C), 33% fresh bracken fern pickled in salt and immersed in water for 17 or 39 weeks (group D), or basal diet alone (controls), and were observed for 70 weeks. Tumours, mostly of the ileum, were observed in 11/14, 3/12, 1/10 and 1/10 rats in groups A, B, C and D (17 weeks), respectively. One rat in group D (39 weeks) developed a reticulum-cell sarcoma of the mesenteric lymph nodes. No tumour was observed in controls (Hirono *et al.*, 1975).

(c) Oral administration of extracts of bracken fern

Rat: Groups of seven to 14 ACI male and female rats, four to six weeks old, received 33% unprocessed bracken fern in the diet for 13 weeks (group A), an aqueous bracken-fern extract (obtained by immersing 60 g dry bracken fern in 2 l boiling water for 3 min) as drinking-water for 70 weeks (group B), another aqueous bracken-fern extract (obtained by immersing 60 g dry bracken fern in 2 l cold water for 72 h) as drinking-water for 70 weeks (group C), a diet containing 33% concentrated boiling-water extract of bracken fern for 70 weeks (group D), or a diet containing 33% of a thrice-extracted boiling-water extract of bracken fern for 72 weeks (group E). All survivors were observed for 70-74 weeks. The numbers of rats with ileal tumours (adenoma, adenocarcinoma and fibrosarcoma) were 13/14, 4/11, 0/12, 6/7 and 8/10 in groups A, B, C, D and E, respectively; the numbers of rats with urinary-bladder tumours (papilloma, transitional-cell carcinoma, squamous-cell carcinoma or leiomyosarcoma) were 1/14, 4/11, 0/12, 7/7 and 9/10, respectively. No tumour was observed in an untreated control group (Hirono *et al.*, 1978).

[The Working Group was aware of a study in rats on tannin isolated from bracken fern and on tannin-free extracts (Pamukcu *et al.*, 1980b). See also monograph on tannins (IARC, 1976).]

Quail: A group of 34 Japanese quail (*Coturnix coturnix japonica*) was fed a hot ethanol extract of dried bracken fern in the diet [details not given] immediately after hatching for 22 weeks. Deaths occurred from 22 weeks of age due to highly malignant adenocarcinomas, predominantly in the caecum and colon and to a lesser extent in the ileum. After 44 weeks, the incidence was 80% compared to 0 in a control group (Evans, 1968).

(*d*)   *Studies with substances isolated from bracken fern*

Mouse: A group of ten male and three female TFI mice, ten weeks of age, received a single intraperitoneal injection of 1-30 mg *shikimic acid* and was observed for up to 70 weeks. A control group of 57 mice was available. Neoplasms of the glandular stomach developed in six treated mice, reticular-cell leukaemia in three and lymphocytic leukaemia in one. No such tumour was reported in the control group (Evans & Osman, 1974). [The Working Group noted the inadequate reporting of the study.]

Rat: A group of six male and six female ACI rats, four weeks old, received 0.1% *shikimic acid* derived from bracken fern in the diet for 142 days and was maintained on basal diet for 70 weeks, at which time all survivors were killed. No tumour was found in treated animals or in an untreated control group (Hirono *et al.*, 1977). [The Working Group noted the small number of animals used.]

Two groups of 12 female CD rats, 25-28 days old, received either 780 mg/kg bw *ptaquiloside* derived from bracken fern by gavage followed by weekly intragastric administration of 100-200 mg/kg bw ptaquiloside for eight consecutive weeks (group 1) or twice-weekly intragastric administrations of 100-150 mg/kg bw ptaquiloside for eight weeks followed by a single administration in week 9 (group 2). Animals were sacrificed 43 weeks after the start of the experiment. Rats surviving more than 24 weeks comprised the effective animals. All seven effective animals in group 1 had mammary tumours (adenocarcinomas and carcinomas); four also had multiple ileal adenocarcinomas. In group 2, 10/11 effective animals had mammary tumours and multiple ileal adenocarcinomas; one animal showed a lung metastasis of a mammary tumour. No tumour was observed in a control group of 15 females (Hirono *et al.*, 1984a).

[See also monographs on kaempferol (IARC, 1983a), quercetin (IARC, 1983b) and tannins (IARC, 1976).]

3.2 Other relevant biological data

(a) *Experimental systems*

Toxic effects

Bracken fern poisoning in cattle and experimental animals has been reviewed (Evans *et al.*, 1954; Yoshihira *et al.*, 1978; Hirono, 1981). Actively growing bracken fern contains toxins that reproduce many of the effects of radiation, and the acute lethal syndrome is radiomimetic (bone-marrow aplasia, haemorrhage and severe gastrointestinal damage) (Evans, 1968).

In cattle, *bracken fern* toxicity can be divided into two categories — enteric and laryngitic. Enteric toxicity, which is more common in adult cattle, induces symptoms of depression, anorexia and enteritis, with frequent blood clots in the faeces. Numerous petechial haemorrhages are visible in the mucous membranes, and there may be bleeding from the nostrils and intestinal and urogenital tracts, especially during the terminal stages, when a high fever (42-43°C) always evolves. Post-mortem examination reveals extensive haemorrhage throughout the body, with numerous ulcers in the digestive tract (Evans *et al.*, 1954).

Laryngitic toxicity is common, but not invariable, in calves suffering from *bracken fern* poisoning. The animals appear dull and listless, with excessive mucous discharge around the nostrils and mouth. Oedema of the throat region, leading to difficulty in breathing and mooing, is characteristic. There is no external sign of bleeding, but high fever usually occurs. On post-mortem examination, petechial haemorrhage may be observed, but there is little evidence of gross internal bleeding (Evans *et al.*, 1954).

Ingestion of *bracken fern* causes B_1 avitaminosis in rats (Weswig *et al.*, 1946) and horses (Roberts *et al.*, 1949), and 'bright blindness' (a primary retinopathy) in sheep (Barnett & Watson, 1970).

Hyperplastic nodules of the liver were induced in CD and ACI rats fed diets containing 30% *bracken fern* for 260 and 180 days, respectively (Hirono *et al.*, 1984c).

Two groups of 12 female Sprague-Dawley rats were given intragastric administrations of *ptaquiloside* derived from bracken fern [purity unspecified], to give total doses of 300 and 339 mg/rat, respectively. In one group, the first dose of 780 mg/kg bw at day 25 after birth was followed by 100-200 mg/kg bw once a week for eight consecutive weeks and resulted in haematuria, urinary incontinence and loss of body weight. Five of the 12 rats died within 12 weeks. In the second group, treated from day 28 after birth with twice-weekly intragastric administrations of 100-150 mg/kg bw ptaquiloside for eight weeks followed by a single administration in week 9, only one of 12 rats died within nine weeks (Hirono *et al.*, 1984a).

Ptaquiloside was isolated from a boiling-water extract of bracken fern and administered by drench to a single calf; dosages given on six days out of seven were: 400 mg/day for 24 days, then 800 mg/day for 14 days and then 1600 mg/day for four days. Granulocytopenia and thrombocytopenia were observed, and the calf was autopsied 86 days after the start of administration: haemorrhage was not observed, but femoral and sternal bone marrows were almost entirely replaced by fat (Hirono *et al.*, 1984d).

Effects on reproduction and prenatal toxicity

Female ICR-JCL mice were fed diets composed of 33% dried Japanese *bracken fern* throughout gestation. Maternal weight gain and serum protein concentration were reduced in comparison to controls; fetuses (eight litters) had lower weights and increased skeletal variations with retarded ossification. The authors suggested that the effects observed were due to the ingested bracken fern and might be related to maternal thiamine deficiency caused by the plant (Yasuda *et al.*, 1974). [The Working Group noted the small number of animals used and the use of a single dose group.]

It was reported in a short communication that groups of seven to 14 pregnant female CF-1 mice were given 0.25 or 1.0 g/kg bw *shikimic acid* in water from day 1-17 of gestation. Although implantations were significantly reduced in treated animals, the number of live fetuses per litter was not significantly reduced as compared to controls. No gross anomaly was detected (O'Donovan *et al.*, 1977).

Absorption, distribution, excretion and metabolism

In cows, toxic components of bracken fern have been demonstrated to pass into the milk, and have been reported to cross the placenta (Evans *et al.*, 1958, 1972; Pamukcu *et al.*, 1978). Maternal passage *via* the placenta and/or milk has also been demonstrated in mice (Evans *et al.*, 1972).

Mutagenicity and other short-term tests

An acetone extract of *bracken fern* was mutagenic to *Salmonella typhimurium* TA98 in the presence of an exogenous metabolic system (White *et al.*, 1983). Light petroleum and methanol extracts of bracken fern that had been activated by alkaline treatment prior to testing were mutagenic to *S. typhimurium* TA98 and/or TA100, in the absence of an exogenous metabolic system, when tested in a preincubation assay; more than 50% of the activity was attributed to the glycoside, ptaquiloside (van der Hoeven *et al.*, 1983).

It was reported in an abstract that rats fed *bracken fern* excreted a urinary fraction that was mutagenic to *S. typhimurium* TA98 and TA100; another fraction was mutagenic to TA100 but not to TA98 (Hatcher *et al.*, 1981). A chloroform:methanol fraction of milk from cows fed bracken fern was mutagenic to TA100 but not to TA98 (Pamukcu *et al.*, 1978). In neither of these studies was the active compound identified.

Ptaquiloside (10^{-6}-10^{-4}M) induced unscheduled DNA synthesis in primary rat-liver hepatocytes (Mori *et al.*, 1985). It was also reported to induce sister chromatid exchanges and HPRT-deficient mutants in Chinese hamster V79 cells and unscheduled DNA synthesis in human fibroblasts and to transform C3H 10T1/2 cells [details not given] (van der Hoeven *et al.*, 1983).

Shikimic acid (tested at up to 2000 μg/plate) was not mutagenic to *S. typhimurium* TA1535, TA1537, TA1538, TA98 or TA100, in the presence or absence of an exogenous metabolic system (S9) from the livers of Aroclor-induced rats (Stavric & Stoltz, 1976; Jacobsen *et al.*, 1978). A number of bacterial and mammalian metabolites of shikimic acid were not mutagenic to *S. typhimurium* TA1535, TA1537, TA98 or TA100, with or without S9 from the livers of Aroclor-induced rats (Jones *et al.*, 1983).

Shikimic acid did not induce chromosomal aberrations in cultured Chinese hamster CHL cells (Ishidate & Odashima, 1977).

Dominant lethal mutations were induced when a group of five TF1 mice were administered 1000 mg/kg bw *shikimic acid* intraperitoneally or 3000 mg/kg by gavage as a single dose and each mated to four virgin females for eight successive weeks (Evans & Osman, 1974). In a later and more substantial study, 500 mg/kg bw shikimic acid were administered intraperitoneally to 15 male Alderly Park mice once a week for eight successive weeks or once only before mating to three females for either two or eight weeks, respectively; no dominant lethal effect was seen. With the same dosage regimen, there was no evidence of heritable translocation (Anderson *et al.*, 1981).

(b) Humans

No data were available to the Working Group.

3.3 Case reports and epidemiological studies of carcinogenicity to humans

Intake of bracken fern, hot tea gruel (*chagayu*), meat and fruit and cigarette smoking were studied in 98 patients with cancer of the oesophagus and 476 control subjects 60 years of age or older in Nara, Wakayama and Mie prefectures of Japan (Hirayama, 1979). The relative risk of cancer of the oesophagus was 2.68 [95% confidence interval, 1.38-5.21] in those who ate bracken fern daily and 1.53 [0.90-2.62] in those who ate it occasionally, in comparison with the incidence in those who ate it rarely or not at all [χ_1^2 for linear trend = 8.04; $p = 0.004$]. The risk gradient appeared to be steeper in females [relative risks, 1.00 (rarely/not at all), 1.65 (occasionally) and 3.67 (daily); χ_1^2 trend = 6.24; $p = 0.012$] than in males [1.00, 1.33, 2.10; χ_1^2 trend = 2.60; $p = 0.11$]. The difference in gradients was not significant, however. When subjects were stratified by intake of hot tea gruel, smoking and intake of meat and fruit, the increase in risk of cancer of the oesophagus associated with consumption of bracken fern appeared to be confined to those who also took hot tea gruel and was greater, relatively, in those who smoked than in those who did not, and in those who did not eat meat or fruit daily compared with those who did. The highest risk of cancer of the oesophagus was in those who smoked and took bracken fern and hot tea gruel daily and did not eat meat or fruit daily. [The Working Group noted the lack of detail in this report, such as information on the source of controls or use of alcohol, which is associated with the occurrence of oesophageal cancer (Tuyns *et al.*, 1979).]

4. Summary of Data Reported and Evaluation

4.1 Exposure

Human exposure to bracken fern and its constituents occurs by direct ingestion of the fronds in some regions of the world, or by ingestion of dairy products from cattle grazing on the fern. In the past, bracken has found other end uses such as in bread flour and medicinals.

4.2 Experimental data

Bracken fern was tested for carcinogenicity by oral administration to mice, rats, guinea-pigs, cows and toads. In all species except cows, bracken fern induced malignant or benign and malignant intestinal tumours, particularly in the small intestine. It also induced bladder carcinomas in rats, guinea-pigs and cows, liver tumours in toads, lymphocytic leukaemias in mice and mammary carcinomas in rats.

Administration in the diet to rats of bracken fern that had been processed as for human consumption produced intestinal tumours, but at a lower incidence than unprocessed bracken fern.

In one study in rats, starch made from bracken fern rhizomes did not produce tumours.

Oral administration of boiling-water extracts of bracken fern to rats induced intestinal and bladder tumours; administration of ethanol extracts to quails produced intestinal tumours.

In studies on the carcinogenicity of substances isolated from bracken fern, oral administration of ptaquiloside to rats produced mammary and intestinal tumours. Shikimic acid has not been adequately studied. Kaempferol, quercetin and tannins, which also occur in bracken fern, were evaluated in previous volumes of *IARC Monographs*.

Administration of bracken fern in the diet in one study in mice at one dose induced maternal toxicity, some embryotoxicity and some minor abnormalities in offspring.

An acetone extract of bracken fern was mutagenic to *Salmonella typhimurium* in the presence of an exogenous metabolic system; light petroleum and methanol extracts of bracken fern activated by alkaline treatment were mutagenic to *S. typhimurium* in the absence of an exogenous metabolic system.

Ptaquiloside induced unscheduled DNA synthesis in primary rat liver hepatocytes.

Shikimic acid was not mutagenic in *Salmonella typhimurium*. It did not induce chromosomal aberrations in cultured Chinese hamster cells. Conflicting results were reported in the dominant lethal test and negative results in the heritable translocation test in mice.

4.3 Human data

One case-control study from Japan has suggested an association between intake of bracken fern and cancer of the oesophagus.

Overall assessment of data from short-term tests: Bracken fern extracts[a]

	Genetic activity			Cell transformation
	DNA damage	Mutation	Chromosomal effects	
Prokaryotes		+		
Fungi/Green plants				
Insects				
Mammalian cells (*in vitro*)				
Mammals (*in vivo*)				
Humans (*in vivo*)				
Degree of evidence in short-term tests for genetic activity: **Inadequate**				Cell transformation: No data

[a]The groups into which the table is divided and the symbol used are defined on pp. 19-20 of the Preamble; the degrees of evidence are defined on pp. 20-21.

Overall assessment of data from short-term tests: Ptaquiloside[a]

	Genetic activity			Cell transformation
	DNA damage	Mutation	Chromosomal effects	
Prokaryotes				
Fungi/Green plants				
Insects				
Mammalian cells (*in vitro*)	+			
Mammals (*in vivo*)				
Humans (*in vivo*)				
Degree of evidence in short-term tests for genetic activity: **Inadequate**				Cell transformation: No data

[a]The groups into which the table is divided and the symbol used are defined on pp. 19-20 of the Preamble; the degrees of evidence are defined on pp. 20-21.

Overall assessment of data from short-term tests: Shikimic acid[a]

	Genetic activity			Cell transformation
	DNA damage	Mutation	Chromosomal effects	
Prokaryotes		−		
Fungi/Green plants				
Insects				
Mammalian cells (*in vitro*)			−	
Mammals (*in vivo*)			?	
Humans (*in vivo*)				
Degree of evidence in short-term tests for genetic activity: **Inadequate**				Cell transformation: No data

[a]The groups into which the table is divided and the symbols used are defined on pp. 19-20 of the Preamble; the degrees of evidence are defined on pp. 20-21.

4.4 Evaluation[1]

There is *sufficient evidence*[2] for the carcinogenicity of bracken fern in experimental animals.

There is *limited evidence* for the carcinogenicity of ptaquiloside derived from bracken fern in experimental animals.

There is *inadequate evidence* for the carcinogenicity of shikimic acid derived from bracken fern in experimental animals.

There is *inadequate evidence* for the carcinogenicity of bracken fern to humans.

5. References

Anderson, D., Hodge, M.C.E., Palmer, S. & Purchase, I.F.H. (1981) Comparison of dominant lethal and heritable translocation methodologies. *Mutat. Res.*, *85*, 417-429

Barnett, K.C. & Watson, W.A. (1970) Bright blindness in sheep. A primary retinopathy due to feeding bracken (*Pteris aquilina*). *Res. vet. Sci.*, *11*, 289-291

---

[1]For definition of the italicized terms, see Preamble, pp. 18 and 22.

[2]In the absence of adequate data in humans, it is reasonable, for practical purposes, to regard chemicals or exposures for which there is *sufficient evidence* of carcinogenicity in animals as if they represented a carcinogenic risk to humans.

Bryan, G.T. & Pamukcu, A.M. (1982) *Sources of carcinogens and mutagens in edible plants: production of urinary bladder and intestinal tumors by bracken fern* (Pteridium aquilinum). In: Stitch, H.F., ed., *Carcinogens and Mutagens in the Environment*, Vol. 1, Boca Raton, FL, CRC Press, pp. 75-82

Carlisle, D.B. & Ellis, P.E. (1968) Bracken and locust ecdysones: their effects on molting in the desert locust. *Science, 159*, 1472-1474

Cooper-Driver, G. (1976) Chemotaxonomy and phytochemical ecology of bracken. *Bot. J. Linn. Soc., 73*, 35-46

El-Mofty, M.M., Sadek, I.A. & Bayoumi, S. (1980) Improvement in detecting the carcinogenicity of bracken fern using an Egyptian toad. *Oncology, 37*, 424-425

Evans, I.A. (1968) The radiomimetic nature of bracken toxin. *Cancer Res., 28*, 2252-2261

Evans, I.A. (1984) *Bracken carcinogenicity*. In: Searle, C.E., ed., *Chemical Carcinogenesis*, 2nd ed. (*ACS Monograph 182*), Vol. 2, Washington DC, American Chemical Society, pp. 1171-1204

Evans, I.A. (1987) Bracken carcinogenicity. *Rev. environ. Health* (in press)

Evans, I.A. & Mason, J. (1965) Carcinogenic activity of bracken. *Nature, 208*, 913-914

Evans, I.A. & Osman, M.A. (1974) Carcinogenicity of bracken and shikimic acid. *Nature, 250*, 348-349

Evans, I.A., Thomas, A.J., Evans, W.C. & Edwards, C.M. (1958) Studies on bracken poisoning in cattle. Part V. *Br. vet. J., 114*, 253-267

Evans, I.A., Jones, R.S. & Mainwaring-Burton, R. (1972) Passage of bracken fern toxicity into milk. *Nature, 237*, 107-108

Evans, W.C., Evans, E.T.R. & Hughes, L.E. (1954) Studies on bracken poisoning in cattle. Part I. *Br. vet. J., 110*, 295-306

Fukuoka, M., Yoshihira, K., Natori, S., Mihashi, K. & Nishi, M. (1983) Carbon-13 nuclear magnetic resonance spectra of pterosin-sesquiterpenes and related indan-1-one derivatives. *Chem. pharm. Bull., 31*, 3113-3128

Gliessman, S.R. (1976) Allelopathy in a broad spectrum of environments as illustrated by bracken. *Bot. J. Linn. Soc., 73*, 95-104

Hatcher, J.F., Pamukcu, A.M. & Bryan, G.T. (1981) Quercetin (Q) and kaempferol (K) content of bracken fern (BF) and mutagenic activity in urine of rats ingesting Q, rutin (R) or BF (Abstract No. 450). *Proc. Am. Assoc. Cancer Res., 22*, 114

Hikino, H., Miyase, T. & Takemoto, T. (1976) Biosynthesis of pteroside B in *Pteridium aquilinum* var. latiusculum, proof of the sesquiterpenoid origin of the pterosides. *Phytochemistry, 15*, 121-123

Hirayama, T. (1979) Diet and cancer. *Nutr. Cancer, 1*, 67-81

Hirono, I. (1981) Natural carcinogenic products of plant origin. *Crit. Rev. Toxicol.*, *8*, 235-277

Hirono, I., Shibuya, C., Fushimi, K. & Haga, M. (1970) Studies on carcinogenic properties of bracken, *Pteridium aquilinum. J. natl Cancer Inst.*, *45*, 179-188

Hirono, I., Fushimi, K., Mori, H., Miwa, T. & Haga, M. (1973) Comparative study of carcinogenic activity in each part of bracken. *J. natl Cancer Inst.*, *50*, 1367-1371

Hirono, I., Sasaoka, I., Shibuya, C., Shimizu, M., Fushimi, K., Mori, H., Kato, K. & Haga, M. (1975) Natural carcinogenic products of plant origin. *Gann Monogr.*, *17*, 205-217

Hirono, I., Fushimi, K. & Matsubara, N. (1977) Carcinogenicity test of shikimic acid in rats. *Toxicol. Lett.*, *1*, 9-10

Hirono, I., Ushimaru, Y., Kato, K., Mori, H. & Sasoaka, I. (1978) Carcinogenicity of boiling water extract of bracken, *Pteridium aquilinum. Gann*, *69*, 383-388

Hirono, I., Aiso, S., Hosaka, S., Yamaji, T. & Haga, M. (1983) Induction of mammary cancer in CD rats fed bracken fern diet. *Carcinogenesis*, *4*, 885-887

Hirono, I., Aiso, S., Yamaji, T., Mori, H., Yamada, K., Niwa, H., Ojika, M., Wakamatsu, K., Kigoshi, H., Niiyama, K. & Uosaki, Y. (1984a) Carcinogenicity in rats of ptaquiloside isolated from bracken. *Gann*, *75*, 833-836

Hirono, I., Yamada, K., Niwa, H., Shizuri, Y., Ojika, M., Hosaka, S., Yamaji, T., Wakamatsu, K., Kigoshi, H., Niiyama, K. & Uosaki, Y. (1984b) Separation of carcinogenic fraction of bracken fern. *Cancer Lett.*, *21*, 239-246

Hirono, I., Aiso, S., Yamaji, T., Niwa, H., Ojika, M., Wakamatsu, K. & Yamada, K. (1984c) Hyperplastic nodules in the liver induced in rats fed bracken diet. *Cancer Lett.*, *22*, 151-155

Hirono, I., Kono, Y., Takahashi, K., Yamada, K., Niwa, H., Ojika, M., Kigoshi, H., Niiyama, K. & Uosaki, Y. (1984d) Reproduction of acute bracken poisoning in a calf with ptaquiloside, a bracken constituent. *Vet. Rec.*, *115*, 375-378

van der Hoeven, J.C.M., Lagerweij, W.J., Posthumus, M.A., van Veldhuizen, A. & Holterman, H.A.J. (1983) Aquilide A, a new mutagenic compound isolated from bracken fern (*Pteridium aquilinum* (L.) Kuhn). *Carcinogenesis*, *4*, 1587-1590

IARC (1976) *IARC Monographs on the Evaluation of Carcinogenic Risk of Chemicals to Man*, Vol. 10, *Some Naturally Occurring Substances*, Lyon, pp. 253-262

IARC (1983a) *IARC Monographs on the Evaluation of the Carcinogenic Risk of Chemicals to Humans*, Vol. 31, *Some Food Additives, Feed Additives and Naturally Occurring Substances*, Lyon, pp. 171-178

IARC (1983b) *IARC Monographs on the Evaluation of the Carcinogenic Risk of Chemicals to Humans*, Vol. 31, *Some Food Additives, Feed Additives and Naturally Occurring Substances*, Lyon, pp. 213-229

Ishidate, M., Jr & Odashima, S. (1977) Chromosome tests with 134 compounds on Chinese hamster cells in vitro — a screening for chemical carcinogens. *Mutat. Res.*, *48*, 337-354

Jacobsen, L.B., Richardson, C.L. & Floss, H.G. (1978) Shikimic acid and quinic acid are not mutagenic in the Ames assay. *Lloydia*, *41*, 450-452

Jarrett, W.F.H. (1978) Transformation of warts to malignancy in alimentary carcinoma in cattle. *Bull. Cancer*, 65, 191-194

Jarrett, W.F.H., McNeil, P.E., Grimshaw, W.T.R., Selman, I.E. & McIntyre, W.I.M. (1978) High incidence area of cattle cancer with a possible interaction between an environmental carcinogen and papilloma virus. *Nature*, 274, 215-217

Jones, C.G. (1983) *Phytochemical variation, colonization, and insect communities: the case of bracken fern (*Pteridium aquilinum). In: Denno, R.F. & McClure, M.S., eds, *Variable Plants and Herbivores in Natural and Managed Systems*, New York, Academic Press, pp. 513-558

Jones, R.S., Ali, M., Ioannides, C., Styles, J.A., Ashby, J., Sulej, J. & Parke, D.V. (1983) The mutagenic and cell transforming properties of shikimic acid and some of its bacterial and mammalian metabolites. *Toxicol. Lett.*, 19, 43-50

Mori, H., Kato, K., Ushimaru, Y., Kato, T. & Hirono, I. (1977) Effect of drying with hot forced draft and of mincing bracken fern on its carcinogenic activity. *Gann*, 68, 517-520

Mori, H., Sugie, S., Hirono, I., Yamada, K., Niwa, H. & Ojika, M. (1985) Genotoxicity of ptaquiloside, a bracken carcinogen, in the hepatocyte primary culture/DNA-repair test. *Mutat. Res.*, 143, 75-78

Niwa, H., Ojika, M., Wakamatsu, K., Yamada, K., Hirono, I. & Matsushita, K. (1983) Ptaquiloside a novel norsesquiterpene glucoside from bracken, *Pteridium aquilinum* var. latiusculum. *Tetrahedron Lett.*, 24, 4117-4120

O'Donovan, M.R., Brewster, D. & Jones, R.S. (1977) Embryotoxic properties of shikimic acid. *Int. Res. Commun. Syst.*, 5, 514

Page, C.N. (1976) The taxonomy and phytogeography of bracken — a review. *Bot. J. Linn. Soc.*, 73, 1-34

Pamukcu, A.M. & Price, J.M. (1969) Induction of intestinal and urinary bladder cancer in rats by feeding bracken fern (*Pteris aquilina*). *J. natl Cancer Inst.*, 43, 275-281

Pamukcu, A.M., Yalçiner, S., Price, J.M. & Bryan, G.T. (1970) Effects of the coadministration of thiamine on the incidence of urinary bladder carcinomas in rats fed bracken fern. *Cancer Res.*, 30, 2671-2674

Pamukcu, A.M., Ertürck, E., Price, J.M. & Bryan, G.T. (1972) Lymphatic leukemia and pulmonary tumors in female Swiss mice fed bracken fern (*Pteris aquilina*). *Cancer Res.*, 32, 1442-1445

Pamukcu, A.M., Price, J.M. & Bryan, G.T. (1976) Naturally occurring and bracken-fern-induced bovine urinary bladder tumors. *Vet. Pathol.*, 13, 110-122

Pamukcu, A.M., Ertürk, E., Yalçiner, S., Milli, U. & Bryan, G.T. (1978) Carcinogenic and mutagenic activities of milk from cows fed bracken fern (*Pteridium aquilinum*). *Cancer Res.*, 38, 1556-1560

Pamukcu, A.M., Yalçiner, S., Hatcher, J.F. & Bryan, G.T. (1980a) Quercetin, a rat intestinal and bladder carcinogen present in bracken fern (*Pteridium aquilinum*). *Cancer Res.*, 40, 3468-3472

Pamukcu, A.M., Wang, C.Y., Hatcher, J. & Bryan, G.T. (1980b) Carcinogenicity of tannin and tannin-free extracts of bracken fern (*Pteridium aquilinum*) in rats. *J. natl Cancer Inst.*, *65*, 131-136

Roberts, H.E., Evans, E.T.R. & Evans, W.C. (1949) The production of bracken staggers in the horse, and its treatment by vitamin B_1 therapy. *Vet. Rec.*, *61*, 549-550

Rymer, L. (1976) The history and ethnobotany of bracken. *Bot. J. Linn. Soc.*, *73*, 151-176

Stavric, B. & Stoltz, D.R. (1976) Shikimic acid. *Food Cosmet. Toxicol.*, *14*, 141-145

Taylor, J.A. (1980) Bracken, an increasing problem and a threat to health. *Outlook Agric.*, *10*, 298-304

Tuyns, A.J., Péquinot, G. & Abbatucci, J.S. (1979) Oesophageal cancer and alcohol consumption; importance of type of beverage. *Int. J. Cancer*, *23*, 443-447

Wang, C.Y., Pamukcu, A.M. & Bryan, G.T. (1976) Bracken fern as a naturally-occurring carcinogen. *Med. Biol. Environ.*, *4*, 567-572

Watson, W.A., Barlow, R.M. & Barnett, K.C. (1965) Bright blindness — a condition prevalent in Yorkshire hill sheep. *Vet. Rec.*, *77*, 1060-1069

Watt, A.S. (1976) The ecological status of bracken. *Bot. J. Linn. Soc.*, *73*, 217-239

Weswig, P.H., Freed, A.M. & Haag, J.R. (1946) Antithiamine activity of plant materials. *J. biol. Chem.*, *165*, 737-738

White, R.D., Krumperman, P.H., Cheeke, P.R. & Buhler, D.R. (1983) An evaluation of acetone extracts from six plants in the Ames mutagenicity test. *Toxicol. Lett.*, *15*, 25-31

Yasuda, Y., Kihara, T. & Nishimura, H. (1974) Embryotoxic effects of feeding bracken fern (*Pteridium aquilinum*) to pregnant mice. *Toxicol. appl. Pharmacol.*, *28*, 264-268

Yoshihira, K., Fukuoka, M., Kuroyanagi, M., Natori, S., Umeda, M., Morohoshi, T., Enomoto, M. & Saito, M. (1978) Chemical and toxicological studies on bracken fern, *Pteridium aquilinum* var. latiusculum. I. Introduction, extraction and fractionation of constituents and toxicological studies including carcinogenicity test. *Chem. pharm. Bull.*, *26*, 2346-2364

CITRININ

1. Chemical and Physical Data

1.1 Synonyms and trade names

Chem. Abstr. Services Reg. No.: 518-75-2

Chem. Abstr. Name: (3*R-trans*)-4,6-Dihydro-8-hydroxy-3,4,5-trimethyl-6-oxo-3*H*-2-benzopyran-7-carboxylic acid

IUPAC Systematic Name: (3*R*,4*S*)-4,6-Dihydro-8-hydroxy-3,4,5-trimethyl-6-oxo-3*H*-2-benzopyran-7-carboxylic acid

1.2 Structural and molecular formulae and molecular weight

$C_{13}H_{14}O_5$ Mol. wt: 250.25

1.3 Chemical and physical properties of the pure substance

(*a*) *Description*: Yellow odourless crystalline solid (IUPAC, 1982); lemon-yellow needles from ethanol (Windholz, 1983); yellow needles (methanol) (Weast, 1985)

(*b*) *Melting-point*: 170-173°C, after drying for 1 h at 60°C (IUPAC, 1982)

(*c*) *Spectroscopy data*: Ultraviolet (IUPAC, 1982), infrared (Pouchert, 1981 [321B[a]]; IUPAC, 1982), proton nuclear magnetic resonance (Barber & Staunton, 1980; IUPAC, 1982), C-13 nuclear magnetic resonance (Barber & Staunton, 1980) and mass spectral data (IUPAC, 1982) have been reported.

---

[a]Spectrum number in Pouchert compilation

(d) *Solubility*: Practically insoluble in water; soluble in ethanol (0.7 g/100 ml), dioxane, dilute alkali (Windholz, 1983), acetone (5 g/100 ml), benzene and chloroform (7.7 g/100 ml) (Ambrose & DeEds, 1946; Weast, 1985)

(e) *Stability*: Decomposes at 178-179°C (Weast, 1985)

1.4 Technical products and impurities

No data were available to the Working Group.

2. Production, Use, Occurrence and Analysis

2.1 Production and use

(a) *Production*

Citrinin was first isolated in 1931 by Hetherington and Raistrick from a culture of *Penicillium citrinum* Thom. A filtrate of the culture solution was acidified to precipitate the crude product; further purification was achieved by recrystallization from boiling absolute ethanol (Hetherington & Raistrick, 1931). More recently, Davis *et al.* (1975) utilized this same procedure to isolate citrinin from *P. citrinum* growing in a sucrose/yeast nutrient solution. The precipitate can be purified by an extraction/filtration sequence with various organic solvents (e.g., chloroform, ethyl acetate) (Scott, 1980). Jackson and Ciegler (1978) described a method for producing citrinin from a solid substrate and isolation involving alternate chloroform/sodium hydrogen carbonate solution extraction steps and final purification from hot absolute ethanol. Betina (1984) has summarized procedures for the isolation and purification of citrinin.

The synthesis of citrinin and dihydrocitrinin was reported by Cartwright *et al.* (1949). Initially, the laevorotatory form of 3-(4,6-dihydroxy-*ortho*-tolyl)butan-2-ol is carboxylated to form the acid. This product is subjected to the Gattermann reaction (conversion of the phenol to the aromatic aldehyde by reaction with hydrogen cyanide/hydrogen chloride in the presence of a zinc chloride catalyst) to produce an intermediate, which is subsequently cyclized with sulphuric acid to form citrinin. The crude product was purified by crystallization from ethanol. An alternative synthetic method involves the conversion of dihydroxycitrinin to citrinin by oxidation with bromine (Warren *et al.*, 1949).

Several authors have described biosynthetic routes for citrinin production. Birch *et al.* (1958) suggested that citrinin produced by *Aspergillus candidus* is derived from the condensation of five acetate groups and three C_1 units. Schwenk *et al.* (1958) demonstrated a similar pathway in *Penicillium citrinum*. This biosynthetic route for citrinin was substantiated by Rodig *et al.* (1966) using radiolabelled glucose. More recently, it was determined that 4,6-dihydroxy-3,5-dimethyl-2-(1-methyl-2-oxopropyl)benzaldehyde is the first enzyme-free aromatic intermediate in the biosynthetic pathway of citrinin in *P. citrinum*. This study also showed that the methylation reactions take place on a polyketide synthetase complex (Barber *et al.*, 1981).

Citrinin is not currently produced in commercial quantities, but small amounts for research purposes are available from four firms in the USA (Baker *et al.*, 1984) and one in Israel (Makor Chemicals Ltd, 1985). No European or Japanese producer has been identified.

(b) Use

Citrinin has been reported to demonstrate antibiotic and bacteriostatic properties. Dilutions of 1:15 000 to 1:50 000 inhibit the growth of Staphylococci and the compound is bacteriocidal at a 1:8000 concentration against *Staphylococcus aureus* and *S. albus* (Ambrose & DeEds, 1946). It has not been developed as a commercial antibiotic because of its reported toxicity in animal tests.

There is no current use for citrinin other than for research purposes. Two firms include purified citrinin in analytical reagent kits for use as a standard for mycotoxins (Makor Chemicals Ltd, 1985; Sigma Chemical Co., 1985).

2.2 Occurrence

(a) Natural occurrence

Citrinin is a toxic secondary metabolite of fungi, first isolated from *P. citrinum* Thom (Hetherington & Raistrick, 1931). It is also produced by several other species of *Penicillium* and *Aspergillus* (Birch *et al.*, 1958; Barber *et al.*, 1981). The citrinin-producing *Penicillium* species include *P. lividum* West, *P. phaeojanthinellum* Biourge, *P. implicatum* Biourge, *P. citreo-sulfuratum* Biourge, *P. chrzaszci* Zaleski, *P. viridicatum* Westling, *P. expansum* Link, *P. steckii* Zaleski, *P. velutinum*, *P. canescens*, *P. purpurescens*, *P. claviforme*, and *P. roqueforti*. The *Aspergillus* species include *A. candidus*, *A. terreus*, and *A. flavipes* (Betina, 1984).

(b) Soil and plants

Citrinin has been found in the leaves of the Australian plant *Crotolaria crispata* (Ewart, 1933). Aoyama *et al.* (1982), who screened 750 samples of filamentous fungi from soil for the presence of antioxidant activity, found that one of two strains selected for further study from 14 positive strains produced citrinin.

(c) Food, beverages and animal feed

Citrinin-producing fungi grow on grains and fruits stored in high humidity; however, the presence of the fungus does not necessarily indicate the presence of the mycotoxin. When samples of wheat, barley, rye and corn from Poland were incubated at 15°C and 25-30% humidity for four weeks, citrinin was observed in 7% of the samples at levels up to 24 mg/kg, in six isolates of *Penicillium* and one of *Aspergillus* (Chelkowski & Goliński, 1983).

Citrinin has been found in rice (National Cancer Institute, 1984). Brown rice stored in two warehouses in Hokkaido, Japan, for seven years under natural conditions was found to contain 700 and 1130 μg/kg citrinin (Sugimoto et al., 1977).

Citrinin was found at a level of 27 μg/kg in one of five samples of corn flour collected in Tokyo between January and April 1980. Resampling showed that one of four corn flour samples had 73 μg/kg citrinin. Eleven corn flour samples prepared from corn imported from Thailand contained 10-98 μg/kg citrinin, while two samples of the raw corn itself contained 174 and 1390 μg/kg citrinin. Corn from Burma had 212 μg/kg citrinin, but corn from Argentina had none. Damaged corn from Thailand (cracked, discoloured or wormy) had 720 μg/kg citrinin, compared to none in normal corn and 174 μg/kg in a random sample of unsorted corn containing both normal and damaged corn (Nishijima, 1984).

Citrinin was found in four of 269 samples of a crop of barley stored in Sweden in 1976 at levels of 30, 50, 170 and 480 μg/kg (Hokby et al., 1979). Of 523 grain samples examined in England and Wales during 1976-1979, 2.1% contained citrinin alone, and 1.7% contained citrinin and other mycotoxins (Buckle, 1983). Following a wet harvest in Saskatchewan in 1968, 11 of 20 samples of naturally heated wheat, rye, barley and oats contained citrinin at levels of 0.07-80 mg/kg (van Walbeek, 1973). When 50 samples of mouldy bread and seven samples of mouldy flour from domestic sources and retail shops were extracted and analysed for mycotoxins, citrinin was detected in one flour sample at a level too low to be measured (Osborne, 1980).

Citrinin occurs naturally in wheat, barley, rye and oats in both Canada and Denmark (Salunkhe et al., 1980). All grains, oilseeds and their meals tested by Bhattacharya and Majumdar (1982) supported the growth of P. citrinum and the production of citrinin in solid-state fermentation; rice, soya bean and groundnut cakes were the most effective substrates.

Citrinin was found in three of 33 samples of barley and oats used for swine feed in three districts of Denmark (Krogh et al., 1973) at levels of 160-2000 μg/kg. Citrinin was extracted from one isolate of P. citrinum obtained from til (sesame seed) (Reddy & Reddy, 1983). Groundnut pods collected in India (Subrahmanyam & Rao, 1974) on the day of harvest in November 1972 were graded into undamaged and damaged pods, and kernel moisture content was determined. High levels of citrinin were associated with kernels that had less than 30% moisture. All damaged kernels contained the toxin.

Citrinin was found in seven of 41 moulds obtained from damaged tomatoes and analysed for mycotoxins, at levels of 0.07-0.76 μg/g (Harwig et al., 1979). Cerutti et al. (1982) found no citrinin in 55 samples of fruit juices, purees and homogenized foods in Italy using an analytical method with a detection limit of 50 ng and a recovery of 50%.

Naturally rotting apples in Canada were found to contain traces of citrinin (Harwig et al., 1973); larger amounts were found when the fungal isolates from these apples were cultured for seven days. Citrinin appears to be unstable in apple juice.

Bullerman (1980) examined retail samples of 75 imported cheeses and 78 domestic cheeses in the USA for moulds. Cultures from four samples produced citrinin.

Of 422 Penicillium cultures isolated from mould-fermented sausage collected in 11

European countries, ten produced citrinin. No citrinin was detected in sausages ripened with mould-producing citrinin for 70 days (Mintzlaff *et al.*, 1972). Country-cured hams from south-eastern USA yielded seven strains of *P. viridicatum*, which produced citrinin on culturing under temperature conditions similar to those in the ageing process used for these products (25-30°C) (Wu *et al.*, 1974). Soya sauce produced by fermentation with *P. citrinum* and *Aspergillus* was analysed by a method able to detect 20 mg/kg citrinin; none was detected (Tu *et al.*, 1984).

2.3 Analysis

Citrinin has been determined by a number of methods, primarily thin-layer chromato-graphy and high-performance liquid chromatography. Nuclear magnetic resonance has usually been used for confirmation of the structure in the presence of other mycotoxins. The sensitivity of methods for citrinin detection can be improved by using chromatographic plates impregnated with oxalic or glycolic acids (Gimeno, 1980, 1984). Clean-up steps are matrix dependent; thus, grain extracts may be easier to analyse than corn or peanuts. Obstacles to citrinin analysis include the fact that it is a chelating agent, its sensitivity to pH, and the effect of temperature on its stability (Stoloff, 1983).

A summary of representative methods is given in Table 1.

3. Biological Data Relevant to the Evaluation of Carcinogenic Risk to Humans

3.1 Carcinogenicity studies in animals

(a) Oral administration

Mouse: Groups of 20 male DDD mice, six weeks of age, were fed diets containing 0, 100 or 200 mg/kg of diet citrinin [purity unspecified] for 70 weeks. The numbers of mice still alive at 40 weeks were 17, 17 and 19 in the three groups, respectively. No renal tumour was reported (Kanisawa, 1984). [The Working Group noted the short duration of the study and the small number of animals used.]

Rat: Groups of 10-20 male Sprague-Dawley rats, eight to ten weeks old, were fed diets containing 0, 0.02 or 0.05% citrinin [purity unspecified] for 48 weeks, at which time survivors were killed. No kidney tumour was observed (Shinohara *et al.*, 1976). [The Working Group noted the short duration of the study.]

Groups of 22 and 50 male Fischer 344 rats, six weeks old, were fed diets containing 0 and 0.1% citrinin (99% pure), respectively, for 80 weeks. At week 32, in 13 treated rats that were sacrificed, the incidence of focal hyperplasia of renal tubular cells was increased. Small adenomas were found in the kidneys of all of eight treated rats sacrificed at week 40. Massive tumours were observed grossly in the kidneys of all treated rats sacrificed at week 60 (17 rats, $p < 0.05$) and at week 80 (ten rats, $p < 0.05$). These tumours were benign and were classified

Table 1. Methods for the analysis of citrinin

Sample matrix	Sample preparation	Assay procedure[a]	Limit of detection	Reference
Standard preparations	Dissolve in chloroform	TLC	10 ng	Reiss (1978)
	Dissolve in chloroform	TLC	0.8 ng	Gimeno (1980)
	Dissolve in chloroform	HPTLC/UV HPTLC/FL	1 ng 0.01 ng	Lee et al. (1980)
	Dissolve in acetone	TLC CT-Chang CT-HEp-2	0.05 ng 100 ng 10 ng	Robb & Norval (1983)
	Dissolve in chloroform	UV or FL	500 ng	Neely et al. (1972)
Fruit juices, fruits, purees	Homogenize sample, extract with acetonitrile/4% KCl	TLC/UV	30-40 ng/g 400 ng/g	Gimeno & Martins (1983) Cerutti et al. (1982)
Processed foods				
mouldy bread, rice and vegetable foodstuffs	Extract with acetonitrile/4% KCl and cyclohexane	TLC/FL (2-D)	100-1000 ng/g	Johann & Dose (1983)
soya sauce		TLC/UV	20 μg/g	Tu et al. (1984)
cheeses	Extract with dichloromethane	HPLC/FL	20 ng/g	Nowotny et al. (1983)
Grains, flours and animal feed	Grind sample, extract with chloroform or acetonitrile/4% KCl, or with acidified acetonitrile/KCl followed by silica gel chromatography	TLC/FL or TLC/UV	80-750 ng/g	Roberts & Patterson (1975); Jackson & Ciegler (1978); Chalam & Stahr (1979); Gimeno (1979); Takeda et al. (1979); Wilson (1982); Goliński & Grabarkiewicz-Szczesna (1984)
	Grind sample, extract with acetonitrile and glycolic acid	TLC/UV	15-20 ng/g	Gimeno (1984)
	Extract with ethyl acetate	PC	20 ng/g	Nakagawa et al. (1982)
	Extract with acidified acetonitrile	HPLC	50 ng/g	Marti et al. (1978)
	Extract with acidified acetonitrile; dissolve in chloroform	FL	100 ng/g	Trantham & Wilson (1984)
	Extract with ethyl acetate/ chloroform; dissolve in methanol/ water	FL	50 ng/g	Nakazato et al. (1981)
Biological fluids	Extract acidified plasma, bile and urine with ethyl acetate; dissolve in acetonitrile	HPLC	10 ng	Phillips et al. (1980)

[a]Abbreviations: TLC, thin-layer chromatography; HPTLC, high-performance thin-layer chromatography; UV, ultraviolet detection; FL, fluorimetry; CT-Chang, cytotoxicity in Chang liver cells; CT-HEp-2, cytotoxicity in HEp-2 cells; 2-D, 2-dimensional; HPLC, high-performance liquid chromatography; PC, reverse-phase ion-pair partition chromatography

as clear-cell adenomas. No renal tumour was seen in the control group (Arai & Hibino, 1983).

Fish: Groups of 50 Medaka fish (*Oryzias latipes*) were fed diets containing 150 or 300 mg/kg citrinin [purity unspecified] for 12, 22 or 24 weeks. (The daily amount of diet given to a group of approximately 50 fish was 800 mg.) An untreated control group was available. Only 1/35 Medaka treated with 150 mg/kg of diet for 24 weeks developed a liver-cell nodule (Hatanaka *et al.*, 1982). [The Working Group noted the short duration of the study.]

(b) Administration with known carcinogens or other chemicals

Mouse: Groups of 20 male DDD mice, six weeks of age, were fed diets containing 25 mg/kg ochratoxin A or 25 mg/kg ochratoxin A plus 200 mg/kg citrinin for 70 weeks. Renal-cell tumours developed in 6/18 mice fed ochratoxin A and in 10/18 mice fed ochratoxin A plus citrinin (Kanisawa, 1984). [The Working Group noted the small number of animals used.]

Rat: Groups of 20 male Sprague-Dawley rats, eight to ten weeks old, were pretreated with 0.05% *N*-nitrosodimethylamine (NDMA) in the diet for two weeks; they then received basal diet for two weeks, followed by diets containing 0.02 or 0.05% citrinin [purity unspecified] for 20 weeks, at which time survivors were sacrificed. A positive control group of 20 rats was fed a diet containing 0.05% NDMA for two weeks and then a basal diet for 22 weeks. The incidence of renal-cell tumours was 18/19 in the low-dose ($p < 0.0001$) and 13/15 in the high-dose ($p < 0.01$) groups. The incidence of embryonal-cell tumours in the kidneys was 14/19 ($p < 0.001$) and 9/15 ($p < 0.01$), respectively. The incidences of renal-cell tumours and embryonal-cell tumours in rats treated with NDMA were 2/14 and 8/14, respectively. When rats were pretreated with 0.5% *N*-(3,5-dichlorophenyl)succinimide for eight weeks followed by treatment with 0.02% citrinin for 20 weeks, 4/18 animals developed renal-cell tumours. *N*-(3,5-Dichlorophenyl)succinimide alone did not produce kidney tumours but caused severe interstitial nephritis (Shinohara *et al.*, 1976).

3.2 Other relevant biological data

(a) Experimental systems

Toxic effects

Subcutaneous or intraperitoneal administration of citrinin (doses ranging from 10 to 50 mg/kg bw) induced hyperaemia of ears and feet, miosis, respiratory stimulation and prostration in rats and rabbits; in mice and guinea-pigs, only effects on respiration were seen. Subcutaneous and intraperitoneal LD_{50} values were reported to be 35 mg/kg bw in mice and 67 mg/kg bw in rats; a subcutaneous LD_{50} of 37 mg/kg bw was reported in guinea-pigs, and an intravenous LD_{50} of 19 mg/kg bw was reported in rabbits (Ambrose & DeEds, 1946).

Mild renal lesions were observed in DDD mice fed diets containing 200 mg/kg citrinin (Kanisawa, 1984). Degeneration of tubular epithelial cells and dilatation of the tubules were observed in kidneys of Sprague-Dawley rats fed 0.02 or 0.05% citrinin (Shinohara et al., 1976).

Fischer rats fed diets containing 0.1% citrinin (99% pure) for 32 weeks showed focal hyperplasia, marked dilatation of proximal convoluted tubules, colloid casts in the tubular lumina and interstitial fibrosis due to nephritis. Focal hyperplasia of renal tubular cells was also observed (Arai & Hibino, 1983).

Repeated administration of citrinin induced nephrotoxic effects in rabbits (20 mg/kg per day intravenously for eight weeks; Ambrose & DeEds, 1946), dogs (20-40 mg/kg per day orally then intraperitoneally for five days; Carlton et al., 1974), pigs (20 mg/kg per day orally for 70 days; Friis et al., 1969) and Wistar rats (14 mg/kg daily orally for 15 days; Krogh et al., 1970). The nephrotoxic effect was characterized by enlarged kidneys, degeneration of tubules with subsequent cortical fibrosis and functional impairment of tubular activity.

Repeated administration of citrinin (six weekly intraperitoneal injections of 20 mg/kg bw) to Swiss mice caused generalized bone-marrow depression (Gupta et al., 1983).

Effects on reproduction and prenatal toxicity

Pregnant Swiss-Webster CD-1 mice received single intraperitoneal injections of 10, 20, 30 or 40 mg/kg bw citrinin in propylene glycol on one of days 6-9 of gestation (five to eight litters per treatment group). With 30 or 40 mg/kg, fetal weight gain was reduced (all treatment days) and fetal lethality increased (treatment days 6, 7 and 9); maternal lethality occurred occasionally. No increase in fetal abnormalities was observed (Hayes et al., 1974; Hood et al., 1976).

Groups of at least ten pregnant Sprague-Dawley CD-1 rats received single subcutaneous injections of 35 mg/kg bw citrinin in 5% sodium bicarbonate on one of days 3-15 of gestation. One-third to one-half of the dams died, and most of the remainder had reduced body-weight gain. Animals exposed on days 8 or 10 produced only 70 or 75% live fetuses; the other groups showed fewer resorptions. Fetal weight was reduced in all exposed groups. Some minor fetal anomalies occurred in all groups (Reddy et al., 1982a). [The Working Group noted that only one dose was used, which was severely toxic to the mothers.]

Groups of six to ten pregnant Sprague-Dawley rats received single subcutaneous injections of 30 mg/kg bw citrinin (from *P. citrinum* NRRL 1842) with or without 1.0 mg/kg bw ochratoxin A on one of gestation days 5-11 or 14. The one control group consisted of nine animals. Dams given citrinin gained body weight normally. Combined treatment on days 5-7 or 14 resulted in 22-40% maternal lethality. Citrinin or ochratoxin A given alone did not influence implantation, fetal weight or resorption rate. No significant change in the incidence of anomalies occurred after treatment with either substance alone, whereas in some groups the combination of citrinin with ochratoxin A increased the occurrence of gross, soft-tissue and skeletal malformations (Mayura et al., 1984). [The Working Group noted that only one dose level of citrinin was used.]

Absorption, distribution, excretion and metabolism

Citrinin (25-50 mg/kg) has been reported to be poorly absorbed from the gastro-intestinal tract of rats and from the mouth of cats (Chu, 1946).

Thirty minutes after intravenous injection of 3 mg/kg bw ^{14}C-citrinin to Sprague-Dawley rats, 15% and 6% of total radioactivity were observed in the liver and kidneys, respectively; these were the sites of major accumulation. By 6 h, the amount had decreased to 8% in the liver and 5% in the kidney. Two plasma elimination rates were observed, with half-lives of 2.6 and 14.9 h, respectively; 74% of the radioactivity appeared in the urine in the first 24 h; 4 and 11% were found in the faeces at 24 and 48 h, respectively (Phillips *et al.*, 1979).

Following subcutaneous injection on day 12 of gestation, ^{14}C-citrinin crossed the placenta in Charles River CD-1 rats (Reddy *et al.*, 1982b).

After subcutanous administration of 35 mg/kg bw ^{14}C-citrinin to pregnant Charles River CD-1 rats on day 12 of gestation, biphasic elimination from plasma was also observed, with half-lives of 2 and 40 h, respectively. High-performance liquid chromatography of maternal plasma extracts revealed the presence of the parent compound and at least one unidentified metabolite, which was more polar than the parent compound; at least two unidentified metabolites were found in urine. Chromatograms of maternal bile samples suggested the presence of at least one metabolite, apart from the parent compound, whereas fetal extracts contained only the parent compound (Reddy *et al.*, 1982b).

Mutagenicity and other short-term tests

In the *Bacillus subtilis rec*$^{+/-}$ citrinin was reported to give both positive (Ueno & Kubota, 1976) and negative (Manabe *et al.*, 1981) results when tested at 20 and 100 μg/disc, and 10 and 100 μg/disc, respectively.

Citrinin was not mutagenic to *Salmonella typhimurium* TA1535, TA1537, TA1538, TA98 or TA100, in the presence or absence of an exogenous metabolic system when tested at up to 400 μg/plate (Engel & von Milczewski, 1976; Kuczuk *et al.*, 1978; Ueno *et al.*, 1978; Wehner *et al.*, 1978).

Concentrations of up to 100 μg citrinin per plate did not induce mitotic gene conversion in *Saccharomyces cerevisiae* D3 in the presence or absence of an exogenous metabolic system (Kuczuk *et al.*, 1978).

Exposure of *Drosophila melanogaster* to aqueous solutions containing up to 8×10^{-2} M citrinin did not induce mitotic recombination measured as somatic mosaicism (Belitsky *et al.*, 1983). [The Working Group noted that this test has not been validated with known mutagens (see Preamble).]

Concentrations of up to 8×10^{-4} M citrinin did not induce unscheduled DNA synthesis in primary cultures of hepatocytes from Wistar rats or in human embryonic hepatocytes *in vitro* (Belitsky *et al.*, 1983).

In Chinese hamster V79 cells in the presence of an exogenous metabolic system from rat or human liver, citrinin was effective in inducing chromosomal aberrations at the only concentration tested, 5×10^{-4}M. Sister chromatid exchanges were not detected (Thust & Kneist, 1979).

(b) Humans

No data were available to the Working Group.

3.3 Case reports and epidemiological studies of carcinogenicity to humans

No data were available to the Working Group.

4. Summary of Data Reported and Evaluation

4.1 Exposure data

Citrinin is produced by various *Penicillium* and *Aspergillus* species that can contaminate foodstuffs, and has been found in some cereals and fruits and peanuts. Thus, human exposure can occur by ingestion of such contaminated products.

4.2 Experimental data

Citrinin was adequately tested for carcinogenicity in one experiment in one strain of male rats by oral administration in the diet; it produced renal tumours. In another experiment in rats, citrinin was administered in the diet after *N*-nitrosodimethylamine or *N*-(3,5-dichlorophenyl)succinimide; an increased incidence of renal tumours was observed as compared to that in animals receiving *N*-nitrosodimethylamine or *N*-(3,5-dichloro-phenyl)succinimide alone.

In rodents, embryotoxicity occurred after injection of maternally toxic doses of citrinin.

Both positive and negative results have been reported with citrinin in the *Bacillus subtilis rec* assay; the compound was not mutagenic in *Salmonella typhimurium* in the presence or absence of an exogenous metabolic system. It did not induce recombination in *Saccharomyces cerevisiae* nor unscheduled DNA synthesis in mammalian cells *in vitro*. Chromosomal aberrations but no sister chromatid exchanges were induced by citrinin in Chinese hamster V79 cells in the presence of an exogenous metabolic system.

4.3 Human data

No case report or epidemiological study of the carcinogenicity of citrinin was available to the Working Group.

Overall assessment of data from short-term tests: Citrinin[a]

	Genetic activity			Cell transformation
	DNA damage	Mutation	Chromosomal effects	
Prokaryotes	?	–		
Fungi/Green plants		–		
Insects				
Mammalian cells (*in vitro*)	–		?	
Mammals (*in vivo*)				
Humans (*in vivo*)				
Degree of evidence in short-term tests for genetic activity: **Inadequate**				Cell transformation: No data

[a]The groups into which the table is divided and the symbols are defined on pp. 19-20 of the Preamble; the degrees of evidence are defined on pp. 20-21.

4.4 Evaluation[1]

There is *limited evidence* for the carcinogenicity of citrinin to experimental animals. No evaluation could be made of the carcinogenicity of citrinin to humans.

5. References

Ambrose, A.M. & DeEds, F. (1946) Some toxicological and pharmacological properties of citrinin. *J. Pharmacol. exp. Ther.*, *88*, 173-186

Aoyama, T., Nakakita, Y., Nakagawa, M. & Sakai, H. (1982) Screening for antioxidants of microbial origin. *Agric. Biol. Chem.*, *46*, 2369-2371

Arai, M. & Hibino, T. (1983) Tumorigenicity of citrinin in male F344 rats. *Cancer Lett.*, *17*, 281-287

Baker, M.J., Gandenberger, C.L., Krohn, C.L., Krohn, D.A., Merz, J.B. & Tedeschi, M.J., eds (1984) *Chem Sources-USA*, 25th ed., Ormand Beach, FL, Directories Publishing Co., p. 152

[1]For definition of the italicized term, see Preamble, p. 18.

Barber, J., Carter, R.H., Garson, M.J. & Staunton, J. (1981) The biosynthesis of citrinin by *Penicillium citrinum*. *J. chem. Soc. Perkin Trans. 1*, *9*, 2577-2583

Belitsky, G.A., Khovanova, E.M., Budunova, I.V. & Sharupich, E.G. (1983) Mycotoxin induction of somatic mutagenesis in *Drosophila* and DNA-repair synthesis in mammalian liver cell cultures (Russ.). *Bull. eksp. Biol. Med.*, *96*, 83-86

Betina, V. (1984) *Citrinin and related substances*. In: Betina, V., ed., *Mycotoxins — Production, Isolation, Separation and Purification*, Amsterdam, Elsevier, pp. 217-236

Bhattacharya, M. & Majumdar, S.K. (1982) Studies on the nutritional requirements of *P. citrinum* for the synthesis of citrinin toxin. *J. Food Sci. Technol.*, *19*, 61-63

Birch, A.J., Fitton, P., Pride, E., Ryan, A.J., Smith, H. & Whalley, W.B. (1958) Studies in relation to biosynthesis. Part XVII. Sclerotiorin, citrinin and citromycetin. *J. chem. Soc.*, 4576-4581

Buckle, A.E. (1983) The occurrence of mycotoxins in cereals and animal feedstuffs. *Vet. Res. Commun.*, *7*, 171-186

Bullerman, L.B. (1980) Incidence of mycotoxic molds in domestic and imported cheeses. *J. Food Saf.*, *2*, 47-58

Carlton, W.W., Sansing, G. & Szczech, G.M. (1974) Citrinin mycotoxicosis in beagle dogs. *Food Cosmet. Toxicol.*, *12*, 479-490

Cartwright, N.J., Robertson, A. & Whalley, W.B. (1949) The chemistry of fungi. Part VII. Synthesis of citrinin and dihydrocitrinin. *J. chem. Soc.*, 1563-1567

Cerutti, G., Finoli, C., Vecchio, A. & Bonolis, M. (1982) Mycotoxins in juices and other fruit products (Ital.). *Tecnol. Aliment.*, *5*, 8-16

Chalam, R.V. & Stahr, H.M. (1979) Thin layer chromatographic determination of citrinin. *J. Assoc. off. anal. Chem.*, *62*, 570-572

Chelkowski, J. & Goliński, P. (1983) Mycotoxins in cereal grain. Part VII. A simple method to assay mycotoxin potential of cereal grain and cereal products. *Nahrung*, *27*, 305-310

Chu, W.-C. (1946) Miscellaneous pharmacologic actions of citrinin. *J. Lab. clin. Med.*, *31*, 72-78

Davis, N.D., Dalby, D.K., Diener, U.L. & Sansing, G.A. (1975) Medium-scale production of citrinin by *Penicillium citrinum* in a semisynthetic medium. *Appl. Microbiol.*, *29*, 118-120

Engel, G. & von Milczewski, K.E. (1976) Evidence of mycotoxins after activation with rat liver homogenates with histidine deficient mutants of *Salmonella typhimurium* (Ger.). *Kieler Milchwirtsch. Forsch.*, *28*, 359-366

Ewart, A.J. (1933) On the presence of citrinin in *Crostolaria crispata*. *Ann. Bot.*, *47*, 913-915

Friis, P., Hasselager, E. & Krogh, P. (1969) Isolation of citrinin and oxalic acid from *Penicillium viridicatum* Westling and their nephrotoxicity in rats and pigs. *Acta pathol. microbiol. scand.*, *77*, 559-560

Gimeno, A. (1979) Thin layer chromatographic determination of aflatoxins, ochratoxins, sterigmatocystin, zearalenone, citrinin, T-2 toxin, diacetoxyscirpenol, penicillic acid, patulin, and penitrem A. *J. Assoc. off. anal. Chem.*, *62*, 579-585

Gimeno, A. (1980) Improved method for thin layer chromatographic analysis of myco-toxins. *J. Assoc. off. anal. Chem.*, *63*, 182-186

Gimeno, A. (1984) Determination of citrinin in corn and barley on thin layer chromato-graphic plates impregnated with glycolic acid. *J. Assoc. off. anal. Chem.*, *67*, 194-196

Gimeno, A. & Martins, M.L. (1983) Rapid thin layer chromatographic determination of patulin, citrinin, and aflatoxins in apples and pears, and their juices and jams. *J. Assoc. off. anal. Chem.*, *66*, 85-91

Goliński, P. & Grabarkiewicz-Szczęsna, J. (1984) Chemical confirmatory tests for ochratoxin A, citrinin, penicillic acid, sterigmatocystin and zearalenone performed directly on thin layer chromatography plates. *J. Assoc. off. anal. Chem.*, *67*, 1108-1110

Gupta, M., Sasmal, D., Bandyopadhyay, S., Bagchi, G., Chatterjee, T. & Dey, S. (1983) Hematological changes produced in mice by ochratoxin A and citrinin. *Toxicology*, *26*, 55-62

Harwig, J., Chen, Y.-K., Kennedy, B.P.C. & Scott, P.M. (1973) Occurrence of patulin and patulin-producing strains of *Penicillium expansum* in natural rots of apples in Canada. *Can. Inst. Food Sci. Technol. J.*, *6*, 22-25

Harwig, J., Scott, P.M., Stoltz, D.R. & Blanchfield, B.J. (1979) Toxins of molds from decaying tomato fruit. *Appl. environ. Microbiol.*, *38*, 267-274

Hatanaka, J., Doke, N., Harada, T., Aikawa, T. & Enomoto, M. (1982) Usefulness and rapidity of screening for the toxicity and carcinogenicity of chemicals in Medaka, *Oryzias latipes*. *Jpn. J. exp. Med.*, *52*, 243-253

Hayes, A.W., Hood, R.D. & Snowden, K. (1974) Preliminary assay for the teratogenicity of mycotoxins (Abstract no. 196). *Toxicol. appl. Pharmacol.*, *29*, 153

Hetherington, A.C. & Raistrick, H. (1931) Study on the biochemistry of micro-organisms. Part XIV. On the production and chemical constitution of a new yellow colouring matter, citrinin, produced from glucose by *Penicillium citrinum* Thom. *Philos. Trans. R. Soc. London, Ser. B*, *220*, 269-295

Hokby, F., Hult, K., Gatenbeck, S. & Rutqvist, L. (1979) Ochratoxin A and citrinin in 1976 crop of barley stored on farms in Sweden. *Acta agric. scand.*, *29*, 174-178 [*Microbiol. Abstr.*, *C8*, 10418]

Hood, R.D., Hayes, A.W. & Scammell, J.G. (1976) Effects of prenatal administration of citrinin and viriditoxin to mice. *Food Cosmet. Toxicol.*, *14*, 175-178

IUPAC (1982) Physicochemical data for some selected mycotoxins. *Pure appl. Chem.*, *54*, 2219-2284

Jackson, L.K. & Ciegler, A. (1978) Production and analysis of citrinin in corn. *Appl. environ. Microbiol.*, *36*, 408-411

Johann, H. & Dose, K. (1983) Multianalytical method for the routine determination of the aflatoxins B1, B2, G1 and G2, and of citrinin, ochratoxin A, patulin, penicillic acid, and sterigmatocystin in molded foods (Ger.). *Fresenius' Z. anal. Chem.*, *314*, 139-142

Kanisawa, M. (1984) Synergistic effect of citrinin on hepatorenal carcinogenesis of ochratoxin A in mice. *Dev. Food Sci.*, *7*, 245-254

Krogh, P., Hasselager, E. & Friis, P. (1970) Studies on fungal nephrotoxicity. 2. Isolation of two nephrotoxic compounds from *Penicillium viridicatum* Westling: citrinin and oxalic acid. *Acta pathol. microbiol. scand.*, *78B*, 401-413

Krogh, P., Hald, B. & Pedersen, E.J. (1973) Occurrence of ochratoxin A and citrinin in cereals associated with mycotoxic porcine nephropathy. *Acta pathol. microbiol. scand.*, *81B*, 689-695

Kuczuk, M.H., Benson, P.M., Heath, H. & Hayes, A.W. (1978) Evaluation of the mutagenic potential of mycotoxins using *Salmonella typhimurium* and *Saccharomyces cerevisiae*. *Mutat. Res.*, *53*, 11-20

Lee, K.Y., Poole, C.F. & Zlatkis, A. (1980) Simultaneous multi-mycotoxin determination by high performance thin-layer chromatography. *Anal. Chem.*, *52*, 837-842

Makor Chemicals Ltd (1985) *Catalogue*, Jerusalem, p. 66

Manabe, M., Goto, T., Tanaka, K. & Matsuura, S. (1981) The capabilities of the *Aspergillus flavus* group to produce aflatoxins and kojic acid (Jpn.). *Rep. natl Food Res. Inst.*, *38*, 115-120

Marti, L.R., Wilson, D.M. & Evans, B.D. (1978) Determination of citrinin in corn and barley. *J. Assoc. off. anal. Chem.*, *61*, 1353-1358

Mayura, K., Parker, R., Berndt, W.O. & Phillips, T.D. (1984) Effect of simultaneous prenatal exposure to ochratoxin A and citrinin in the rat. *J. Toxicol. environ. Health*, *13*, 553-561

Mintzlaff, H.-J., Ciegler, A. & Leistner, L. (1972) Potential mycotoxin problems in mould-fermented sausage. *Z. Lebensmittel-Untersuch. Forsch.*, *150*, 133-137

Nakagawa, T., Kawamura, T., Fujimoto, Y. & Tatsuno, T. (1982) Determination of citrinin in grain by reverse-phase ion-pair partition chromatography (Jpn.). *Shokuhin Eiseigaku Zasshi*, *23*, 297-301 [*Chem. Abstr.*, *98*, 33188u]

Nakazato, M., Kanmuri, M., Nakazawa, K., Ariga, T., Fujinuma, K., Nishijima, M. & Naoi, Y. (1981) Mycotoxins in food. XV. Fluorometric determination of citrinin in cereals (Jpn.). *Shokuhin Eiseigaku Zasshi*, *22*, 391-396 [*Chem. Abstr.*, *96*, 33458r]

National Cancer Institute (1984) *Data Bank on Environmental Agents. Selected Contaminants and Toxicants in Foods and Diets.* Vol. 1 (*Contract NO1-CP-26003*), Bethesda, MD

Neely, W.C., Ellis, S.P., Davis, N.D. & Diener, U.L. (1972) Spectroanalytical parameters of fungal metabolites. I. Citrinin. *J. Assoc. off. anal. Chem.*, *55*, 1122-1127

Nishijima, M. (1984) Survey for mycotoxins in commercial foods. *Dev. Food Sci.*, *7*, 172-181

Nowotny, P., Baltes, W., Kroenert, W. & Weber, R. (1983) Study of commercial cheese samples for the mycotoxins sterigmatocystin, citrinin, and ochratoxin A (Ger.). *Lebensmittelchem. Gerichtl. Chem.*, *37*, 71-72

Osborne, B.G. (1980) The occurrence of ochratoxin A in mouldy bread and flour. *Food Cosmet. Toxicol.*, *18*, 615-617

Phillips, R.D., Berndt, W.O. & Hayes, A.W. (1979) Distribution and excretion of [14C]citrinin in rats. *Toxicology*, *12*, 285-298

Phillips, R.D., Hayes, A.W. & Berndt, W.O. (1980) High-performance liquid chromatographic analysis of the mycotoxin citrin and its application to biological fluids. *J. Chromatogr.*, *190*, 419-427

Pouchert, C.J., ed. (1981) *The Aldrich Library of Infrared Spectra*, 3rd ed., Milwaukee, WI, Aldrich Chemical Co., p. 321B

Reddy, A.S. & Reddy, S.M. (1983) Elaboration of mycotoxins by fungi associated with til (*Sesamun indicum* L.). *Curr. Sci.*, *52*, 613-614

Reddy, R.V., Mayura, K., Hayes, A.W. & Berndt, W.O. (1982a) Embryocidal teratogenic and fetotoxic effects of citrinin in rats. *Toxicology*, *25*, 151-160

Reddy, R.V., Hayes, A.W. & Berndt, W.O. (1982b) Disposition and metabolism of [14C]citrinin in pregnant rats. *Toxicology*, *25*, 161-174

Reiss, J. (1978) Semiquantitative estimation of the mycotoxins citrinin, ochratoxin A, aflatoxin Ml, and penicillic acid on thin-layer chromatograms with a grey scale. *Fresenius' Z. anal. Chem.*, *293*, 138-140

Robb, J. & Norval, M. (1983) Comparison of cytotoxicity and thin-layer chromatography methods for detection of mycotoxins. *Appl. environ. Microbiol.*, *46*, 948-950

Roberts, B.A. & Patterson, D.S.P. (1975) Detection of twelve mycotoxins in mixed animal feedstuffs, using a novel membrane cleanup procedure. *J. Assoc. off. anal. Chem.*, *58*, 1178-1181

Rodig, O.R., Ellis, L.C. & Glover, I.T. (1966) The biosynthesis of citrinin from *Penicillium citrinum*. II. Tracer studies on the formation of citrinin. *Biochemistry*, *5*, 2458-2462

Salunkhe, D.K., Wu, M.T., Do, J.Y. & Maas, M.R. (1980) *Mycotoxins in foods and feeds*. In: Gordon, H.D., ed., *The Safety of Foods*, 2nd ed., Westport, CT, AVI Publishing Co., p. 215

Schwenk, E., Alexander, G.J., Gold, A.M. & Stevens, D.F. (1958) Biogenesis of citrinin. *J. biol. Chem.*, *233*, 1211-1213

Scott, P.M. (1980) Penicillium *mycotoxins*. In: Wyllie, T.D. & Morehouse, L.G., eds, *Mycotoxic Fungi, Mycotoxins, Mycotoxicoses, An Encyclopedic Handbook*, Part 2, *Chemistry of Mycotoxins*, New York, Marcel Dekker, pp. 283-356

Shinohara, Y., Arai, M., Hirao, K., Sugihara, S., Nakanishi, K., Tsonoda, H. & Ito, N. (1976) Combination effect of citrinin and other chemicals on rat kidney tumorigenesis. *Gann*, *67*, 147-155

Sigma Chemical Co. (1985) *Biochemical and Organic Compounds for Research and Diagnostic Clinical Reagents: Sigma Price List Feb. 1985*, St Louis, MO, p. 1105

Stoloff, L. (1983) Report on mycotoxins. General referee reports. *J. Assoc. off. anal. Chem.*, *66*, 355-363

Subrahmanyam, P. & Rao, A.S. (1974) Occurrence of aflatoxins and citrinin in groundnut (*Arachis hypogaeal* L.) at harvest in relation to pod condition and kernel moisture content. *Curr. Sci.*, *43*, 707-710

Sugimoto, T., Minamisawa, M., Takano, K., Sasamura, Y. & Tsuruta, O. (1977) Detection of ochratoxin A, citrinin, and sterigmatocystin in stored rice contaminated by a natural occurrence of *Penicillium vindicatum* and *Aspergillus versicolo*r (Jpn.). *Shokuhin Eiseigaku Zasshi*, *18*, 176-181 [*Chem. Abstr.*, *87*, 166168g]

Takeda, Y., Isohata, E., Amano, R. & Uchiyama, M. (1979) Simultaneous extraction and fractionation and thin layer chromatographic determination of 14 mycotoxins in grains. *J. Assoc. off. anal. Chem.*, *62*, 573-578

Thust, R. & Kneist, S. (1979) Activity of citrinin metabolized by rat and human microsome fractions in clastogenicity and SCE assays on Chinese hamster V79-E cells. *Mutat. Res.*, *67*, 321-330

Trantham, A.L. & Wilson, D.M. (1984) Fluorometric screening method for citrinin in corn, barley, and peanuts. *J. Assoc. off. anal. Chem.*, *67*, 37-38

Tu, C., Zhang, S. & Fang, Z. (1984) Detection of citrinin in soy sauce produced by mixed fermentation (Chin.). *Shipin Yu Fajiao Gongye*, *5*, 24-27 [*Chem. Abstr.*, *102*, 44471h]

Ueno, Y. & Kubota, K. (1976) DNA-attacking ability of carcinogenic mycotoxins in recombination-deficient mutant cells of *Bacillus subtilis*. *Cancer Res.*, *36*, 445-451

Ueno, Y., Kubota, K., Ito, T. & Nakamura, Y. (1978) Mutagenicity of carcinogenic mycotoxins in *Salmonella typhimurium*. *Cancer Res.*, *38*, 536-542

van Walbeek, W. (1973) Fungal toxins in foods, *Can. Inst. Food Sci. Technol. J.*, *6*, 96-105

Warren, H.H., Dougherty, G. & Wallis, E.S. (1949) The synthesis of dihydrocitrinin and citrinin. *J. Am. chem. Soc.*, *71*, 3422-3423

Weast, R.C., ed. (1985) *CRC Handbook of Chemistry and Physics*, 66th ed., Boca Raton, FL, CRC Press, p. C-213

Wehner, F.C., Thiel, P.G., van Rensburg, S.J. & Demasius, I.P.C. (1978) Mutagenicity to *Salmonella typhimurium* of some *Aspergillus* and *Penicillium* mycotoxins. *Mutat. Res.*, *58*, 193-203

Wilson, D.M. (1982) *Analytical method. Qualitative determination of citrinin.* In: Egan, H., Stoloff, L., Castegnaro, M., O'Neill, I.K., Scott, P. & Bartsch, H., eds, *Environmental Carcinogens. Selected Methods of Analysis*, Vol. 5, *Some Mycotoxins* (*IARC Scientific Publications No. 44*), Lyon, International Agency for Research on Cancer, pp. 353-364

Windholz, M., ed. (1983) *The Merck Index*, 10th ed., Rahway, NJ, Merck & Co., p. 331

Wu, M.T., Ayres, J.C. & Koehler, P.E. (1974) Production of citrinin by *Penicillium viridicatum* on country-cured ham. *Appl. Microbiol.*, *27*, 427-428

PATULIN

This substance was considered by a previous Working Group, in October 1975 (IARC, 1976). Since that time, new data have become available, and these have been incorporated into the monograph and taken into consideration in the present evaluation.

1. Chemical and Physical Data

1.1 Synonyms and trade names

Chem. Abstr. Services Reg. No.: 149-29-1

Chem. Abstr. Name: 4-Hydroxy-4*H*-furo[3,2-*c*]pyran-2(6*H*)-one

IUPAC Systematic Name: 4-Hydroxy-4*H*-furo[3,2-*c*]pyran-2(6*H*)-one

Synonyms: Clairformin; clavacin; clavatin; claviformin; (2,4-dihydroxy-2*H*-pyran-3-(6*H*)ylidene)acetic acid, 3,4-lactone; expansin; expansine; mycoin; mycoin C; mycoin C3; patuline; penicidin; terinin

1.2 Structural and molecular formulae and molecular weight

$C_7H_6O_4$ Mol. wt: 154.12

1.3 Chemical and physical properties of the pure substance

(*a*)   *Description*: White, odourless crystalline solid (IUPAC, 1982); compact prisms or thick plates from ether or chloroform (Windholz, 1983; Weast, 1985)

(*b*)   *Melting-point*: 105-108°C, after drying for 1 h at 60°C (IUPAC, 1982); 111°C (Windholz, 1983; Weast, 1985)

(c) *Spectroscopy data*: Ultraviolet, infrared, proton nuclear magnetic resonance (IUPAC, 1982) and mass spectral data (IUPAC, 1982; ICIS Chemical Information System, 1984 [MSSS]) have been reported.

(d) *Solubility*: Soluble in water, ethanol, diethyl ether, acetone, benzene and ethyl or amyl acetate (Windholz, 1983; Weast, 1985)

(e) *Stability*: Unstable in alkali with loss of biological activity (Windholz, 1983)

2. Production, Use, Occurrence and Analysis

2.1 Production and use

(a) Production

The synthesis of patulin was first reported by Woodward and Singh (1949, 1950) starting with tetrahydro-γ-pyrone.

The isolation and purification of patulin have been described by a number of investigators. It was initially called claviformin, following its isolation from *Penicillium claviforme* by Chain *et al.* (1942), and was later called patulin, following its isolation from *P. patulum* by Birkinshaw *et al.* (1943). The structure of patulin, however, was not established until 1949 (Woodward & Singh, 1949). Patulin can be isolated from apple juice by ethyl acetate extraction and silica gel column chromatography (Scott & Kennedy, 1973; Ware *et al.*, 1974; Stray, 1978) and from potato-glucose broth inoculated with *P. urticae* by ethyl acetate extraction and alumina column chromatography (Norstadt & McCalla, 1969).

Several investigators have studied the biosynthesis of patulin. Using ^{14}C-labelled 6-methylsalicylic acid as a precursor, Bu'Lock and Ryan (1958) and Tannenbaum and Bassett (1959) demonstrated oxidative fission of the aromatic ring and rearrangement to produce patulin. Scott *et al.* (1973) fed deuterated precursors to cultures of *P. patulum* to elucidate further the metabolic conversion of 6-methylsalicylic acid to patulin. Two mechanisms —dioxygenase-catalysed cleavage of *meta*-hydroxybenzaldehyde with subsequent rearrangement, and dioxygenase-promoted cleavage of gentisaldehyde with subsequent reduction and rearrangement — were proposed as the final steps in the formation of patulin. Zamir (1980) speculated that the latter pathway is more likely, since the enzyme that catalyses the conversion of gentisaldehyde to patulin has been isolated.

Patulin is not currently available in bulk commercial quantities. It is available from several US and European producers in small quantities for research purposes.

(b) Use

There is no current use for patulin, other than for experimental purposes. Two firms include purified patulin in an analytical reagent kit for use as a standard for mycotoxins (Makor Chemicals Ltd, 1985; Sigma Chemical Co., 1985).

Gye (1943) and Hopkins (1943) tested the clinical effectiveness of patulin as an antibiotic for the treatment of the common cold. Although it reportedly has bacteriostatic activity against various Gram-positive and Gram-negative bacteria (Hopkins, 1943), testing was discontinued because of undesirable side-effects and lack of efficacy (Rodericks & Pohland, 1981; Pohland & Thorpe, 1982). Patulin was also used at one time as an antibiotic cream for topical application, but was found to cause dermal irritation (Rodericks & Pohland, 1981).

(c) Regulatory status and guidelines

The maximum tolerable level of patulin in foods is regulated in five countries (Belgium, Norway, Sweden, Switzerland and the USSR) at 50 μg/kg or less (Schuller et al., 1982).

2.2 Occurrence

Patulin is one of several mycotoxins produced by certain fungi on fruit, grains and other foods. The fungal species include *Penicillium claviforme, P. chrysogenum, P. cyclopium, P. divergens, P. equinum, P. expansum, P. griseofulvum, P. lapidosum, P. leucopus, P. melinii, P. novaezielandiae, P. patulum, P. roqueforti, P. rugulosum, P. urticae, P. variabile, Aspergillus clavatus, A. giganteus, A. terreus* and *Byssochlamys nivea* (Pohland et al., 1970; Gorst-Allman & Steyn, 1979).

Patulin has been detected in numerous mouldy fruits, vegetables, cereals and animal feeds. It has been found following natural infection or inoculation with *Penicillium* species or *Byssochlamys nivea* in apples, peaches, pears, tomatoes, apricots, bananas, pineapples, grapes, greengages, strawberries, honeydew melons, red and green paprika, cucumbers and carrots. A number of other vegetables, including aubergines, cauliflower, celeriac, courgettes, kohlrabi, horseradish, radish, red cabbage, onions and potatoes, did not support the growth of patulin-producing moulds (Frank, 1977). Patulin is not detectable in sound fruit with no apparent fungal contamination (Stray, 1978; Cerutti et al., 1984).

The presence of fungi on food does not mean *a priori* that mycotoxins are being produced. Mintzlaff et al. (1972) isolated *Penicillium* cultures from commercial European mould-ripened sausages, which produced mycotoxins, including patulin, in culture but not apparently during growth on the sausage. Patulin was detected in blue cheese starter broth containing *P. roqueforti* but not in the final product (Engel & Prokopek, 1980). Although it has been found in processed fruit and vegetable products, patulin was not found in fermented products (e.g., apple wine, cider and fruit vinegar) (Woller & Majerus, 1982).

Levels of patulin measured in various natural and processed products are summarized in Table 1.

2.3 Analysis

A number of analytical methods have been described for the isolation and detection of patulin in apple juice and, after adaptation with appropriate clean-up procedures, for use on

Table 1. Levels of patulin found in natural and processed products

Sample	Sampling period	Country	No. of samples analysed	Percent positive samples	Concentration (μg/g)	Reference
Apples	–	USSR	30	7	0.021-0.031	Dvali et al. (1985)
Apples (puree)	1976-1981	France	64	100	1-4.8	Jacquet et al. (1983)
Apples (rotten)	1978-1982	Federal Republic of Germany	16	6.3	–	Woller & Majerus (1982)
	–	Italy	–	–	0.2-1.6	Cerutti et al. (1984)
	–	Portugal	~30	67	0.8-100	Gimeno & Martins (1983)
Apple juice	1980-1981	Federal Republic of Germany	50	64	0.002-0.042	Geipel et al. (1981)
	1978-1982	Federal Republic of Germany	172	17	0.024	Woller & Majerus (1982)
	1982	Federal Republic of Germany	33	3	0.052	Bergner-Lang et al. (1983)
Home-made Commercial Concentrate	1976	Finland	20 24 71	40 0 21	0.03-16.4 – 0.05-1.45	Lindroth & Niskanen (1978)
	1976-1981	France	20	30	0.001-1.2	Jacquet et al. (1983)
	1975-1980	German Democratic Republic	609	94 74	<0.4 <0.1	Meyer (1982)
	–	Mexico	34	24	0.009-0.04	Guzmán-Robles et al. (1983)
	–	Norway	140	~80	0.009-0.22	Stray (1978)
	1975-1976	Sweden	66	44	0.005-0.054	Josefsson & Andersson (1977)
	–	USA	13	62	0.044-0.309	Ware et al. (1974)
	–	USSR	47	17	0.054	Dvali et al. (1985)
Baby food (apples)	1976-1981	France	42	26	0.01-0.1	Jacquet et al. (1983)
Beetroots (fodder, mouldy)	1980	Poland	20	60	0.012-3.7	Wisniewska & Piskorska-Pliszczynska (1982)
Bread (mouldy)	–	Federal Republic of Germany	21	24	0.1-0.3	Reiss (1972)

Table 1 (contd)

Sample	Sampling period	Country	No. of samples analysed	Percent positive samples	Concentration (μg/g)	Reference
	–	Finland	23	91	0.02-0.16	Tyllinen et al. (1977)
Cherry juice	–	USSR	7	14	0.062	Dvali et al. (1985)
Mandarines	–	USSR	17	12	0.032	Dvali et al. (1985)
Peach juice	–	USSR	6	17	0.030	Dvali et al. (1985)
Pear juice	1982	Federal Republic of Germany	4	25	0.024	Bergner-Lang et al. (1983)
	–	USSR	10	10	0.031	Dvali et al. (1985)
Plum juice	–	USSR	33	9	0.021-0.04	Dvali et al. (1985)
Rhubarb sauce	1978-1982	Federal Republic of Germany	2	50	2.3	Woller & Majerus (1982)
Silage	1976-1979	UK	451	2	–	Buckle (1983)

other substrates. These include high-performance liquid chromatography (HPLC), reverse-phase HPLC, gas chromatography (GC), GC combined with mass spectrometry (GC/MS) and thin-layer chromatography (TLC). Several reagents have been applied to TLC plates to enhance visualization of sample spots and thereby increase sensitivity. The method of the Association of Official Analytical Chemists for determination of patulin in apple juice involves use of TLC (Stoloff & Scott, 1984), and that of the Federal Commission for the Swiss Food Manual for juices and jellies includes use of HPLC (Eidgenössischen Lebensmittelbuch-Kommission, 1984). Methods for the isolation and analysis of patulin have been reviewed by Engel and Teuber (1984). Representative methods for the analysis of patulin in various matrices are summarized in Table 2.

3. Biological Data Relevant to the Evaluation of Carcinogenic Risk to Humans

3.1 Carcinogenicity studies in animals

(a) Oral administration

Mouse: Two groups of 12 pregnant Swiss mice, weighing 28 g each, received by gavage on days 14-20 of gestation two daily doses of 0 (control) or 2 mg/kg bw patulin (98% pure by gas chromatography and infrared spectroscopy) in distilled water containing 0.05% lactic

Table 2. Methods for the analysis of patulin

Sample matrix	Sample preparation	Assay procedure[a]	Limit of detection	Reference
Apple juice	Ethyl acetate extraction; silica gel column clean-up	TLC/MBTH/UV	20 μg/l	Scott (1982); Stoloff & Scott (1984)
	Ethyl acetate extraction; acetylation	GC/FID	700 μg/l	Pohland et al. (1970)
	Ethyl acetate extraction; silylation	GC/MS	0.2-5 μg/l	Price (1979)
	Ethyl acetate extraction; acetylation	TLC/GC/MS	1 μg/l	Bergner-Lang et al. (1983)
	Ethyl acetate extraction	HPLC/UV	11 μg/l	Ware et al. (1974)
	Ethyl acetate extraction	HPLC/UV	1-5 μg/l	Eidgenössischen Lebens-mittelbuch-Kommission (1984)
Bread and rice	Ethyl ether extraction	TLC/PH	1000 μg/kg	Subramanian (1982)
Cheese	Sodium chloride/ methanol, acetone extraction	TLC/DEA	20 μg/kg	Siriwardana & Lafont (1979)
Food grain	Acetonitrole extraction; silica gel column clean-up	HPLC/UV	5 μg/kg	Hunt et al. (1978)
	Acetonitrile/water extraction	TLC/UV	400-1000 μg/kg	Stoloff et al. (1971)
	Ethyl acetate extraction; silylation	GC/EC	20 μg/kg	Fujimoto et al. (1975)

[a]Abbreviations: TLC, thin-layer chromatography; MBTH, 3-methyl-2-benzothiazolinone; UV, ultraviolet detection; GC, gas chromatography; FID, flame-ionization detection; MS, mass spectrometry; HPLC, high-performance liquid chromatography; PH, phenylhydrazine; DEA, diethylamine; EC, electron capture detection

acid to avoid the possibility of partial decomposition of patulin. The dams and offspring were observed throughout life. Of the dams, 2/12 controls and 5/11 of the effective treated animals developed various malignant and benign tumours. In the F_1 generation, 22/40 control males and 23/54 control females, and 12/35 effective treated males and 18/41 effective treated females developed various malignant tumours; the tumour types did not differ between control and treated groups of either sex (Osswald et al., 1978). [The Working Group noted the small number of animals used.]

Rat: Two groups of 50 female Sprague-Dawley rats, weighing 40 g each, received by gavage twice weekly at 72-h intervals 0 or 1 mg/kg bw patulin (purity, 98% by gas chromatography and infrared spectroscopy) dissolved in distilled water containing 0.05% lactic acid. After four weeks, the concentration of patulin was increased to 2.5 mg/kg bw for the subsequent 60 weeks. Rats were observed for approximately 110 weeks. Both control and treated animals developed various malignant neoplasms (controls: 13/50; treated: 12/50), but the tumour types did not differ in incidence between the groups (Osswald *et al.*, 1978). [The Working Group noted that only one dose was used.]

Groups of 70 male and 70 female Wistar rats, 28 days old, which were the offspring of rats exposed by gavage to 0.1, 0.5 or 1.5 mg/kg bw patulin (>95% pure by high-performance liquid chromatography with ultraviolet detection) for four weeks before mating and throughout mating, gestation and lactation, received thrice-weekly administrations of 0.1, 0.5 or 1.5 mg/kg bw patulin by gavage for six, 12, 18 or 24 months. A group of 110 male and 110 female offspring served as controls. No difference in tumour incidence was described (Becci *et al.*, 1981). [The Working Group noted that specific data on the incidence and types of tumours in control and treated groups were not provided in the report.]

(b)   Subcutaneous administration

Rat: Two groups of five male Wistar rats, weighing 100 g each, were given twice-weekly subcutaneous injections of 0.2 mg/rat patulin (melting-point, 109-111°C; purity unspecified) in 0.5 ml arachis oil for 61 and 64 weeks, respectively. In the group treated for 61 weeks, all of four rats surviving at the appearance of the first tumour (58 weeks) developed local sarcomas before 69 weeks; no tumour was observed at other sites. In the second group, two of four rats surviving at the appearance of the first tumour (62 weeks) developed local sarcomas by 64 weeks (end of experiment). No local tumour occurred in 16 controls injected with 0.5 ml arachis oil and surviving 54-107 weeks (Dickens & Jones, 1961). [The Working Group noted the small number of animals used.]

3.2 Other relevant biological data

(a)   Experimental systems

Toxic effects

The oral LD_{50} of patulin was reported to be 32.5 mg/kg bw in Sprague-Dawley rats and 170 mg/kg bw in White Leghorn cockerels (Dailey *et al.*, 1977a). The 14-day LD_{50} for patulin when dissolved in saline (pH 7.2) and administered intraperitoneally was 7.6 mg/kg bw in ICR mice and 5.9 mg/kg bw in weanling Sprague-Dawley rats; when administered by gavage, the LD_{50}s were 17 mg/kg bw and 108-118 mg/kg bw, respectively. The 14-day oral LD_{50} in neonatal Sprague-Dawley rats was 6.8 mg/kg bw. No change in the intraperitoneal LD_{50} of patulin was observed in mice pretreated with 3-methylcholanthrene, but pretreatment with a known inhibitor of cytochrome P450, SKF-525A, reduced the LD_{50} from 7.6 to 2.3 mg/kg bw. Following pretreatment of mice with an intraperitoneal injection of 75 mg/kg bw pentobarbital, the LD_{50} of patulin was 8.5 mg/kg bw (Hayes *et al.*, 1979).

Subcutaneous injection into mice of 1.25 mg/kg bw patulin twice daily produced induration and tenderness at the site of injection within 1 h. Generalized subcutaneous oedema was seen at an unspecified time. Injection of 0.5 mg/kg bw per day for 11 days led to the development of hard patches and adhesions at the injection site during a subsequent seven days' observation. Doses of 2.0-10.0 mg/kg bw patulin produced subcutaneous necrosis and inflammation within one to two days in guinea-pigs (Broom *et al.*, 1944).

Administration of patulin (4 mg/kg) in the diet for six weeks to male Fischer 344 rats significantly increased the number of hyperplastic liver nodules induced by partial hepatectomy at week 1 and subsequent (weeks 7-9) exposure to 2-acetylaminofluorene in the diet in combination with a single intragastric dose of carbon tetrachloride (Imaida *et al.*, 1982).

Patulin non-competitively inhibited the activity of rabbit muscle aldolase ($K_i = 1.3 \times 10^{-5}$ M) and competitively inhibited the activity of lactic dehydrogenase ($K_i = 6.2 \times 10^{-6}$ M) *in vitro* (Ashoor & Chu, 1973a,b).

Effects on reproduction and prenatal toxicity

Male and female Sprague-Dawley rats were administered 1.5 mg/kg bw patulin (98.7% pure) in 1 mM aqueous citrate buffer by gavage on five days per week for at least seven weeks before mating. During gestation, females (30 per group) were treated on seven days per week. At this dose, no sign of maternal toxicity was seen and no treatment-related teratogenicity was observed. Owing to severe maternal and embryotoxicity, higher doses could not be tested (Dailey *et al.*, 1977a).

Groups of 15 and ten pregnant female CD-1 rats were administered 1.5 and 2.0 mg/kg bw patulin [purity unspecified], respectively, intraperitoneally from days 5-16 of gestation. At the low dose, there was a reduction in fetal weight; at the high dose, all implanted embryos were resorbed (Reddy *et al.*, 1978). [The Working Group noted that no information on maternal toxicity was given.]

Absorption, distribution, excretion and metabolism

Adult male and female Sprague-Dawley rats were given a single oral dose of ^{14}C-patulin; approximately 49% of the radioactivity was excreted in the faeces and 36% in the urine within seven days, and 1-2% was recovered as $^{14}CO_2$ from expired air. Radioactivity was measured throughout the seven-day period in various tissues and organs; the most significant retention site was red-blood cells (Dailey *et al.*, 1977b).

Mutagenicity and other short-term tests

Patulin (20 and 100 μg/plate) was mutagenic in the *Bacillus subtilis rec*$^{+/-}$ assay (Ueno & Kubota, 1976; Manabe *et al.*, 1981) but not in the *Escherichia coli polA*$^{+/-}$ assay in a plate test (3-50 μg/disc) or liquid incubation assay (1-10 μg/ml) (Lindroth & von Wright, 1978).

Patulin was not mutagenic to *Salmonella typhimurium* TA1535, TA1537, TA1538, TA98 or TA100 when tested at up to 250 μg/plate, in the presence or absence of an exogenous metabolic system (Engel & von Milczewski, 1976; Kuczuk *et al.*, 1978; Ueno *et al.*, 1978; Wehner *et al.*, 1978; von Wright & Lindroth, 1978).

In host-mediated assays, a single oral administration of 10 or 20 mg/kg bw patulin, or three intramuscular injections of 0.5 mg patulin combined with intraperitoneal administration of *S. typhimurium* TA1950, TA1951 or *his*G46 to mice did not induce mutagenic activity (Gabridge & Legator, 1969; von Wright & Lindroth, 1978).

Concentrations of 50 or 100 μg patulin, in the presence or absence of an exogenous metabolic system, did not induce mitotic recombination in a diploid strain of *Saccharomyces cerevisiae* (Kuczuk *et al.*, 1978). In a haploid strain of *S. cerevisiae*, doses of 20-70 μg/ml patulin increased the frequency of cytoplasmic petite mutants (Mayer & Legator, 1969).

A small but significant increase in the incidence of somatic mosaicism was reported in *Drosophila melanogaster* administered 3.2×10^{-3} M patulin, but not with doses of 4×10^{-4} or 3.2×10^{-2} M (Belitsky *et al.*, 1983). [The Working Group noted that this test system is not validated (see Preamble).]

Patulin induced single- and double-strand breaks in DNA of HeLa cells (Umeda *et al.*, 1972). Concentrations of up to 6×10^{-4} M patulin did not induce unscheduled DNA synthesis in primary hepatocytes from rats or mice (Mori *et al.*, 1984) nor in cultured rat liver or human embryonic liver cells tested with up to 1.6×10^{-3} M (Belitsky *et al.*, 1983).

It was reported in an abstract that 0.5-2 μg/ml patulin increased the incidence of sister chromatid exchanges in primary cultures of Chinese hamster cells (Kubiak & Kosz-Vnenchak, 1983). The incidence of sister chromatid exchanges was also increased in human lymphocytes treated with 0.1 and 0.2 μg/ml patulin (Cooray *et al.*, 1982), but not in Chinese hamster V79 cells treated with up to 10^{-5} M patulin, in the presence or absence of an exogenous metabolic system. Chromosomal aberrations were induced by 2.5×10^{-6} M patulin only in the absence of an exogenous metabolic system (Thust *et al.*, 1982). Patulin (3.5×10^{-6} M) induced chromosomal aberrations in cultured human peripheral leucocytes (Withers, 1966).

Patulin induced mutations to 8-azaguanine resistance and chromosomal aberrations in cultured CH3 mouse mammary carcinoma cells (Umeda *et al.*, 1977). [The Working Group noted the inadequate experimental design.]

Oral administration of two doses of up to 20 mg/kg bw patulin did not induce sister chromatid exchanges in the bone-marrow cells of Chinese hamsters, but 10 and 20 mg/kg bw significantly increased the incidence of chromosomal aberrations (Korte *et al.*, 1979; Korte, 1980; Korte & Rückert, 1980).

Administration of 1.5, 7.5 or 15 mg/kg bw patulin to male rats by gavage on five days per week for 10 or 11 weeks, followed by mating for three successive weeks, did not induce dominant lethal mutations (Dailey *et al.*, 1977a); negative results were also obtained in mice receiving a single intraperitoneal injection of up to 3 mg/kg bw patulin and mated for eight successive weeks (Epstein *et al.*, 1972; Reddy *et al.*, 1978).

(b) *Humans*

No data were available to the Working Group.

3.3 Case reports and epidemiological studies of carcinogenicity to humans

No data were available to the Working Group.

4. Summary of Data Reported and Evaluation

4.1 Exposure data

Patulin is produced by various *Penicillium*, *Aspergillus* and *Byssochlamys* fungi that can contaminate many common fruits and some vegetables. Human exposure may occur if these contaminated foods are consumed.

4.2 Experimental data

Patulin was tested for carcinogenicity in one experiment in mice and in two experiments in two strains of rats by oral administration. The study in mice and one of the studies in rats involved treatment of pregnant dams and the continued treatment of offspring of the F_1 generation. In one study, subcutaneous injection of patulin produced local sarcomas in rats. The studies were considered to be inadequate for evaluation.

No adequate data were available to evaluate the reproductive effects or prenatal toxicity of patulin to experimental animals.

Patulin induced DNA damage in *Bacillus subtilis*, but not in *Escherichia coli*. It was not mutagenic to *Salmonella typhimurium*. Patulin induced petite mutants but not mitotic recombination in *Saccharomyces cerevisiae*. The compound induced DNA strand breaks in HeLa cells, but not unscheduled DNA synthesis in cultured mammalian cells. It induced sister chromatid exchanges in cultured mammalian cells. Patulin induced chromosomal aberrations but not sister chromatid exchanges in the bone-marrow cells of Chinese hamsters treated *in vivo*. It did not induce dominant lethal mutations in rats or mice.

Overall assessment of data from short-term tests: Patulin[a]

	Genetic activity			Cell transformation
	DNA damage	Mutation	Chromosomal effects	
Prokaryotes	?	–		
Fungi/Green plants		?		
Insects				
Mammalian cells (*in vitro*)	?		+	
Mammals (*in vivo*)			?	
Humans (*in vivo*)				
Degree of evidence in short-term tests for genetic activity: **Inadequate**				Cell transformation: No data

[a]The groups into which the table is divided and the symbols used are defined on pp. 19-20 of the Preamble; the degrees of evidence are defined on pp. 20-21.

4.3 Human data

No case report or epidemiological study of the carcinogenicity of patulin was available to the Working Group.

4.4 Evaluation[1]

There is *inadequate evidence* for the carcinogenicity of patulin in experimental animals. No evaluation could be made of the carcinogenicity of patulin to humans.

5. References

Ashoor, S.H. & Chu, F.S. (1973a) Inhibition of alcohol and lactic acid dehydrogenases by patulin and penicillic acid *in vitro*. *Food Cosmet. Toxicol.*, *11*, 617-624

Ashoor, S.H. & Chu, F.S. (1973b) Inhibition of muscle aldolase by penicillic acid and patulin *in vitro*. *Food Cosmet. Toxicol.*, *11*, 995-1000

Becci, P.J., Hess, F.G., Johnson, W.D., Gallo, M.A., Babish, J.G., Dailey, R.E. & Parent, R.A. (1981) Long-term carcinogenicity and toxicity studies of patulin in the rat. *J. appl. Toxicol.*, *1*, 256-261

Belitsky, G.A., Khovanova, E.M., Budunova, I.V. & Sharupich, E.G. (1983) Mycotoxin induction of somatic mutagenesis in *Drosophila* and DNA-repair synthesis in mammalian liver cell cultures (Russ.). *Bull. exp. Biol. Med.*, *96*, 83-86

Bergner-Lang, B., Kächele, M. & Stengel, E. (1983) Analyzing patulin in fruit juices and fruit products (Ger.). *Dtsch. Lebensmittel.-Rundsch.*, *79*, 400-404

Birkinshaw, J.H., Michael, S.E., Bracken, A. & Raistrick, H. (1943) Patulin in the common cold. Collaborative research on a derivative of *Penicillium patulum* Bainier. II. Biochemistry and chemistry. *Lancet*, *ii*, 625-630

Broom, W.A., Bülbring, E., Chapman, C.J., Hampton, J.W.F., Thomson, A.M., Ungar, J., Wien, R. & Woolfe, G. (1944) The pharmacology of patulin. *Br. J. exp. Pathol.*, *25*, 195-207

Buckle, A.E. (1983) The occurrence of mycotoxins in cereals and animal feedstuffs. *Vet. Res. Comm.*, *7*, 171-186

Bu'Lock, J.D. & Ryan, A.J. (1958) The biogenesis of patulin. *Proc. chem. Soc. Lond.*, 222-223

Cerutti, G., Finoli, C., Vecchio, A. & Volonterio, A. (1984) Formation and presence of patulin in apples and their products (Ital.). *Tecnol. Aliment.*, *7*, 19-25

Chain, E., Florey, H.W. & Jennings, M.A. (1942) An antibacterial substance produced by *Penicillium claviforme*. *Br. J. exp. Pathol.*, *23*, 202-205

---

[1]For definition of the italicized term, see Preamble, p. 18.

Cooray, R., Kiessling, K.-H. & Lindahl-Kiessling, K. (1982) The effects of patulin and patulin-cysteine mixtures on DNA synthesis and the frequency of sister chromatid exchanges in human lymphocytes. *Food Chem. Toxicol.*, *20*, 893-898

Dailey, R.E., Brouwer, E., Blaschka, A.M., Reynaldo, E.F., Green, S., Monlux, W.S. & Ruggles, D.I. (1977a) Intermediate-duration toxicity study of patulin in rats. *J. Toxicol. environ. Health*, *2*, 713-725

Dailey, R.E., Blaschka, A.M. & Brouwer, E.A. (1977b) Absorption, distribution, and excretion of [^{14}C]patulin by rats. *J. Toxicol. environ. Health*, *3*, 479-489

Dickens, F. & Jones, H.E.H. (1961) Carcinogenic activity of a series of reactive lactones and related substances. *Br. J. Cancer*, *15*, 85-100

Dvali, G.N., Maximenko, L.V., Eller, K.I. & Tutelyan, V.A. (1985) Study of food contamination with patulin (Russ.). *Vopr. Pitan*, *1*, 45-48

Eidgenössischen Lebensmittelbuch-Kommission (1984) Official methods of analysis for patulin (Ger.). *Mitt. Geb. Lebensmitteluntersuch. Hyg.*, *75*, 506-513

Engel, G. & von Milczewski, K.E. (1976) Detection of mycotoxins after activation with rat-liver homogenates with *Salmonella typhimurium* histidine-deficient mutants (Ger.). *Kieler Milchwirtsch. Forsch.*, *28*, 359-365

Engel, G. & Prokopek, D. (1980) No detection of patulin and penicillinic acid in cheese produced by *Penicillium roqueforti*-strains forming patulin and penicillinic acid (Ger.). *Milchwissenschaft*, *35*, 218-220

Engel, G. & Teuber, M. (1984) *Patulin and other small lactones*. In: Betina, V., ed., *Mycotoxins — Production, Isolation, Separation and Purification*, Amsterdam, Elsevier, pp. 291-314

Epstein, S.S., Arnold, E., Andrea, J., Bass, W. & Bishop, Y. (1972) Detection of chemical mutagens by the dominant lethal assay in the mouse. *Toxicol. appl. Pharmacol.*, *23*, 288-325

Frank, H.K. (1977) Occurrence of patulin in fruits and vegetables. *Ann. Nutr. Aliment.*, *31*, 459-465

Fujimoto, Y., Suzuki, T. & Hoshino, Y. (1975) Determination of penicillic acid and patulin by gas-liquid chromatography with an electron-capture detector. *J. Chromatogr.*, *105*, 99-106

Gabridge, M.G. & Legator, M.S. (1969) A host-mediated microbial assay for the detection of mutagenic compounds. *Proc. Soc. exp. Biol. Med.*, *130*, 831-834

Geipel, M., Baltes, W., Kröenert, W. & Weber, R. (1981) Determination of patulin in apple products by high performance liquid chromatography (Ger.). *Chem. Mikrobiol.*, *7*, 93-96

Gimeno, A. & Martins, M.L. (1983) Rapid thin-layer chromatographic determination of patulin, citrinin, and aflatoxin in apples and pears, and their juices and jams. *J. Assoc. off. anal. Chem.*, *66*, 85-91

Gorst-Allman, C.P. & Steyn, P.S. (1979) Screening methods for the detection of thirteen common mycotoxins. *J. Chromatogr.*, *175*, 325-331

Guzmán-Robles, M.R., González-Pérez, J. & González-Pérez, A. (1983) Quantitative patulin determination in commercial pear and apple juices and nectars. *Tecnol. Aliment.*, *18*, 16-20

Gye, W.E. (1943) Patulin in the common cold. III. Preliminary trial in the common cold. *Lancet*, *ii*, 630-631

Hayes, A.W., Phillips, T.D., Williams, W.L. & Ciegler, A. (1979) Acute toxicity of patulin in mice and rats. *Toxicology*, *13*, 91-100

Hopkins, W.A. (1943) Patulin in the common cold. IV. Biological properties: extended trial in the common cold. *Lancet*, *ii*, 631-634

Hunt, D.C., Bourdon, A.T. & Crosby N.T. (1978) Use of high performance liquid chromatography for the identification and estimation of zearalenone, patulin and penicillic acid in food. *J. Sci. Food Agric.*, *29*, 239-244

IARC (1976) *IARC Monographs on the Evaluation of Carcinogenic Risk of Chemicals to Man*, Vol. 10, *Some Naturally Occurring Substances*, Lyon, pp. 205-210

ICIS Chemical Information System (1984) *Carbon-13 NMR Spectral Search System* (CNMR), *Mass Spectral Search System* (MSSS), *Infrared Spectral Search System* (IRSS), *Information System for Hazardous Organics in Water* (ISHOW), and *Environmental Fate* (ENVIROFATE), Washington DC, Information Consultants, Inc.

Imaida, K., Hirose, M., Ogiso, T., Kurata, Y. & Ito, N. (1982) Quantitative analysis of initiating and promoting activities of five mycotoxins in liver carcinogenesis in rats. *Cancer Lett.*, *16*, 137-143

IUPAC (1982) Physicochemical data for some selected mycotoxins. *Pure appl. Chem.*, *54*, 2219-2284

Jacquet, J., Lafonte, J. & Vilette, O. (1983) Contamination of apples and apple products by patulin (Fr.). *Microbiol. Aliments Nutr.*, *1*, 127-131

Josefsson, E. & Andersson, A. (1977) Analysis of patulin in apple beverages sold in Sweden. *Arch. Inst. Pasteur Tunis*, *54*, 261-267

Korte, A. (1980) Comparative analysis of chromosomal aberrations and sister chromatid exchanges in bone-marrow cells of Chinese hamsters after treatment with aflatoxin B_1, patulin and cyclophosphamide (Abstract No. 24). *Mutat. Res.*, *74*, 164

Korte, A. & Rückert, G. (1980) Chromosomal analysis in bone-marrow cells of Chinese hamsters after treatment with mycotoxins. *Mutat. Res.*, *78*, 41-49

Korte, A., Slacik-Erben, R. & Obe, G. (1979) The influence of ethanol treatment on cytogenetic effects in bone marrow cells of Chinese hamsters by cyclophosphamide, aflatoxin B_1 and patulin. *Toxicology*, *12*, 53-61

Kubiak, R. & Kosz-Vnenchak, M. (1983) Mutagenic properties of mycotoxins as naturally occurring mutagens: chromosome aberrations and SCEs induced by patulin (Abstract No. 84). *Mutat. Res.*, *113*, 273

Kuczuk, M.H., Benzon, P.M., Heath, H. & Hayes, A.W. (1978) Evaluation of the mutagenic potential of mycotoxins using *Salmonella typhimurium* and *Saccharomyces cerevisiae*. *Mutat. Res.*, *53*, 11-20

Lindroth, S. & Niskanen, A. (1978) Comparison of potential patulin hazard in home-made and commercial apple products. *J. Food Sci.*, *43*, 446-448

Lindroth, S. & von Wright, A. (1978) Comparison of the toxicities of patulin and patulin adducts formed with cysteine. *Appl. environ. Microbiol.*, *35*, 1003-1007

Makor Chemicals Ltd (1985) *Catalogue*, Jerusalem, p. 69

Manabe, M., Goto, T., Tanaka, K. & Matsuura, S. (1981) The capabilities of the *Aspergillus flavus* group to produce aflatoxins and kojic acid (Jpn). *Rep. natl Food Res. Inst.*, *38*, 115-120

Mayer, V.W. & Legator, M.S. (1969) Production of petite mutants of *Saccharomyces cerevisiae* by patulin. *J. agric. Food Chem.*, *17*, 454-456

Meyer, R.A. (1982) Determination of patulin in foods — proposal of a standard method (Ger.). *Nahrung*, *26*, 337-342

Mintzlaff, H.J., Ciegler, A. & Leistner, L. (1972) Potential mycotoxin problems in mould-fermented sausage. *Z. Lebensmittel.-Untersuch. Forsch.*, *150*, 133-137

Mori, H., Kawai, K., Ohbayashi, F., Kuniyasu, T., Yamazaki, M., Hamasaki, T. & Williams, G.M. (1984) Genotoxicity of a variety of mycotoxins in the hepatocyte primary culture/DNA repair test using rat and mouse hepatocytes. *Cancer Res.*, *44*, 2918-2923

Norstadt, F.A. & McCalla, T.M. (1969) Patulin production by *Penicillium urticae* Bainier in batch culture. *Appl. Microbiol,*, *17*, 193-196

Osswald, H., Frank, H.K., Komitowski, D. & Winter, H. (1978) Long-term testing of patulin administered orally to Sprague-Dawley rats and Swiss mice. *Food Cosmet. Toxicol.*, *16*, 243-247

Pohland, A.E. & Thorpe, C.W. (1982) *Mycotoxins*. In: Bowman, M.C., ed., *Handbook of Carcinogens and Hazardous Substances: Chemical and Trace Analysis*, New York, Marcel Dekker, pp. 303-390

Pohland, A.E., Sanders, K. & Thorpe, C.W. (1970) Determination of patulin in apple juice. *J. Assoc. off. anal. Chem.*, *53*, 692-695

Price, K.R. (1979) A comparison of two quantitative mass spectrometric methods for the analysis of patulin in apple juice. *Biomed. Mass Spectrom.*, *6*, 573-574

Reddy, C.S., Chan, P.K. & Hayes, A.W. (1978) Teratogenic and dominant lethal studies of patulin in mice. *Toxicology*, *11*, 219-223

Reiss, J. (1972) Occurrence of patulin in spontaneously mouldy bread and pastry. Mycotoxins in food supplies. II. (Ger.). *Naturwissenschaften*, *59*, 37

Rodericks, J.V. & Pohland, A.E. (1981) *Food hazards of natural origin*. In: Roberts, H.R., ed., *Food Safety*, New York, Wiley-Interscience, pp. 181-237

Schuller, P.L., Stoloff, L. & van Egmond, M.P. (1982) *Limits and regulations in environmental carcinogens.* In: Stoloff, L., Scott, P., Castegnaro, M., O'Neill, I.K. & Bartsch, H., eds, *Environmental Carcinogens. Selected Methods of Analysis,* Vol. 5, *Some Mycotoxins (IARC Scientific Publications No. 44)*, Lyon, International Agency for Research on Cancer, pp. 107-116

Scott, A.I., Zamir, L., Phillips, G.T. & Yalpani, M. (1973) The biosynthesis of patulin. *Bioorg. Chem.*, *2*, 124-139

Scott, P.M. (1982) *Thin-layer chromatographic determination of patulin in apple juice.* In: Stoloff, L., Scott, P., Castegnaro, M., O'Neill, I.K. & Bartsch, H., eds, *Environmental Carcinogens. Selected Methods of Analysis,* Vol. 5, *Some Mycotoxins (IARC Scientific Publications No. 44)*, Lyon, International Agency for Research on Cancer, pp. 317-327

Scott, P.M. & Kennedy, B.P.C. (1973) Improved method for the thin layer chromatographic determination of patulin in apple juice. *J. Assoc. off. anal. Chem.*, *56*, 813-816

Sigma Chemical Co. (1985) *Biochemical and Organic Compounds for Research and Diagnostic Clinical Reagents: Sigma Price List Feb. 1985*, St Louis, MO, p. 1105

Siriwardana, M.G. & Lafont, P. (1979) Determination of mycophenolic acid, penicillic acid, patulin, sterigmatocystin, and aflatoxins in cheese. *J. Dairy Sci.*, *62*, 1145-1148

Stoloff, L. & Scott, P.M. (1984) *Natural poisons.* In: Williams, S., ed., *Official Methods of Analysis of the Association of Official Analytical Chemists*, 14th ed., Arlington, VA, Association of Official Analytical Chemists, pp. 496-497

Stoloff, L., Nesheim, S., Yin, L., Rodricks, J.V., Stack, M. & Campbell, A.D. (1971) A multimycotoxin detection method for aflatoxins, ochratoxins, zearalenone, sterigmatocystin, and patulin. *J. Assoc. off. anal. Chem.*, *54*, 91-97

Stray, H. (1978) High pressure liquid chromatographic determination of patulin in apple juice. *J. Assoc. off. anal. Chem.*, *61*, 1359-1362

Subramanian, T. (1982) Colorimetric determination of patulin produced by *Penicillium patulum. J. Assoc. off. anal. Chem.*, *65*, 5-7

Tannenbaum, S.W. & Bassett, E.W. (1959) The biosynthesis of patulin. III. Evidence for a molecular rearrangement of the aromatic ring. *J. biol. Chem.*, *234*, 1861-1866

Thust, R., Kneist, S. & Mendel, J. (1982) Patulin, a further clastogenic mycotoxin, is negative in the SCE assay in Chinese hamster V79-E cells *in vitro. Mutat. Res.*, *103*, 91-97

Tyllinen, H., Raevuori, M., Karppanen, E. & Garry-Andersson, A.-S. (1977) A study on the toxicity of spontaneously moulded bread. *Nord. Veterinaermed.*, *29*, 546-551

Ueno, Y. & Kubota, K. (1976) DNA-attacking ability of carcinogenic mycotoxins in recombination-deficient mutant cells of *Bacillus subtilis. Cancer Res.*, *36*, 445-451

Ueno, Y., Kubota, K., Ito, T. & Nakamura, Y. (1978) Mutagenicity of carcinogenic mycotoxins in *Salmonella typhimurium. Cancer Res.*, *38*, 536-542

Umeda, M., Yamamoto, T. & Saito, M. (1972) DNA-strand breakage of HeLa cells induced by several mycotoxins. *Jpn. J. exp. Med., 42,* 527-535

Umeda, M., Tsutsui, T. & Saito, M. (1977) Mutagenicity and inducibility of DNA single-strand breaks and chromosome aberrations by various mycotoxins. *Gann, 68,* 619-625

Ware, G.M., Thorpe, C.W. & Pohland, A.E. (1974) Liquid chromatographic method for the determination of patulin in apple juice. *J. Assoc. off. anal. Chem., 57,* 1111-1113

Weast, R.C., ed. (1985) *CRC Handbook of Chemistry and Physics,* 66th ed., Boca Raton, FL, CRC Press, p. C-390

Wehner, F.C., Thiel, P.G., van Rensburg, S.J. & Demasius, I.P.C. (1978) Mutagenicity to *Salmonella typhimurium* of some *Aspergillus* and *Penicillium* mycotoxins. *Mutat. Res., 58,* 193-203

Windholz, M., ed. (1983) *The Merck Index,* 10th ed., Rahway, NJ, Merck & Co., p. 1012

Wisniewska, H. & Piskorska-Pliszczynska, J. (1982) Natural occurrence of patulin in fodder beetroots. *Bull. vet. Inst. Pulawy, 25,* 38-42

Withers, R.F.J. (1966) *The action of some lactones and related compounds on human chromosomes.* In: Landa, Z., ed., *Mechanism of Mutation and Inducing Factors,* Prague, Academia, pp. 359-364

Woller, R. & Majerus, P. (1982) Patulin in fruit and fruit products — properties, formation, and occurrence. *Fluess. Obst., 49,* 564-570

Woodward, R.B. & Singh, G. (1949) The structure of patulin. *J. Am. chem. Soc., 71,* 758-759

Woodward, R.B. & Singh, G. (1950) The synthesis of patulin. *J. Am. chem. Soc., 72,* 1428

von Wright, A. & Lindroth, S. (1978) The lack of mutagenic properties of patulin and patulin adducts formed with cysteine in *Salmonella* test systems. *Mutat. Res., 58,* 211-215

Zamir, L.O. (1980) *The biosynthesis of patulin and penicillic acid.* In: Steyn, P.S., ed., *The Biosynthesis of Mycotoxins,* New York, Academic Press, pp. 223-268

RUGULOSIN

1. Chemical and Physical Data

1.1 Synonyms and trade names

Chem. Abstr. Services Reg. No.: 23537-16-8

Chem. Abstr. Name: Rugulosin

IUPAC Systematic Name: (5a*S*,6*R*,13a*S*,14*R*,17*S*,18*R*,19*R*,20*S*)-1,7,9,15,17,20-Hexa-hydroxy-3,11-dimethyl-5*H*,6*H*-6,13a,5a,14-[1,2,3,4]butanetetraylcycloocta[1,2-*b*:5,6-*b'*]dinaphthalene-5,8,13,16(14*H*)-tetrone

Synonyms: 1,7,9,15,17,20-Hexahydroxy-3,11-dimethyl-5*H*,6*H*-6,13a,5a,14-[1,2,3,4]-butanetetraylcycloocta[1,2-*b*:5,6-*b'*]dinaphthalene-5,8,13,16(14*H*)-tetrone; (5a*S*-(5a*R**,6*S**,13a*R**,14*S**,17*R**,18*S**,19*S**,20*R**))-1,7,9,15,17,20-hexahydroxy-3,11-dimethyl-5*H*,6*H*-6,13a,5a,14-(1,2,3,4)butanetetraylcycloocta(1,2-*b*:5,6-*b'*)dinaphtha-lene-5,8,13,16(14*H*)-tetrone

1.2 Structural and molecular formulae and molecular weight

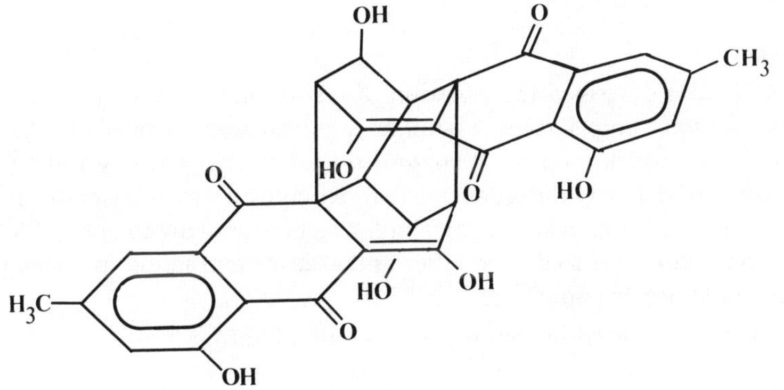

$C_{30}H_{22}O_{10}$

Mol. wt: 542.50

—99—

1.3 Chemical and physical properties of the pure substance

(a) *Description*: With retention of solvent of crystallization: large dull-yellow cubes (ethanol), bright yellow blunt-ended prisms and rods (ether or acetone), yellow rosettes of elongated prisms (methanol) (Breen *et al.*, 1955); fine pale-yellow needles (methanol) or rods (acetone) (Ueno *et al.*, 1971); without solvent of crystallization: yellow powder (Breen *et al.*, 1955)

(b) *Melting-point*: ~ 290°C (decomposition) (Breen *et al.*, 1955; Shibata *et al.*, 1968)

(c) *Spectroscopy data*: Ultraviolet, infrared, proton nuclear magnetic resonance (Pham Van Chuong *et al.*, 1973; Bouhet *et al.*, 1976), C-13 nuclear magnetic resonance (Toma *et al.*, 1975) and mass spectral data and circular dichroism (Bouhet *et al.*, 1976) have been reported.

(d) *Solubility*: Soluble in acetone, dioxane, pyridine, ethyl acetate, glacial acetic acid and aqueous alkalis, including sodium bicarbonate and ammonia; moderately soluble in methanol, ethanol, diethyl ether, chloroform, butanol and benzene; almost insoluble in light petroleum and water (Breen *et al.*, 1955); soluble in dimethyl sulphoxide and tetrahydrofuran (Bouhet *et al.*, 1976)

(e) *Optical rotation*: α_D^{20} +466° (0.5% in dioxane) (Ueno *et al.*, 1971)

(f) *Stability*: Hygroscopic and light-sensitive; readily loses solvent of crystallization on exposure to air, vacuum or dessication (Breen *et al.*, 1955; Bouhet *et al.*, 1976)

2. Production, Use, Occurrence and Analysis

2.1 Production and use

(a) *Production*

Breen *et al.* (1955) described the isolation of a substance they named rugulosin from *Penicillium rugulosum* Thom. Crude, crystalline rugulosin was obtained by ether extraction of the dried, defatted mycelium from *P. rugulosum*; additional washing and crystallization procedures were used to purify the crude product. Rugulosin was also isolated from a strain of *Penicillium wortmanni* Klöcker, using similar techniques (Breen *et al.*, 1955). Acidification of the mycelium prior to diethyl ether and acetone extraction has been reported to increase yields significantly (Bouhet *et al.*, 1976).

Rugulosin is not produced in commercial or bulk quantities.

(b) *Use*

Rugulosin is not known to be used commercially. It has been reported to have antibacterial and antifungal activity (Breen *et al.*, 1955; Ueno *et al.*, 1971).

2.2 Occurrence

Rugulosin, a yellow fungal pigment, is synthesized by *Penicillia* that can contaminate rice, maize and other cereal grains. It has been detected in cultures of *Penicillium rugulosum* Thom, and also in cultures of *P. brunneum*, *P. wortmanni*, *P. tardum*, *P. variabile*, *Sepedonium ampullosporum*, in various species of *Endothia* and a lichen, *Acroscyphus sphaerophoroides* (Breen *et al.*, 1955; Takeda *et al.*, 1973; Bouhet *et al.*, 1976; Roane & Stipes, 1978; Sankawa *et al.*, 1978; Stark *et al.*, 1978). The mycelium of *P. rugulosum* may contain as much as 5% (dry weight) rugulosin (Bouhet *et al.*, 1976).

2.3 Analysis

Rugulosin has been separated from other mycotoxins by column chromatography on silica gel and further purified and identified by thin-layer chromatography. The lowest level detected in grains using this method is 0.1 $\mu g/g$ (Takeda *et al.*, 1979).

3. Biological Data Relevant to the Evaluation of Carcinogenic Risk to Humans

3.1 Carcinogenicity studies in animals

Oral administration

Mouse: A group of 30 male DDD mice, seven weeks old, was fed a diet containing 1.5 mg/mouse per day (+)-rugulosin (>98% pure) for 22 days followed by basal diet for 692 days. A control group of nine mice received basal diet only for 715 days. Between days 21-42, 16 rugulosin-treated mice died; histopathology revealed liver lesions characterized by fatty degeneration, necrosis and nuclear damage of liver cells. Average survival in controls was 412 ± 133 days and that in treated mice 252 ± 268 days. Among 14 treated survivors, one mouse had a well-differentiated hepatocellular carcinoma at 481 days and another a lymphocytic leukaemia at 688 days. One control mouse developed a lung adenoma at 652 days (Ueno *et al.*, 1980). [The Working Group noted the small number of animals used and the incomplete reporting of the results.]

Groups of 14-16 male ddYS mice, seven weeks old, were fed diets containing 0, 0.30 or 0.75 mg/mouse per day (+)-rugulosin (>98% pure) for over 800 days. Average survival was approximately 580 days. In the high-dose group, 4/16 developed hyperlastic nodules in the liver (days 542, 664, 726 and 833), and one had a hepatocellular adenoma (day 540). One mouse in the control group developed leukaemia (day 477) (Ueno *et al.*, 1980). [The Working Group noted the small number of animals used and the incomplete reporting of the results.]

3.2 Other relevant biological data

(a) Experimental systems

Toxic effects

A single oral dose of 4 g/kg (+)-rugulosin caused no fatality in mice (Sato *et al.*, 1977). Intraperitoneal LD_{50} values (with olive oil as the solvent) were 55 mg/kg bw in mice and 44 mg/kg bw in rats (Ueno *et al.*, 1971).

Following intraperitoneal administration of (+)-rugulosin to mice and rats, diffuse fatty degeneration of parenchymal cells and centrilobular liver-cell necrosis were observed (Ueno *et al.*, 1971). Subcutaneous administration of (+)-rugulosin daily for three days to mice resulted in elevation of serum transaminase levels (Sato *et al.*, 1977). Exposure of male mice to (+)-rugulosin in the diet (1.5 mg/mouse per day for 22 days or 0.30, 0.75 mg/mouse per day for over 800 days) induced liver injury and weight loss (Ueno *et al.*, 1980).

Administration of (+)-rugulosin (100 mg/kg) in the diet for six weeks to male Fischer 344 rats increased by three fold the number of hyperplastic liver nodules induced by partial hepatectomy at week 1 and subsequent (weeks 7-9) exposure to 2-acetylaminofluorene in the diet in combination with a single intragastric dose of carbon tetrachloride (Imaida *et al.*, 1982).

Ribonucleic acid polymerase of rat liver and *Escherichia coli* and nuclear ribonuclease H of rat liver and *Tetrahymena pyriformis* were strongly inhibited by (+)-rugulosin (Tashiro *et al.*, 1979).

Effects on reproduction and prenatal toxicity
No data were available to the Working Group.

Absorption, distribution, excretion and metabolism
No data were available to the Working Group.

Mutagenicity and other short-term tests

(+)-Rugulosin gave positive results in the *Bacillus subtilis rec⁺/⁻* assay (Ueno & Kubota, 1976).

(+)-Rugulosin (at concentrations up to 100 μg/plate) was not mutagenic to *Salmonella typhimurium* TA98, TA100 or TA2637, in the presence or absence of an exogenous metabolic system (S9), with or without preincubation (Stark *et al.*, 1978; Ueno *et al.*, 1978; Mori *et al.*, 1983; Tikkanen *et al.*, 1983). However, a weak mutagenic response was reported in *S. typhimurium* TM677 in a forward mutation assay, in a spot test and in a prolonged suspension test (Stark *et al.*, 1978). (+)-Rugulosin was not mutagenic to *Escherichia coli* WP2 *uvr*A or WP2 *uvr*A/pKM 101 at concentrations of 0.01-100 μg/plate, in the presence or absence of Aroclor- or 5,6-benzoflavone-induced rat or hamster S9 (Tikkanen *et al.*, 1983).

(+)-Rugulosin induced cytoplasmic petite mutations in *Saccharomyces cerevisiae* (Ueno & Nakajima, 1974).

It did not induce unscheduled DNA synthesis in primary cultured hepatocytes of mice and rats when tested at concentrations of up to 10^{-4}M (Mori *et al.*, 1983, 1984), or in cultured human fibroblasts when tested at concentrations of up to 10^{-2}M (San & Stich, 1975).

(*b*) *Humans*

No data were available to the Working Group.

3.3 Case reports and epidemiological studies of carcinogenicity to humans

No data were available to the Working Group.

4. Summary of Data Reported and Evaluation

4.1 Exposure data

Rugulosin is a mycotoxin produced by certain fungal species that can contaminate cereal grains. Human exposure may occur by the ingestion of contaminated grain products.

4.2 Experimental data

Rugulosin was tested for carcinogenicity in two experiments in male mice by oral administration in the diet. Both experiments were considered to be inadequate for evaluation.

No data were available to evaluate the reproductive effects or prenatal toxicity of rugulosin.

Rugulosin induced DNA damage in *Bacillus subtilis*. It did not induce reverse mutations in *Salmonella typhimurium* but was reported to induce forward mutations. It did not induce mutations in *Escherichia coli*. It induced cytoplasmic petite mutations in yeast. Rugulosin did not induce unscheduled DNA synthesis in mammalian cells *in vitro*.

4.3 Human data

No case report or epidemiological study of the carcinogenicity of rugulosin was available to the Working Group.

4.4 Evaluation[1]

There is *inadequate evidence* for the carcinogenicity of rugulosin in experimental animals.

No evaluation could be made of the carcinogenicity of rugulosin to humans.

---

[1]For definition of the italicized term, see Preamble, p. 18.

Overall assessment of data from short-term tests: Rugulosin[a]

	Genetic activity			Cell transformation
	DNA damage	Mutation	Chromosomal effects	
Prokaryotes	+	?		
Fungi/Green plants		+		
Insects				
Mammalian cells (*in vitro*)	–			
Mammals (*in vivo*)				
Humans (*in vivo*)				
Degree of evidence in short-term tests for genetic activity: **Limited**				Cell transformation: No data

[a]The groups into which the table is divided and the symbols used are defined on pp. 19-20 of the Preamble; the degrees of evidence are defined on pp. 20-21.

5. References

Bouhet, J.C., Pham Van Chuong, P., Toma, F., Kirszenbaum, M. & Fromageot, P. (1976) Isolation and characterization of luteoskyrin and rugulosin, two hepatotoxic anthraquinonoids from *Penicillium islandicum* Sopp. and *Penicillium rugulosum* Thom. *J. agric. Food Chem.*, *24*, 964-972

Breen, J., Dacre, J.C., Raistrick, H. & Smith, G. (1955) Studies in the biochemistry of micro-organisms. 95. Rugulosin, a crystalline colouring matter of *Penicillium rugulosum* Thom. *Biochem. J.*, *60*, 618-626

Imaida, K., Hirose, M., Ogiso, T., Kurata, Y. & Ito, N. (1982) Quantitative analysis of initiating and promoting activities of five mycotoxins in liver carcinogenesis in rats. *Cancer Lett.*, *16*, 137-143

Mori, H., Kawai, K., Ohbayashi, F., Kitamura, J. & Nozawa, Y. (1983) Genotoxicity of quinone pigments from pathogenic fungi. *Mutat. Res.*, *122*, 29-34

Mori, H., Kawai, K., Ohbayashi, F., Kuniyasu, T., Yamazaki, M., Hamasaki, T. & Williams, G.M. (1984) Genotoxicity of a variety of mycotoxins in the hepatocyte primary culture/DNA repair test using rat and mouse hepatocytes. *Cancer Res.*, *44*, 2918-2923

Pham Van Chuong, P., Bouhet, J.C., Thiery, J. & Fromageot, P. (1973) Conformations of luteoskyrin and rugulosin in solution. *Tetrahedron, 29*, 3533-3538

Roane, M.K. & Stipes, R.J. (1978) Pigments in the fungal genus *Endothia. Virginia J. Sci., 29*, 137-141

San, R.H.C. & Stich, H.F. (1975) DNA repair synthesis of cultured human cells as a rapid bioassay for chemical carcinogens. *Int. J. Cancer, 16*, 284-291

Sankawa, U., Shimada, H. & Yamasaki, K. (1978) Acetate-[2-^{13}C,2-^{2}H$_3$] as a precursor in polyketide biosynthesis: detection of deuterium incorporation with ^{13}C-NMR. *Tetrahedron Lett., 36*, 3375-3378

Sato, N., Ueno, Y. & Ueno, I. (1977) Hepatic injury and hepato-accumulation of (+)-rugulosin in mice. *J. toxicol. Sci., 2*, 261-271

Shibata, S., Ogihara, Y., Kobayashi, N., Seo, S. & Kitagawa, I. (1968) The revised structures of luteoskyrin, rubroskyrin and rugulosin. *Tetrahedron Lett., 27*, 3179-3184

Stark, A.A., Townsend, J.M., Wogan, G.N., Demain, A.L., Manmade, A. & Ghosh, A.C. (1978) Mutagenicity and antibacterial activity of mycotoxins produced by *Penicillium islandicum* Sopp. and *Penicillium rugulosum. J. environ. Pathol. Toxicol., 2*, 313-324

Takeda, N., Seo, S., Ogihara, Y., Sankawa, U., Iitaka, I., Kitagawa, I. & Shibata, S. (1973) Studies on fungal metabolites — XXXI. Anthraquinonoid colouring matters of *Penicillium islandicum* Sopp. and some other fungi. (−)Luteoskyrin, (−)rubroskyrin, (+)rugulosin and their related compounds. *Tetrahedron, 29*, 3703-3719

Takeda, Y., Isohata, E., Armano, R. & Uchiyama, M. (1979) Simultaneous extraction and fractionation and thin-layer chromatography determination of 14 mycotoxins in grains. *J. Assoc. off. anal. Chem., 62*, 573-578

Tashiro, F., Hirai, K. & Ueno, Y. (1979) Inhibitory effects of carcinogenic mycotoxins on deoxyribonucleic acid-dependent ribonucleic acid polymerase and ribonuclease H. *Appl. environ. Biol., 38*, 191-196

Tikkanen, L., Matsushima, T. & Natori, S. (1983) Mutagenicity of anthraquinones in the Salmonella preincubation test. *Mutat. Res., 116*, 297-304

Toma, F., Bouhet, J.C., Pham Van Chuong, P., Fromageot, P., Haar, W., Rüterjans, H. & Maurer, W. (1975) Carbon-13 NMR spectroscopy of the biological pigments luteoskyrin and rugulosin and some polyhydroxyanthraquinone analogues. *Org. magn. Resonance, 7*, 496-503

Ueno, Y. & Kubota, K. (1976) DNA-attacking ability of carcinogenic mycotoxins in recombination-deficient mutant cells of *Bacillus subtilis. Cancer Res., 36*, 445-451

Ueno, Y. & Nakajima, M. (1974) Production of respiratory-deficient mutants of *Saccharomyces cerevisiae* by (−)luteoskyrin and (+)rugulosin. *Chem. pharm. Bull., 22*, 2258-2262

Ueno, Y., Ueno, I., Sato, N., Iitoi, Y., Saito, M., Enomoto, M. & Tsunoda, H. (1971) Toxicological approach to (+)-rugulosin, an anthraquinoid mycotoxin of *Penicillium rugulosum* Thom. *Jpn. J. exp. Med.*, *41*, 177-188

Ueno, Y., Kubota, K., Ito, T. & Nakamura, Y. (1978) Mutagenicity of carcinogenic mycotoxins in *Salmonella typhimurium*. *Cancer Res.*, *38*, 536-542

Ueno, Y., Sato, N., Ito, T., Ueno, I., Enomoto, M. & Tsunoda, H. (1980) Chronic toxicity and hepatocarcinogenicity of (+)rugulosin, an anthraquinoid mycotoxin from Penicillium species: preliminary surveys in mice. *J. toxicol. Sci.*, *5*, 295-302

FOOD ADDITIVES

BENZYL ACETATE

1. Chemical and Physical Data

1.1 Synonyms and trade names

Chem. Abstr. Services Reg. No.: 140-11-4

Chem. Abstr. Name: Acetic acid, phenylmethyl ester

IUPAC Systematic Name: Benzyl acetate

Synonyms: Acetic acid, benzyl ester; (acetoxymethyl)benzene; α-acetoxytoluene; benzyl ethanoate; phenylmethyl acetate

1.2 Structural and molecular formulae and molecular weight

$$CH_2-O-\overset{\displaystyle O}{\underset{\displaystyle \|}{C}}-CH_3$$

$C_9H_{10}O_2$ Mol. wt: 150.18

1.3 Chemical and physical properties of the pure substance

(a) *Description*: Colourless liquid with a jasmine-like odour (PPF Norda, 1980); liquid with a pear-like odour (Windholz, 1983)

(b) *Boiling-point*: 215.5°C (Weast, 1985)

(c) *Melting-point*: −51.3°C (Weast, 1985)

(d) *Density*: d_4^{20} 1.0550 (Weast, 1985)

(e) *Spectroscopy data*: Ultraviolet (Sadtler Research Laboratories, 1980 [260[a]]), infrared (Sadtler Research Laboratories, 1980, prism [859], grating [167]; Pouchert, 1981 [1018c[b]]; ICIS Chemical Information System [IRSS], 1984), proton nuclear magnetic resonance (Sadtler Research Laboratories, 1980 [1022, V530]; Pouchert, 1983 [269A]), C-13 nuclear magnetic resonance (Sadtler Research Laboratories, 1980 [138]; ICIS Chemical Information System [CNMR], 1984) and mass spectral data (ICIS Chemical Information System [MSSS], 1984) have been reported.

(f) *Solubility*: Slightly soluble in water (Hawley, 1981); soluble in diethyl ether and acetone; very soluble in ethanol (Weast, 1985)

(g) *Volatility*: Vapour pressure, 1 mm Hg at 45°C; relative vapour density (air = 1), 5.1 (Sax, 1984)

(h) *Stability*: Flash-point, 102°C (closed-cup) (Hawley, 1981; Windholz, 1983)

(i) *Octanol water/partition coefficient (P)*: log P, 1.96 (Hansch & Leo, 1979; ICIS Chemical Information System [ISHOW, ENVIROFATE], 1984)

(j) *Conversion factor in air*: mg/m³ = 6.14 × ppm[c]

1.4 Technical products and impurities

The Food Chemicals Codex (National Research Council, 1981) specifies that food grade benzyl acetate must have a purity of at least 98% with an acid value of not more than 1.0. The product should also be free of chlorinated compounds. One firm based in France and the USA offers four grades of benzyl acetate, differentiated by their odour quality, with the same food-grade specifications as the Food Chemicals Codex (Givaudan, 1979). Benzyl alcohol has been detected as an impurity in food-grade benzyl acetate (National Toxicology Program, 1986).

2. Production, Use, Occurrence and Analysis

2.1 Production and use

(a) *Production*

Hennis *et al.* (1967) reported the preparation of benzyl acetate from sodium acetate, benzyl chloride and triethylamine catalyst. Other previously reported synthetic methods

---

[a]Spectrum number in Sadtler compilation

[b]Spectrum number in Pouchert compilation

[c]Calculated from: mg/m³ = (molecular weight/24.45) × ppm, assuming standard temperature (25°C) and pressure (760 mm Hg)

include the acetylation of benzyl alcohol or the reaction of benzaldehyde and acetic acid with zinc dust (Furia & Bellanca, 1975).

Benzyl acetate is currently available in commercial quantities from four major producers (US International Trade Commission, 1983) and a number of smaller producers in the USA. The US International Trade Commission (1981) reported the production of 640 thousand kg of benzyl acetate in the USA in 1980 and 700 thousand kg in 1977 (US International Trade Commission, 1978). US imports in 1983 were 436 thousand kg (US International Trade Commission, 1984).

Five producers of benzyl acetate were identified in France, five in the UK, four in Spain, and one each in The Netherlands and in the Federal Republic of Germany. It is also made available by 12 producers in Japan (The Chemical Daily Co., 1980).

(b) Use

Benzyl acetate has been in commercial use since the 1900s, primarily as a flavouring ingredient and a component of perfumes (Opdyke, 1973). For use as a flavouring component, benzyl acetate is formulated in a number of imitation flavours, such as apple, apricot, banana, cherry, peach, pear, plum, pineapple, quince, raspberry and strawberry (PPF Norda, 1980). As a food additive, it has been reported to be used in nonalcoholic beverages, ice cream, ices, sweets, baked goods, gelatins, puddings and chewing-gum (Furia & Bellanca, 1975).

Benzyl acetate is widely used as a fragrance for soaps because of its jasmine-like odour. It may be present in 30-40% of all laundry detergents, soaps and incense fragrances (Anon., 1983).

Benzyl acetate has also been used, to a lesser degree, as a solvent for cellulose acetate, cellulose nitrate and natural and synthetic resins. It may be used as a component of oils, lacquers, polishes, printing inks and varnish removers (Hawley, 1981).

(c) Regulatory status and guidelines

The US Food and Drug Administration (1984) specifies that benzyl acetate may be used safely as a synthetic flavouring substance for food. The Joint FAO/WHO Expert Committee on Food Additives recommended in 1967 that the average daily intake (ADI) of benzyl acetate in humans be limited to 0-5 mg/kg body weight as total benzoic acid from all food additive sources (WHO, 1968). In 1983, this Committee changed the ADI to a temporary status at the same level (WHO, 1983), and the status was extended in 1985 (WHO, 1986).

Exposure limits for workplace concentrations of benzyl acetate in air have been set at 94 mg/m^3 by the Council of Europe and at 50 mg/m^3 (average) and 100 mg/m^3 (maximum) in Romania (International Labour Office, 1980).

2.2 Occurrence

(a) Natural occurrence

Examples of natural products in which benzyl acetate occurs are presented in Table 1. It is found in a variety of plants and fruits and is a main constituent of a number of essential oils and flower absolutes, including *Jasminium grandiflorum* L. (jasmine), *Hyacinthus orientalis* (hyacinth), *Gardenia jasminoides* (gardenia), *Polianthes tuberosa* (tuberose),

Table 1. Occurrence of benzyl acetate in natural products

Source	Sample	Concentration in sample	Reference
Jasmine (*Jasminium grandiflorum* L.)	Jasmine absolute	10.7% French oil 25.1 % Italian oil 8.5% Algerian oil	Verzele *et al.* (1981)
Alfalfa (*Medicago sativa* L.)	Essential oil	2%	Kami (1983)
Bael fruit (fruit of *Aegle marmelos*)	Aroma concentrate	~5%	Tokitomo *et al.* (1982)
Fruit of cherimoya (*Annona cherimolia* Mill.)	Pulp extract	<10 μg/kg pulp	Idstein *et al.* (1984)
Ylang-ylang (*Cananga odorata*)	Essential oil	26.2%	Ross (1978)
Passion fruit Purple Yellow Hybrid	Volatiles from pulp juice	0.06 mg/kg pulp 0.06 mg/kg pulp 0.10 mg/kg pulp	Chen *et al.* (1982)
Mushroom (*Agaricus subrufecens*)	Volatile extract	0.3%	Chen & Wu (1984)
Clover — red, alsike, white	Flower extract	Trace	Honkanen *et al.* (1969)
Jasmine tea	Aroma concentrate	Predominant component (not otherwise quantified)	Yamanishi (1978)
Quince (*Cydonia vulgaris*)	Volatile extract	Minor component (not otherwise quantified)	Schreyen *et al.* (1979)
Apples and apple products	Aroma concentrate	Present	Pudil *et al.* (1983)
Muscadine grapes (*Vitis rotundifolia*)	Volatile extract Oil extract	Present Present	Welch *et al.* (1982) Horvat & Senter (1984)
Grenache grapes (*Vitis vinifera* L.)	Oil extract from juice	Present	Stevens *et al.* (1967)
Kogyoku apples	Juice and peel extracts	Present	Yajima *et al.* (1984)

Cananga odorata (ylang-ylang) and *Citrus aurantium* (neroli) (Furia & Bellanca, 1975). Concentrations are highest in essential oil extracts and are generally very low in juice and pulp extracts of the fruit.

(b) Food and beverages

Benzyl acetate is considered one of the most important volatile components for enhancing fruit flavours (Ahmed, 1981). It is reported to occur at a concentration of 4750 mg/kg as a constituent of imitation jasmine flavouring mixtures for food (Merory, 1968). Approximate concentrations of benzyl acetate in various foods have been reported as follows: chewing-gum, 760 mg/kg; sweets, 34 mg/kg; puddings and gelatins, 23 mg/kg; baked goods, 22 mg/kg; ice cream, 14 mg/kg; nonalcoholic beverages, 7.8 mg/kg (Furia & Bellanca, 1975).

(c) Consumer products

Usual and maximal percentages of benzyl acetate in various commercial products have been reported to be as follows: soap, 0.05 and 0.36%; detergent, 0.005 and 0.036%; creams and lotions, 0.015 and 0.15%; and perfume, 0.54 and 3.0%, respectively (Opdyke, 1973). A typical formulated fragrance used in the manufacture of these products contained 30% benzyl acetate by weight (James, 1975).

2.3 Analysis

Gas chromatography with flame ionization detection or mass spectrometry has been used to analyse for benzyl acetate in volatile mixtures (Habboush & Al-Rubaie, 1978; Korte, 1981; Healey & Carnevale, 1984; Horvat & Senter, 1984). Combined gas chromatography/mass spectrometry has also been used to detect benzyl acetate at trace levels in mouse urine (Miyashita & Robinson, 1980).

Leahy and Reineccius (1984) compared various methods for the sampling of volatiles in foods and found that headspace concentration (Tenax adsorbent) and solvent extraction (dichloromethane) techniques were most effective for sampling benzyl acetate. Junk *et al.* (1974) developed a procedure for the extraction of trace impurities, including benzyl acetate, from water at levels of 10-100 μg/l using XAD-2, a macroreticular low polarity resin.

3. Biological Data Relevant to the Evaluation of Carcinogenic Risk to Humans

3.1 Carcinogenicity studies in animals

Oral administration

Mouse: Groups of 50 male and 50 female B6C3F$_1$ mice, eight weeks old, received 0 (vehicle controls), 500 (low dose) or 1000 (high dose) mg/kg bw benzyl acetate (>99% pure;

benzyl alcohol and two to three unidentified impurities were found in the two lots used) in corn oil by gavage on five days per week for 103 weeks. Surviving animals were killed at 104-106 weeks, at which time 38/50 (76%), 33/50 (66%) and 39/50 (78%) males and 15/50 (30%), 18/50 (36%) and 30/50 (60%) females were still alive in the control, low- and high-dose groups, respectively. At 87 weeks, more than 50% of all female mice were still alive (control: 28/50, 56%; low-dose: 29/50, 58%; high-dose: 36/50, 72%). An infection in the genital tract was probably responsible for the death of 26/35 control, 14/32 low-dose and 8/20 high-dose females that died before the end of the study. A significant dose-related increase in the incidence of hepatocellular adenomas was observed in the treated mice: males — control, 0/50; low-dose 5/49 (13%, age-adjusted); high-dose, 13/50 (33%, age-adjusted); $p < 0.001$; females — control, 0/50; low-dose, 0/50; high-dose, 6/50 (17%, age-adjusted); incidental tumour test for trend, $p = 0.002$. The incidence of hepatocellular carcinomas was: males — control, 10/50 (24%, age-adjusted); low-dose, 14/49 (36%, age-adjusted); and high-dose, 12/50 (26%, age-adjusted); females — control, 1/50 (7%, age-adjusted); low-dose, 0/50; and high-dose, 4/50 (13%, age-adjusted); no statistically significant difference was observed. The incidence of adenomas and carcinomas of the liver combined showed a significant positive trend in animals of each sex and was significantly ($p < 0.02$) increased in each sex in the high-dose groups compared to controls: males — control, 10/50 (24%, age-adjusted); low-dose, 18/49 (45%, age-adjusted); high-dose, 23/50 (50%, age-adjusted); females — control, 1/50 (7%, age-adjusted); low-dose, 0/50; high-dose, 10/50 (29%, age-adjusted). Incidences of hepatocellular adenomas in high-dose animals of each sex were also increased in comparison to historical vehicle controls: males — adenomas, 140/1091; carcinomas, 238/1091; combined, 357/1091; females — adenomas, 41/1092; carcinomas, 34/1092; combined, 74/1092. An increased ($p < 0.04$) incidence of squamous-cell papillomas of the forestomach was observed in males: control, 3/49 (8%, age-adjusted); low-dose, 3/48 (9%, age-adjusted); high-dose, 9/49 (23%, age-adjusted); and in females: control, 0/50; low-dose, 0/50; high-dose, 4/48 (13%, age-adjusted; $p = 0.054$). The incidences of forestomach carcinomas in males were 1/49, 1/48 and 2/49 in the three groups, respectively; no such tumour was observed in females. The combined incidence of squamous-cell papillomas and carcinomas of the forestomach was increased ($p < 0.05$) with dose in males: control, 4/49 (10%, age-adjusted); low-dose, 4/48 (11%, age-adjusted); high-dose, 11/49 (28%, age-adjusted) (Abdo et al., 1985; National Toxicology Program, 1986).

Rat: Groups of 50 male and 50 female Fischer 344 rats, seven weeks old, received 0 (vehicle controls), 250 (low dose) or 500 (high dose) mg/kg bw benzyl acetate (>99% pure; benzyl alcohol and two to three unidentified impurities were found in the two lots used) in corn oil by gavage on five days per week for 103 weeks. Survival rates at the end of the study (104-107 weeks) were 38/50 (76%), 46/50 (92%) and 40/50 (80%) males and 40/50 (80%), 36/50 (72%) and 36/50 (72%) females in the control, low- and high-dose groups, respectively. A significant increase (incidental tumour test for trend, $p = 0.001$) in the incidence of acinar-cell adenomas of the pancreas was found in low-dose (27/50; 59%, age-adjusted) and high-dose (37/49; 82%, age-adjusted) males in comparison to vehicle controls (22/50; 54%, age-adjusted). Multiple adenomas of the pancreas occurred more frequently in high-dose male rats (control, 10/50, 20%; low-dose, 12/50, 24%; high-dose, 22/49, 45%). No pancreatic tumour was found in female rats. [These incidences were calculated on the basis of serial sections of the entire pancreas.] Preputial-gland cystadenocarcinomas, adenocarcinomas or adenocarcinomas plus carcinomas occurred with a positive trend ($p < 0.05$) in male rats: cystadenocarcinoma — control, 0/50; low-dose, 0/50; high-dose, 3/50 (7.5%, age-adjusted); adenocarcinoma — control, 0/50; low-dose, 1/50 (2%, age-adjusted); high-dose, 4/50 (10%, age-adjusted); adenocarcinoma and carcinoma combined — control, 1/50 (3%, age-adjusted); low-dose, 1/50 (2%, age-adjusted); high-dose, 6/50 (14%, age-adjusted). The combined incidence of preputial-gland adenoma, adenocarcinoma and carcinoma was not statistically significantly different from that in controls: control, 2/50 (4%); low-dose, 1/50 (2%); high-dose, 6/50 (12%). There was also one preputial sarcoma in the high-dose group. In females, a statistically nonsignificant increase in the incidence of clitoral-gland tumours (adenomas or carcinomas) was observed: control, 2/50 (4%); low-dose, 0/50; high-dose, 5/50 (10%) (Abdo *et al.*, 1985; National Toxicology Program, 1986).

3.2 Other relevant biological data

(a) Experimental systems

Toxic effects

The oral LD_{50} for benzyl acetate was 3690 mg/kg bw in rats and 2640 mg/kg bw in rabbits (Graham-Kuizenga, 1945).

Intravenous, intramuscular or intraperitoneal administration of benzyl acetate (~40 mg/kg bw) to rabbits and dogs caused hypotension and rapid diuresis (Gruber, 1924). Exposure of dogs to a flowing 'vapour-air mixture' containing 0.5 mg/l (81.5 ppm) benzyl acetate over several days was reported to produce central nervous system depression and death. Central nervous system depression, convulsions and some deaths were observed in mice exposed to 1.3 mg/l (212 ppm) for 7-13 h. Cats exposed similarly to 1.1 mg/l (180 ppm) showed only moderate irritation, but after exposure to 1.5 mg/l (245 ppm) they developed central nervous system depression and death. Repeated exposure of cats to concentrations of 1.1-1.5 mg/l (180-245 ppm) for 8-10 h daily for seven days produced marked salivation, especially at the beginning of exposure, somnolence and, later, moderate albuminuria (von Oettingen, 1960).

Benzyl acetate was administered in corn oil by gavage to male and female Fischer 344/N rats at 250-4000 mg/kg bw as a single dose or daily on 14 consecutive days or at doses of 62.5-1000 mg/kg bw on five days per week for 13 weeks. In the single-dose study, all rats receiving 4000 mg/kg were inactive within 2 h after dosing, and 4/5 males and 2/5 females in these groups died. In the 14-day study, all rats receiving 4000 mg/kg died by day 2, and all rats receiving 2000 mg/kg died by day 5. In the 13-week study, 2/10 male rats and 1/10 females receiving 1000 mg/kg died on day 86; final mean body weight in male rats receiving 1000 mg/kg was about 12% lower than that in the control group. Compound-related clinical signs (trembling, ataxia and sluggishness) were observed in male and female rats receiving

1000 mg/kg and in females receiving 500 mg/kg; thickened stomach walls were observed in 2/9 males and 4/10 females receiving 1000 mg/kg. No compound-related histopathological effect was observed (National Toxicology Program, 1986).

Benzyl acetate was administered in corn oil by gavage to male and female B6C3F$_1$ mice at single doses of 250-4000 mg/kg bw or at doses of 125-2000 mg/kg bw daily for 14 days or on five days per week for 13 weeks. In the single-dose study, all mice receiving 4000 mg/kg and females receiving 2000 mg/kg benzyl acetate were inactive immediately after dosing. All mice receiving 4000 mg/kg and 1/5 males and 2/5 females receiving 2000 mg/kg died on day 2. In the 14-day study, all male mice receiving 2000 mg/kg were dead by day 3; no dose-related change in weight was seen. Compound-related clinical signs were observed in high-dose males (ruffled fur, ataxia) and in high-dose females (laboured breathing, hyperactivity). The mucosa in the cardiac region of the stomach was roughened in 2/5 males and 5/5 females receiving 2000 mg/kg and in 1/5 females receiving 1000 mg/kg. In the 13-week study, 7/9 female mice receiving 2000 mg/kg died. Compound-related clinical signs observed in high-dose mice included trembling, inactivity, laboured breathing and depressed body temperature. No compound-related gross or microscopic pathological effect was observed. In the two-year studies (see section 3.1), hyperplasia was found in the forestomach of both male and female B6C3F$_1$ mice receiving 500 and 1000 mg/kg bw (National Toxicology Program, 1986).

Effects on reproduction and prenatal toxicity
No data were available to the Working Group.

Absorption, distribution, excretion and metabolism
Benzyl acetate is absorbed from the gastrointestinal tract and lungs, and through the skin of numerous species, including dogs, rats, mice, rabbits and cats (Graham & Kuizenga, 1945; von Oettingen, 1960; Abdo et al., 1985; National Toxicology Program, 1986). It is hydrolysed to benzyl alcohol; the benzyl radical is oxidized to benzoic acid and excreted primarily in the urine as hippuric and benzylmercapturic acids (von Oettingen, 1960; Abdo et al., 1985; National Toxicology Program, 1986). In Fischer 344/N rats given single doses of 5-500 mg/kg bw or doses of 500 mg/kg bw per day for 14 days and in B6C3F$_1$ mice given single doses of 10-1000 mg/kg bw or 1000 mg/kg bw per day orally for 14 days, no residual benzyl acetate was detected in the urine or any of the tissues 24 h later. More than 90% of the activity from the ^{14}C-ring-labelled benzyl acetate was recovered in the urine and ≤1% in the faeces; >95% was hippuric acid, <1% benzyl alcohol and 0.3-3% unidentified; in rats, 1-3% was mercapturic acid. There was no evidence of saturation of the absorption, distribution, metabolism or excretion pathways in either species (Abdo et al., 1985; National Toxicology Program, 1986).

Mutagenicity and other short-term tests
Benzyl acetate was reported to give negative results in the Bacillus subtilis rec$^{+/-}$ assay when tested at 21 μg/disc (Oda et al., 1978). It was not mutagenic to Salmonella typhimurium TA1535, TA1537, TA98 or TA100 when tested at up to 10 000 μg/plate in a preincubation assay in the presence or absence of a metabolic system (S9) from the liver of

Aroclor-induced rats or Syrian hamsters (Mortelmans *et al.*, 1986; National Toxicology Program, 1986). Florin *et al.* (1980) also reported negative results in a spot test (3 μmol/disc) in strains TA1535, TA1537, TA98 and TA100, in the presence or absence of an exogenous metabolic system.

It was reported in an abstract that benzyl acetate did not induce unscheduled DNA synthesis in rat hepatocytes *in vitro* or *in vivo* (Mirsalis *et al.*, 1983).

Benzyl acetate (up to 5000 μg/ml) did not induce sister chromatid exchanges or chromosomal aberrations in cultured Chinese hamster ovary cells in the presence or absence of Aroclor-induced rat-liver S9 (National Toxicology Program, 1986). Benzyl acetate (tested at up to 1.25 μl/ml) was reported to be mutagenic in the mouse lymphoma L5178Y/TK$^{+/-}$ assay in the presence, but not in the absence of Aroclor-induced rat-liver S9 (National Toxicology Program, 1986).

(b)   Humans

Toxic effects
Benzyl acetate has been reported to cause irritation in the upper respiratory tract and to the eyes (Opdyke, 1973).

Effects on reproduction and prenatal toxicity
No data were available to the Working Group.

Absorption, distribution, excretion and metabolism
After oral doses of 2 g benzyl acetate, at least 80% was rapidly excreted as hippuric acid in the urine (Snapper *et al.*, 1925).

Mutagenicity and chromosomal effects
No data were available to the Working Group.

3.3 Case reports and epidemiological studies of carcinogenicity to humans

No data were available to the Working Group.

4. Summary of Data Reported and Evaluation

4.1 Exposure data

Benzyl acetate has been identified in several fruits, such as bael fruit (from the *Aegle marmelos* tree) and quince (*Cydonia vulgaris*), and in a mushroom (*Agaricus* species). It is a major volatile constituent of the flowers of a number of plants, including jasmine (*Jasminum grandiflorum* L.), hyacinth (*Hyacinthus orientalis*), gardenia (*Gardenia jasminoides*), ylang-ylang (*Cananga odorata*), alfalfa (*Medicago sativa* L.) and others. It has been used as a food additive in fruit flavours and as a component of perfumes since the early 1900s and is widely used as a fragrance in soaps, detergents and incense. There is widespread human exposure to benzyl acetate by ingestion, skin application and inhalation.

4.2 Experimental data

Benzyl acetate was tested for carcinogenicity by oral intubation in one experiment in mice of both sexes and in one experiment in rats of both sexes. In the study in mice, increased incidences of liver adenomas and of combined liver adenomas and carcinomas were observed in animals of each sex; the incidence of carcinomas of the liver alone was not statistically significantly increased in animals of either sex. An increased incidence of forestomach tumours was observed in mice of each sex. An increased incidence of acinar-cell adenomas of the pancreas was observed in male rats.

No data were available to evaluate the reproductive effects or prenatal toxicity of benzyl acetate to experimental animals.

Benzyl acetate was reported to give negative results in the *Bacillus subtilis rec* assay. It was not mutagenic to *Salmonella typhimurium* in the presence or absence of an exogenous metabolic system and did not induce sister chromatid exchanges or chromosomal aberrations in Chinese hamster ovary cells in the presence or absence of a metabolic system. Benzyl acetate was reported to be mutagenic in mouse lymphoma L5178Y cells in the presence of a metabolic system.

Overall assessment of data from short-term tests: Benzyl acetate[a]

	Genetic activity			Cell transformation
	DNA damage	Mutation	Chromosomal effects	
Prokaryotes	?	—		
Fungi/Green plants				
Insects				
Mammalian cells (*in vitro*)		?	—	
Mammals (*in vivo*)				
Humans (*in vivo*)				
Degree of evidence in short-term tests for genetic activity: **Inadequate**				Cell transformation: No data

[a]The groups into which the table is divided and the symbols used are defined on pp. 19-20 of the Preamble; the degrees of evidence are defined on pp. 20-21.

4.3 Human data

No case report or epidemiological study of the carcinogenicity of benzyl acetate was available to the Working Group.

4.4 Evaluation[1]

There is *limited evidence* for the carcinogenicity of benzyl acetate to experimental animals.

No evaluation could be made of the carcinogenicity of benzyl acetate to humans.

5. References

Abdo, K.M., Huff, J.E., Haseman, J.K., Boorman, G.A., Eustis, S.L., Matthews, H.B., Burka, L.T., Prejean, J.D. & Thompson, R.B. (1985) Benzyl acetate carcinogenicity, metabolism, and disposition in Fischer 344 rats and B6C3F$_1$ mice. *Toxicology, 37,* 159-170

Ahmed, M. (1981) *Organic compounds, inorganic salts and processing reactions as means of enhancing fruit flavors in desserts.* In: Charalambous, G. & Inglett, G., eds, *The Quality of Foods and Beverages: Chemical Technology,* 2nd ed., Vol. 2, New York, Academic Press, pp. 47-56

Anon. (1983) Benzyl acetate apparently weathers questions raised by cancer study. *Chem. Mark. Rep., 224,* 4, 20

The Chemical Daily Co. (1980) *JCW Chemicals Guide,* Tokyo, p. 59

Chen, C.-C. & Wu, C.-M. (1984) Volatile components of mushroom (*Agaricus subrufecens*). *J. Food Sci., 49,* 1208-1209

Chen, C.-C., Kuo, M.-C., Hwang, L.S., Wu, J.S.-B. & Wu, C.-M. (1982) Headspace components of passion fruit juice. *J. agric. Food Chem., 30,* 1211-1215

Florin, I., Rutberg, L., Curvall, M. & Enzell, C.R. (1980) Screening of tobacco smoke constituents for mutagenicity using the Ames' test. *Toxicology, 18,* 219-232

Furia, T.E. & Bellanca, N. (1975) *Fenaroli's Handbook of Flavor Ingredients,* 2nd ed., Vol. II, Cleveland, OH, Chemical Rubber Co., pp. 44, 655

Givaudan (1979) *Benzyl acetate.* In: *The Givaudan Index,* Dubendorf-Zurich, p. 68

Graham, B.E. & Kuizenga, M.H. (1945) Toxicity studies of benzyl benzoate and related benzyl compounds. *J. Pharmacol. exp. Ther., 84,* 358-362

---

[1]For definition of the italicized term, see Preamble, p. 18.

Gruber, C.M. (1924) The pharmacology of benzyl alcohol and its esters. IV. The diuretic effect of benzyl alcohol, benzyl acetate and benzyl benzoate. *J. Lab. clin. Med.*, *10*, 284-294

Habboush, A.E. & Al-Rubaie, A.Z. (1978) Separation of benzyl compounds by gas-liquid chromatography. *J. Chromatogr.*, *157*, 409-411

Hansch, C. & Leo, A. (1979) *Substituent Constants for Correlation Analysis in Chemistry and Biology*, New York, John Wiley & Sons, p. 242

Hawley, G.G., ed. (1981) *The Condensed Chemical Dictionary*, 10th ed., New York, Van Nostrand Reinhold, pp. 120-121

Healey, K.W. & Carnevale, J. (1984) Determination of volatile fatty acids in molasses by gas-liquid chromatography of their benzyl esters. *J. agric. Food Chem.*, *32*, 1363-1366

Hennis, H.E., Easterly, J.P., Jr, Collins, L.R. & Thompson, L.R. (1967) Esters from the reactions of alkyl halides and salts of carboxylic acids. *Ind. Eng. chem. Prod. Res. Dev.*, *6*, 193-195

Honkanen, E., Moisio, T. & Karvonen, P. (1969) Studies on the volatile flavour substances in some clover species. *Suom. Kemistil.*, B*42*, 448-451

Horvat, R.J. & Senter, S.D. (1984) Identification of the volatile constituents from scuppernong berries (*Vitis rotundifolia*). *J. Food Sci.*, *49*, 64-66, 81

ICIS Chemical Information System (1984) *Carbon-13 NMR Spectral Search System* (CNMR), *Mass Spectral Search System* (MSSS), *Infrared Spectral Search System* (IRSS), *Information System for Hazardous Organics in Water* (ISHOW), and *Environmental Fate* (ENVIROFATE), Washington DC, Information Consultants

Idstein, H., Herres, W. & Schreier, P. (1984) High-resolution gas chromatography-mass spectrometry and -Fourier transform infrared analysis of cherimoya (*Annona cherimolia* Mill.) volatiles. *J. agric. Food Chem.*, *32*, 383-389

International Labour Office (1980) *Occupational Exposure Limits for Airborne Toxic Substances*, 2nd (rev.) ed. (*Occupational Safety and Health Series No. 37*), Geneva, pp. 50-51

James, R.W. (1975) *Fragrance Technology. Synthetic and Natural Perfumes*, Park Ridge, NJ, Noyes Data Corp., p. 108

Junk, G.A., Richard, J.J., Grieser, M.D., Witiak, D., Witiak, J.L., Arguello, M.D., Vick, R., Svec, H.J., Fritz, J.S. & Calder, G.V. (1974) Use of macroreticular resins in the analysis of water for trace organic contaminants. *J. Chromatogr.*, *99*, 745-762

Kami, T. (1983) Composition of the essential oil of alfalfa. *J. agric. Food Chem.*, *31*, 38-41

Korte, W.D. (1981) Alternate procedure for the preparation and separation of benzyl derivatives of organic acids. *J. Chromatogr.*, *214*, 131-134

Leahy, M.M. & Reineccius, G.A. (1984) *Comparison of methods for the isolation of volatile compounds from aqueous model systems*. In: Schreier, P., ed., *Analysis of Volatiles: Methods and Applications*, Berlin (West), de Gruyter, pp. 19-47

Merory, J. (1968) *Food Flavorings: Composition, Manufacture, and Use*, 2nd ed., Westport, CT, AVI Publishing Co., p. 200

Mirsalis, J., Tyson, K., Beck, J., Loh, F., Steinmetz, K., Contreras, C., Austere, L., Martin, S. & Spalding, J. (1983) Induction of unscheduled DNA synthesis (UDS) in hepatocytes following in vitro and in vivo treatment (Abstract No. Ef-5). *Environ. Mutagenesis, 5*, 482

Miyashita, K. & Robinson, A.B. (1980) Identification of compounds in mouse urine vapor by gas chromatography and mass spectrometry. *Mech. Ageing Dev., 13*, 177-184

Mortelmans, K., Haworth, S., Lawlor, T., Speck, W., Tainer, B. & Zeiger, E. (1986) *Salmonella* mutagenicity tests: II. Results from the testing of 270 chemicals. *Environ. Mutagenesis, 8* (Suppl. 7), 1-119

National Research Council (1981) *Benzyl acetate.* In: *Food Chemicals Codex*, 3rd ed., Washington DC, National Academy of Sciences, pp. 358-359

National Toxicology Program (1986) *Toxicology and Carcinogenesis Studies of Benzyl Acetate (CAS No. 140-11-4) in F344/N rats and B6C3F1 mice (Gavage Studies)* (Technical Report Series No. 250), Research Triangle Park, NC (in press)

Oda, Y., Hamano, Y., Inoue, K., Yamamoto, H., Niihara, T. & Kunita, N. (1978) Mutagenicity of food flavours in bacteria (1st report) (Jpn.). *Osaka Pref. Inst. publ. Health, ED Food Microbiol., 9*, 177-181

von Oettingen, W.F. (1960) The aliphatic acids and their esters: toxicity and potential dangers. *Arch. ind. Health, 21*, 28-65

Opdyke, D.L.J. (1973) Monographs on fragrance raw materials: benzyl acetate. *Food Cosmet. Toxicol., 11*, 875-876

Pouchert, C.J., ed. (1981) *The Aldrich Library of Infrared Spectra*, 3rd ed., Milwaukee, WI, Aldrich Chemical Co., p. 1018

Pouchert, C.J., ed. (1983) *The Aldrich Library of NMR Spectra*, 2nd ed., Milwaukee, WI, Aldrich Chemical Co., p. 269

PPF Norda (1980) *Benzyl Acetate FCC: Technical Bulletin*, East Hanover, NJ

Pudil, F., Viden, I., Velisek, J. & Davidek, J. (1983) The volatile components of an industrial apple aroma concentrate. *Z. Lebensmittel.-Untersuch. Forsch., 177*, 181-185

Ross, M.S.F. (1978) Application of high-performance liquid chromatography to the analysis of volatile oils. *J. Chromatogr., 160*, 199-204

Sadtler Research Laboratories (1980) *The Sadtler Standard Spectra, Cumulative Index*, Philadelphia, PA

Sax, N.I. (1984) *Dangerous Properties of Industrial Materials*, 6th ed., New York, Van Nostrand Reinhold, p. 399

Schreyen, L., Dirinck, P., Sandra, P. & Schamp, N. (1979) Flavor analysis of quince. *J. agric. Food Chem., 27*, 872-876

Snapper, J., Grünbaum, A. & Sturkop, S. (1925) Cleavage and oxidation of benzyl alcohol and benzyl esters in humans (Ger.). *Biochem. Z., 155*, 163-173

Stevens, K.L., Bomben, J.L. & McFadden, W.H. (1967) Volatiles from grapes. *Vitis vinifera* (Linn.) cultivar Grenache. *J. agric. Food Chem.*, *15*, 378-380

Tokitomo, Y., Shimono, Y., Kobayashi, A. & Yamanishi, T. (1982) Aroma components of baelfruit (*Aegle marmelos* Correa). *Agric. Biol. Chem.*, *46*, 1873-1877

US Food and Drug Administration (1984) Food and drugs. *US Code fed. Regul.*, *Title 21*, Part 172.515, p. 48

US International Trade Commission (1978) *Synthetic Organic Chemicals, US Production and Sales, 1977 (USITC Publ. No. 920)*, Washington DC, US Government Printing Office, p. 193

US International Trade Commission (1981) *Synthetic Organic Chemicals, US Production and Sales, 1980 (USITC Publ. No. 1183)*, Washington DC, US Government Printing Office, p. 143

US International Trade Commission (1983) *Synthetic Organic Chemicals, US Production and Sales, 1982 (USITC Publ. No. 1422)*, Washington DC, US Government Printing Office, pp. 125, 127

US International Trade Commission (1984) *Imports of Benzenoid Chemicals and Products, 1983 (USITC Publ. No. 1548)*, Washington DC, US Government Printing Office, p. 91

Verzele, M., Maes, G., Vuye, A., Godefroot, M., Van Alboom, M., Vervisch, J. & Sandra, P. (1981) Chromatographic investigation of jasmine absolutes. *J. Chromatogr.*, *205*, 367-386

Weast, R.C., ed. (1985) *CRC Handbook of Chemistry and Physics*, 66th ed., Boca Raton, FL, CRC Press, p. C-47

Welch, R.C., Johnston, J.C. & Hunter, G.L.K. (1982) Volatile constituents of the muscadine grape (*Vitis rotundifolia*). *J. agric. Food Chem.*, *30*, 681-684

WHO (1968) *Specifications for the Identity and Purity of Food Additives and Their Toxicological Evaluation: Some Flavouring Substances and Non-nutritive Sweetening Agents. 11th Report of the Joint FAO/WHO Expert Committee on Food Additives (Tech. Rep. Ser. No. 383)*, Geneva, p. 18

WHO (1983) *Evaluation of Certain Food Additives and Contaminants. Twenty-seventh Report of the Joint FAO/WHO Expert Committee on Food Additives (Tech. Rep. Ser. No. 696*, Geneva, pp. 17-18

WHO (1986) *Evaluation of Certain Food Additives and Contaminants. Twenty-ninth Report of the Joint FAO/WHO Expert Committee on Food Additives (Tech. Rep. Ser. No. 733)*, Geneva, pp. 21-22

Windholz, M., ed. (1983) *The Merck Index*, 10th ed., Rahway, NJ, Merck & Co., p. 161

Yajima, I., Yanai, T., Nakamura, M., Sakakibara, H. & Hayashi, K. (1984) Volatile flavor components of Kogyoku apples. *Agric. Biol. Chem.*, *48*, 849-855

Yamanishi, T. (1978) Flavor of green tea. *Jpn. agric. Res. Q.*, *12*, 205-210

BUTYLATED HYDROXYANISOLE (BHA)

1. Chemical and Physical Data

1.1 Synonyms and trade names

Chem. Abstr. Services Reg. No.: 25013-16-5

Chem. Abstr. Name: (1,1-Dimethylethyl)-4-methoxyphenol

IUPAC Systematic Name: tert-Butyl-4-methoxyphenol

Synonyms: Butylhydroxyanisole; tert-butylhydroxyanisole; tert-butyl-para-hydroxy-anisole; tert-butyl-4-hydroxyanisole; 2(3)-tert-butyl-4-hydroxyanisole; EEC No. E320

Trade Names: Antioxyne B; Antrancine 12; Embanox; Protex; Sustan 1F; Sustane 1F; Tenox BHA

1.2 Structural and molecular formulae and molecular weight

Mixture of:

3-tert-Butyl-4-hydroxyanisole
(3-BHA)

2-tert-Butyl-4-hydroxyanisole
(2-BHA)

$C_{11}H_{16}O_2$ Mol. wt: 180.25

1.3 Chemical and physical properties of the commercial mixture (unless otherwise specified)

(a)   *Description*: White or slightly yellow waxy solid (Hawley, 1981; Windholz, 1983)

(b)   *Boiling-point*: 264-270°C at 733 mm Hg (Windholz, 1983)

(c)   *Melting-point*: 48-63°C (Hawley, 1981); 48-55°C (Windholz, 1983)

(d)   *Spectroscopy data*: Infrared (Sadtler Research Laboratories, 1980: [2-BHA] prism [25091[a]], grating [1066]; [3-BHA] prism [25090], grating [1065]; ICIS Chemical Information System, 1984 [IRSS]) and mass spectral data (ICIS Chemical Information System, 1984 [MSSS]) have been reported.

(e)   *Solubility*: Insoluble in water; soluble in petroleum ether (Skellysolve H), 50% ethanol, propylene glycol, alcohols, fats and oils (Windholz, 1983)

(f)   *Stability*: Flash-point, 156°C (Eastman Chemical Products, Inc., 1982; Chemical Dynamics Corp., undated); degrades following prolonged exposure to sunlight (Cosmetic Ingredient Review Expert Panel, 1984)

(g)   *Reactivity*: Exhibits antioxidant properties as a scavenger of free radicals (Cosmetic Ingredient Review Expert Panel, 1984).

1.4 Technical products and impurities

Commercially available food-grade BHA is generally a mixture containing >85% 3-*tert*-butyl-4-hydroxyanisole (3-BHA) and <15% of the 2-*tert*-butyl isomer (2-BHA) (Branen, 1975; Lam *et al.*, 1979). Depending on the intended use, BHA may be combined with other synthetic antioxidants, such as butylated hydroxytoluene (see monograph, p. 161), *tert*-butylhydroquinone, propyl gallate and citric acid (Eastman Chemical Products, Inc., 1982). The Food Chemicals Codex (National Research Council, 1981) specifies that food-grade BHA contain not less than 98.5% w/w BHA; impurities present in this food-grade product are allowed at limits of 3 ppm (mg/kg) arsenic (see IARC, 1982a) and 10 ppm (mg/kg) heavy metals (as lead). Food-grade BHA is reported to contain 0.5% max hydroxyanisole and 0.6% max hydroquinone (see IARC, 1977) (Cosmetic Ingredient Review Expert Panel, 1984).

Cosmetic-grade BHA has been reported to contain 90% min 3-BHA and approximately 8% 2-BHA, and the following impurities: 4-hydroxyanisole, 0.5% max; 1-*tert*-butyl-2,5-dimethoxybenzene, 0.5% max; 2,5-di-*tert*-butylhydroxyanisole, 0.2% max; hydroquinone dimethyl ether, 0.1% max; lead (see IARC, 1982b), 20 ppm (mg/kg) max; and arsenic, 3 ppm (mg/kg) max (Cosmetic Ingredient Review Expert Panel, 1984).

---

[a]Spectrum number in Sadtler compilation

2. Production, Use, Occurrence and Analysis

2.1 Production and use

(a) Production

Several methods are used for the commercial production of BHA. Methylation of hydroquinone yields an intermediate that gives a mixture of 3-BHA and 2-BHA upon treatment with *tert*-butyl alcohol and phosphoric acid. Butylation of hydroquinone and subsequent methylation with dimethyl sulphate (see IARC, 1982c) and sodium hydroxide can also be used to produce a mixture of the two BHA isomers (Verma *et al.*, 1970). In addition, BHA can be synthesized by the *tert*-butylation of 4-methoxyphenol over silica or alumina at 150°C (Keeley, 1980).

A method for synthesizing the 2-*tert*-butyl isomer has been described by Lam *et al.* (1979), in which 2-*tert*-butyl-4-[(dimethyl-*tert*-butylsilyl)oxy]phenol is methylated with dimethyl sulphate and the intermediate converted to 2-BHA by acid hydrolysis.

There are two major producers of BHA in the USA (Giragosian, 1982). In addition, there are two firms in the UK and one in The Netherlands. In 1980, eight Japanese manufacturers were identified as producers of BHA (The Chemical Daily Co., 1980).

(b) Use

Foods: BHA has been used as an antioxidant in fat-containing foods and in edible fats and oils since 1947 (Lam *et al.*, 1979). It prevents foods from becoming rancid and developing objectionable odours (Freydberg & Gortner, 1982). It may be used as a food additive in butter, lard, meats, cereals, baked goods, sweets and beer (Keeley, 1980). It is used in vegetable oils, potato crisps (Freydberg & Gortner, 1982), snack foods, nuts, dehydrated potatoes and flavouring materials (Eastman Chemical Products, Inc., 1982).

The estimated US consumption of BHA in foods increased from 170 thousand kg in 1960 to approximately 300 thousand kg per year during the period 1970-1982 (Anon., 1983).

Cosmetics: BHA is reportedly used as a preservative and antioxidant in cosmetic formulations. Companies participating in a US Food and Drug Administration-sponsored cosmetic registration programme in 1981 indicated that BHA was used in 3217 of 21 279 cosmetic formulations. Of the 1914 formulations in which the concentration of BHA was reported, the majority (88%) had levels ⩽0.1%; only one product in the survey, a lipstick, contained >10% BHA. Of the cosmetics reported in the survey, lipstick formulations represented the greatest use (1256 products), followed by eye shadow (410 products) (Cosmetic Ingredient Review Expert Panel, 1984). A widely used antioxidant mixture for cosmetic use contains 20% BHA, 6% propyl gallate, 4% citric acid and 70% propylene glycol (Isacoff, 1979).

(c) Regulatory status and guidelines

Approximately 50 countries reportedly permit the use of BHA as a food additive (International Life Sciences Institute, 1984).

BHA is classified as Generally Recognized As Safe (GRAS) by the US Food and Drug Administration (1984a) when the total content of antioxidants represents not more than 0.02% w/w of the total fat or oil content of the food. It is also permitted at maximum levels of 0.001-0.02% in other specific products including sausage, poultry and meat products, breakfast cereals, potato flakes or granules, dry mixes for beverages or desserts, glazed fruits, emulsion stabilizers for shortenings, and food packaging materials. BHA also may be used in chewing gum (0.1% total antioxidant), active dry yeast (0.1%), flavouring substances (0.5% of essential oil content) and defoaming agents for the processing of beet sugar and yeast at levels not to exceed 0.1% of the defoamer (US Department of Agriculture, 1984; US Food and Drug Administration, 1984b-h).

The Commission of the European Communities (1978) established a temporary acceptable daily intake (ADI) of 30 mg/adult for BHA or BHA combined with butylated hydroxytoluene (see monograph, p. 161). The Joint FAO/WHO Expert Committee on Food Additives decided to retain a temporary ADI of 0-0.5 mg/kg bw for BHA or combined BHA, butylated hydroxytoluene and *tert*-butylhydroquinone (WHO, 1983).

2.2 Occurrence

(a) Natural occurrence

BHA in not known to occur as a natural product.

(b) Food

The average daily intake of BHA in the diet of individuals in the USA in 1975 was estimated to be 4.3 mg, or <0.1 mg/kg bw for a person weighing 60 kg (Freydberg & Gortner, 1982). BHA has been detected at 7-22 mg/kg in flour mixes and cereals, and vegetable and animal fats and oils have been reported to contain levels of 19-91 mg/kg (Kline *et al.*, 1978; Page, 1979). Analysis of chewing-gum samples gave values of 92 and 121 mg/kg in two of nine samples (Pellerin *et al.*, 1982).

2.3 Analysis

The analytical methods described for BHA include gas chromatography (GC), paper chromatography, thin-layer chromatography, colorimetric techniques, fluorimetric techniques, nuclear magnetic resonance, voltametric techniques, gel permeation chromatography, high-performance liquid chromatography (HPLC), polarographic techniques, lipophilic gel chromatography, spectrophotometry and densitometric techniques (Cosmetic Ingredient Review Expert Panel, 1984). Representative methods for various matrices are summarized in Table 1.

There is an International Union for Pure and Applied Chemistry (IUPAC)-Food and Drug Administration (FDA)-Association of Official Analytical Chemists (AOAC) Method (HPLC/ultraviolet spectrometry) (US Food and Drug Administration, 1983a; Fazio, 1984a) for the determination of BHA in oils and lard, an FDA-AOAC Method (vacuum sublimation/GC) (US Food and Drug Administration, 1983b) for BHA in lard, and an AOAC Method (GC/flame ionization detection) (Fazio, 1984b) for BHA in cereals.

Table 1. Methods for the analysis of BHA

Sample matrix	Sample preparation	Assay procedure[a]	Reference
Separation of (1:1) BHA isomers	Chloroform-cyclohexane eluant	C on Sephadex LH20	Kauffman (1977)
Soft drinks	Extractive accumulation at carbon paste electrode; BHT not accumulated	V	Wang & Freiha (1983); Wang & Luo (1984)
Plasma and urine	Petroleum ether extraction	GC/FID	El-Rashidy & Niazi (1979)
Edible oils and fats	n-Hexane-ethanol extraction	TLC	McKone (1976)
	Acetonitrile extraction; silyl derivative	GC/FID	Senten et al. (1977); Wyatt (1981)
	Partition from hexane-oil into acetonitrile; reverse-phase gradient elution	HPLC	Page (1979)
	Dilute into tetrahydrofuran or chloroform	GPC/UV	Majors & Johnson (1978); Doeden et al. (1979)
	Dilute with hexane; extract with acetonitrile	HPLC/UV	US Food and Drug Administration (1983a); Fazio (1984a)
	Sublime under vacuum	GC	US Food and Drug Administration (1983b)
Foods	Steam distill from matrices	SF	Dilli & Robards (1977)
	Steam distill from foods; dichloromethane extraction of distillate	GC	Isshiki et al. (1980)
	Extract with carbon disulphide	GC/FID	Fazio (1984b)
Yeast	Determine samples directly	MS	McClusky et al. (1978)
Foods, fats and oils	Glass-wool precolumn	GC	Kline et al. (1978)
	Chromatograph extracts directly; BHT not detected	LC/ECD	King et al. (1980)
Chewing-gum	Extract with hexane, alkaline dimethyl sulphoxide	HPLC/UV	Pellerin et al. (1982)
Rubber	Acetone extract; visualize with sulphanilic acid	TLC	Gedeon et al. (1983)

[a]Abbreviations: C, chromatography; V, voltammetry; GC, gas chromatography; FID, flame-ionization detection; TLC, thin-layer chromatography; HPLC, high-performance liquid chromatography; GPC, gel permeation chromatography; UV, ultraviolet detection; SF, spectrofluorimetry; MS, mass spectrometry; LC, liquid chromatography; ECD, electrochemical detection

3. Biological Data Relevant to the Evaluation of Carcinogenic Risk to Humans

3.1 Carcinogenicity studies in animals

Several reviews discuss carcinogenicity studies on BHA in experimental animals (WHO, 1974; International Programme on Chemical Safety, 1983; WHO, 1983; Kahl, 1984; Ito *et al.*, 1985).

(a) Oral administration

Mouse: [The Working Group noted that several studies are available in which BHA-treated mice were included as control groups for studies on the modulating effects of this chemical on the actions of carcinogens and in which the effect of BHA was examined for a shorter period than the standard two years (Wattenberg *et al.*, 1979; Witschi, 1981; Witschi & Doherty, 1984; Jones *et al.*, 1984). These studies could not be used to evaluate the carcinogenicity of BHA alone, but the study of Witschi (1981) is considered in section 3.1(*e*).]

Rat: Groups of 51-52 male and 51 female Fischer 344 rats, six weeks of age, were fed pelleted diets containing 0 (control), 0.5 (low dose) or 2.0% (high dose) additive- (or reagent-) grade BHA (98.8% pure) *ad libitum* for 104 weeks and maintained on basal diet for a further eight weeks, at which time all animals were sacrificed. The first tumour, a pituitary-gland tumour in a female in the low-dose group, occurred at 41 weeks, at which time all animals except one were still alive. Survival at 112 weeks was >65% in all groups. In the high-dose group, there were significantly increased incidences of papillomas of the forestomach: males — control, 0/51 *versus* high-dose, 52/52 ($p < 0.001$); females — control, 0/51 *versus* high-dose, 49/51 (96%) ($p < 0.001$) and of squamous-cell carcinomas of the forestomach: males — control, 0/51 *versus* high-dose, 18/52 (34.6%) ($p < 0.001$), the first carcinoma appearing at week 59; females — control, 0/51 *versus* high-dose, 15/51 (29.4%) ($p < 0.001$), the first carcinoma appearing at week 82. No such increase in incidence was observed in low-dose rats of either sex (Ito *et al.*, 1982, 1983a).

Groups of 50 male Fischer 344 rats, six weeks of age, were fed powdered diets containing 0, 0.125, 0.25, 0.5, 1 or 2% food additive-grade BHA (containing >98% 3-BHA and <2% 2-BHA) for 104 weeks, at which time all animals were killed. Survival at 104 weeks was >70% in all groups. A significantly increased incidence of papillomas of the forestomach was observed in the two higher-dose groups: control, 0/50; 1% BHA, 10/50 ($p < 0.01$); 2% BHA, 50/50 ($p < 0.001$). An increase in the incidence of squamous-cell carcinomas of the forestomach occurred in the highest-dose group (control, 0/50; 2% BHA, 11/50), which was statistically significant ($p < 0.001$) (Ito *et al.*, 1986).

[The Working Group noted that several studies are available in which BHA-treated rats were used as control groups for studies on the modulating effects of this chemical on the actions of carcinogens and in which the effect of BHA was examined for a shorter period than the standard two years (Pamukcu *et al.*, 1977; Imaida *et al.*, 1983; Ito *et al.*, 1983b; Rao *et al.*, 1984; Shirai *et al.*, 1984). These studies could not be used to evaluate the carcinogenicity of BHA alone, but some of them are considered in section 3.1(*e*).]

Hamster: Groups of ten male Syrian golden hamsters, six weeks of age, were fed diets containing 0, 1 (powdered diet) or 2% (pelleted diet) [subsequently analysed as 1% and 1.94%, respectively] food additive-grade BHA for 24 weeks, at which time all of the 30 surviving animals were killed. There was a significantly increased incidence of papillomas of the forestomach (10/10, high-dose; 10/10, low-dose) in all BHA-treated animals in comparison to controls (0/10; $p < 0.001$). Submucosal growth was found in 10/10 lesions in animals in the high-dose group and in 7/10 lesions in animals in the low-dose group (Ito *et al.*, 1983c). [The Working Group interpreted submucosal growth as evidence of malignancy.]

Groups of 26-32 male Syrian golden hamsters, seven weeks of age, were fed powdered diets containing 0, 1% crude BHA ('food-additive grade', containing >98% 3-BHA), 1% 2-BHA (purity, >99.9%) or 1% 3-BHA (purity, >99.9%) for 16 weeks. Three animals from each group were killed at weeks 1, 2, 3 and 4; the remainder were killed in week 16. Papillomas of the forestomach were found in animals fed 3-BHA at week 3 or food-grade BHA at week 4; no such neoplasm was observed in animals receiving 2-BHA or in controls. At 16 weeks, there were 0.5 ± 0.5 papillomas per animal fed 3-BHA and 0.29 ± 0.17 in those fed food-grade BHA. Severe hyperplasia of the forestomach occurred within the first week of feeding food-grade BHA or 3-BHA, which became more severe at week 4 but decreased at week 16 (Ito *et al.*, 1984; Hirose *et al.*, 1986).

In a study reported only as an abstract[1], a total of 210 hamsters [sex unspecified] were fed diets containing 0, 1 or 2% BHA. Groups of animals [numbers unspecified] were killed at eight, 16, 24, 32, 40, 48 and 104 weeks, and the forestomach and other major organs were examined grossly and histologically. Forestomach papillomas were found in all hamsters fed 2% BHA in the diet and killed from 16 to 104 weeks. Forestomach carcinomas were not reported in the group fed 2% BHA. Of hamsters fed 1% BHA in the diet and killed at 104 weeks, 92.3% had forestomach papillomas and 7.7% had forestomach carcinomas (Masui *et al.*, 1985).

Dog: Groups of one or two male and one or two female young adult beagle dogs were fed diets containing 0 or 50% BHA (70 or 96% 3-BHA) in propylene glycol, to give daily doses of 0, 0.3, 3.0, 30 or 100 mg/kg bw, for one year. One group of three dogs was given 30 mg/kg bw BHA in propylallate-citric acid-propylene glycol. All animals survived to the end of the study period. No effect was reported (Hodge *et al.*, 1964). [The Working Group noted the short duration of the experiment, the small number of animals used and the inadequate reporting.]

---

[1]Subsequent to the meeting, a full report of this study became available (Masui *et al.*, 1986). In addition to the tumours reported in the abstract, carcinomas of the forestomach were found in 10% (4/40) of hamsters given the 2% dose. In the full paper, data are also presented on forestomach tumours in rats and mice given oral doses of BHA. In rats, 75.5% of the group given the 1% dose developed papillomas, but no carcinoma of the forestomach was seen; in the group given the 2% dose, 91.5% had papillomas and 13.9% had carcinomas of the forestomach. In mice, 13.5% of the group given the 0.5% dose had papillomas and 2.7% had carcinomas of the forestomach; in mice given the 1% dose, 14.3% had papillomas and 4.7% had carcinomas of the forestomach.

[The Working Group was aware of short-term studies in animals without forestomachs, such as monkeys and pigs, designed to study the effect of BHA on the stomach (Olsen, 1983; Iverson *et al.*, 1985). [See section 3.2(*a*).]

(*b*) Skin application

Mouse: Groups of 50 male and 50 female C3H/Anf mice, two to four months of age, received weekly topical applications of 0, 0.1 or 10 mg BHA [purity unspecified] in 0.2 ml acetone on shaved skin for life. Survival was 267-401 days after the start of the study for females and 385-548 days for males and was not related to treatment. No skin tumour was observed at the site of application in any of the 13-21 mice per group that were examined histologically (Hodge *et al.*, 1966). [The Working Group noted the small number of animals examined histologically.]

(*c*) Subcutaneous administration

Mouse: Groups of 50 male and 50 female C3H/Anf mice, two to four months old, received a single subcutaneous injection of 0 or 10 mg BHA [purity unspecified] in 0.2 ml trioctanoin. Survival of females was 251-525 days after treatment and that of males was 411-667 days and was not related to treatment. No tumour was observed in the 13-29 mice examined histologically (Hodge *et al.*, 1966). [The Working Group noted that only a single administration was given.]

(*d*) Intraperitoneal administration

Mouse: In a screening assay based on the production of lung tumours in strain A/He mice, groups of 15 male and 15 female mice, six to eight weeks old, received thrice-weekly intraperitoneal injections of BHA [purity unspecified] in 0.1 ml tricaprylin for eight weeks (total doses, 0, 1.2 or 6 g/kg bw). All animals were killed after 24 weeks. All BHA-treated mice survived to the end of the experimental period. No difference in the incidence or multiplicity of lung tumours was observed between BHA-treated and control mice (approximately 0.3 lung tumours/mouse compared with about 10 lung tumours/mouse in urethane-treated positive controls) (Stoner *et al.*, 1973).

(*e*) Administration with known carcinogens

(i) Sequential exposure

Mouse: Groups of 30 female CD-1 mice, six to eight weeks of age, received a single skin application of 200 nmol 7,12-dimethylbenz[*a*]anthracene (DMBA) on the shaven skin on the back. One group subsequently received twice-weekly applications of 1 mg BHA in acetone for 30 weeks. No skin papilloma occurred in mice treated with DMBA alone, with DMBA and BHA or with BHA alone whereas treatment with DMBA and 12-*O*-tetradecanoylphorbol 13-acetate produced skin papillomas in 92% of mice (Berry *et al.*, 1978).

Groups of 20-30 male A/J mice, six to eight weeks of age, were given a single intraperitoneal injection of 500 mg/kg bw urethane in saline. Beginning one week later, mice were treated with weekly intraperitoneal injections of 150, 300 or 500 mg/kg bw BHA for eight weeks. Four months after administration of urethane, the incidence of lung tumours was 96-100% in all groups; BHA did not increase the number of tumours per mouse (Witschi et al., 1981).

Groups of 30 male A/J mice, six to eight weeks of age, were given a single intraperitoneal injection of 500 mg/kg bw urethane and one week or one day later were fed a diet containing 0.75% BHA on one day a week for eight weeks or continuously for eight weeks, respectively, after which they were maintained on basal diet until four months after urethane treatment. Neither intermittent nor continuous BHA exposure altered the incidence of lung tumours due to urethane (Witschi, 1981).

Rat: Groups of 25-26 male Fischer 344 rats, six weeks of age, were given drinking-water containing 0.01 or 0.05% N-butyl-N-(4-hydroxybutyl)nitrosamine for four weeks after which they were fed either basal diet alone or basal diet containing 2% BHA for 32 weeks. Increased incidences of bladder hyperplasia, papillomas and carcinomas were observed in the group given the high dose of nitrosamine plus BHA. The incidence of bladder cancer was 5/26 in rats fed nitrosamine alone and 19/25 in those fed nitrosamine followed by BHA ($p <$ 0.001). BHA alone did not produce bladder lesions, but forestomach papillomas were reported to have occurred in animals fed BHA alone or with nitrosamine (Imaida et al., 1983).

Groups of 25 female Sprague-Dawley rats, 50 days old, were administered a single dose of 8 mg DMBA intragastrically and were fed diets containing 0.25 or 0.5% BHA from one week after DMBA treatment until the end of the study (210 days). Only the high dose of BHA significantly inhibited mammary carcinogenesis induced by DMBA (McCormick et al., 1984).

Two groups of 20 male Fischer 344 rats, six weeks of age, were given a single dose of 150 mg/kg bw N-methyl-N'-nitro-N-nitrosoguanidine (MNNG) in dimethyl sulphoxide by intragastric intubation. One week later, one group was fed a diet containing 0.5% BHA for 51 weeks. The incidence of squamous-cell carcinomas of the forestomach was 9/20 (45%) in the group receiving MNNG plus BHA compared to 2/18 (11%) in that receiving MNNG alone. There was no difference between the groups in the incidence of carcinomas of the glandular stomach (3/20 compared to 3/18) (Shirai et al., 1984).

Groups of 25 male Fischer 344 rats [age unspecified] were given four intraperitoneal injections of 50 mg/kg bw N-methyl-N-nitrosourea (MNU) at four-day intervals; approximately one week after the last injection, one group was fed 1% BHA (food-additive grade) in the diet for 22 weeks. The incidence of squamous-cell carcinomas of the forestomach was 2/17 (11.8%) in the group receiving MNU alone and 15/18 (83.3%) in that receiving MNU plus BHA. The incidence of papillomas or carcinomas of the urinary bladder was not increased in animals receiving MNU plus BHA (Tsuda et al., 1984).

Groups of 20 male Fischer 344 rats, six weeks old, received weekly subcutaneous injections of 20 mg/kg bw 1,2-dimethylhydrazine (DMH) in 0.9% saline for four weeks. One week after the last DMH treatment, groups were fed basal diet containing 0.5% BHA or basal diet alone for 36 weeks. At the end of this period, 1/20 animals in the group treated with DMH only had adenomas and 6/20 had adenocarcinomas of the colon; of the animals treated with DMH and BHA, 2/20 had adenomas and 8/20 adenocarcinomas of the colon. The differences between the two groups were not significant (Shirai *et al.*, 1985).

Groups of 30 male Fischer 344 rats, six weeks old, received twice-weekly intraperitoneal injections of 20 mg/kg bw MNU (4 mg/ml in citrate buffer) or citrate buffer alone (controls) for four weeks, after which they were fed a basal diet containing 0 or 2% BHA for 32 weeks; all animals were killed at 36 weeks. The incidences of papillomas of the urinary bladder were 0/21 in rats treated with MNU only and 10/24 ($p < 0.01$) in rats receiving MNU followed by BHA; the incidences of carcinomas of the urinary bladder were 0/21 and 4/24 ($p < 0.01$), respectively. No such tumour was observed in animals receiving BHA treatment alone. Treatment with MNU or BHA alone induced forestomach papillomas (8/22 and 29/30, respectively) but not carcinomas. In rats treated with MNU followed by BHA, the incidence of forestomach papillomas (23/25) was not greater than that with BHA alone, but the incidence of carcinomas of the forestomach was higher (22/25; $p < 0.001$) (Imaida *et al.*, 1984).

(ii)   *Prior or concomitant exposure*

Mouse: Groups of 29 female Swiss ICR/Ha mice [age unspecified] were fed basal diet containing 0.375 or 0.5% BHA for one week prior to a single subcutaneous injection of 100 mg 3,4,9,10-dibenzopyrene (dibenzo[*a,i*]pyrene; DBP) in 0.2 ml tricaprylin and were observed until termination of the experiment at one year. A control group of 68 mice was fed basal diet only. Mortality due to all tumours [unspecified] at one year was 95% in the group receiving DBP alone, 89% in the group receiving the low dose of BHA plus DBP and 96% in the group receiving the high dose of BHA plus DBP. In a second experiment, neither 0.25% or 0.5% BHA had an inhibitory effect on the carcinogenicity of DBP (Epstein *et al.*, 1967).

Groups of 12-19 female Ha/ICR mice, nine to ten weeks of age, were fed diets containing 0.03% benzo[*a*]pyrene (BaP) alone or with 1.0% BHA for 28 days and were subsequently maintained on basal diet until 28-38 weeks of age. The incidences of forestomach tumours were 13/19 (68%) in the group fed BaP alone and 4/18 (22%) in the group fed BaP plus BHA. BHA also inhibited the incidence of DMBA-induced forestomach tumours (100% with DMBA alone, 58% with DMBA plus BHA). Similar groups of female A/HeJ mice, aged nine to ten weeks, were fed diets containing 0.1% BaP alone or with 0.5% BHA for two weeks. At 21 weeks, the incidences of forestomach tumours were 12/12 (100%) in the group receiving BaP alone and 2/12 (17%) in that receiving BaP plus BHA (Wattenberg, 1972).

Groups of 11-12 female A/HeJ mice, eight or nine weeks of age, were fed diets containing 0 or 0.5% BHA for three weeks. On days 4 and 18 after the beginning of treatment, groups were given a single dose of 3 mg BaP or 0.75 mg DMBA by oral intubation. Three weeks after the beginning of treatment, all mice were fed basal diet and maintained for a further 17 weeks. The numbers of pulmonary adenomas per mouse were 5.3 in the group receiving BaP alone compared to 2.5 in the group receiving BHA plus BaP, and 28.2 in the group receiving DMBA alone compared to 12.7 in the group receiving DMBA plus BHA. In other experiments, BHA reduced the multiplicity of pulmonary adenomas induced by intraperitoneal injection of urethane or by oral administration of uracil mustard. Administration of BHA in conjunction with dibenz[a,h]anthracene or 7-hydroxymethyl-12-methylbenz[a]anthracene in the diet also inhibited the pulmonary tumour formation induced by those compounds (Wattenberg, 1973).

Two groups of 30 female Charles River CD-1 mice, seven to nine weeks of age, received a single topical application of 2.56 μg DMBA on an area of shaved skin; one group was treated 5 min previously with a topical application of 1 mg BHA. One week later, both groups received twice-weekly promoting applications of 10 μg 12-O-tetradecanoylphorbol 13-acetate for 20 weeks. The incidences of skin papillomas were approximately 80% in mice receiving applications of DMBA alone and 70% in those receiving DMBA plus BHA pretreatment (Slaga & Bracken, 1977).

Groups of about 20 female Ha:ICR mice, 11 weeks of age, were fed diets containing 0 or 0.5% BHA. Ten days after the beginning of treatment, groups were given 1 μmol of either BaP or ($\pm$)-trans-7,8-dihydroxy-7,8-dihydrobenzo[a]pyrene by oral intubation three times a week for six weeks. Administration of BHA in the diet was discontinued three days after the last intubation. The experiment was terminated after 30 weeks. The incidences of forestomach tumours were 71% in mice exposed to BaP alone and 17% in those exposed to BaP and BHA, and 100% in mice exposed to the dihydrodiol compared to 60% in those exposed to the dihydrodiol and fed BHA. Administration of BHA also reduced the occurrence of dihydrodiol-induced pulmonary adenomas and lymphomas (Wattenberg et al., 1979).

Two groups of 40 and 20 female CF-1 mice, eight weeks of age, were fed diets containing 0 or 0.5% BHA. Nine days after the beginning of treatment, the groups received twice-weekly subcutaneous injections of 0.3 mg methylazoxymethanol (MAM) acetate in water for three weeks. BHA treatment was discontinued after the last injection, and all animals were maintained on basal diet until 46 weeks of age, at which time the experiment was terminated. The incidences of neoplasms of the large intestine were 41% in mice receiving MAM acetate alone and 5% in those fed BHA concomitantly. A second study confirmed this finding and revealed complete inhibition of carcinogenesis in the large intestine with administration of a diet containing 1.0% BHA (Wattenberg & Sparnins, 1979).

Groups of about 20 female ICR/Ha mice, nine weeks of age, were fed diets containing 0, 0.03 or 0.06 mmol/g of diet [$\sim$ 0.5 or 1.0%] 2-BHA or 3-BHA. On day 8 of the study, the mice were given twice-weekly administrations of 1 mg BaP in corn oil by oral intubation for four weeks. BHA administration was continued for a further three days after the last intubation; mice were then maintained on basal diet for 113 days and then killed. The incidences of tumours of the forestomach were 90-94% in mice receiving BaP alone and 60-65% in those receiving BaP and 2-BHA (the number of tumours per mouse was more than halved). 3-BHA reduced the number of mice with tumours to 79% and almost halved the number of tumours per mouse (Wattenberg et al., 1980).

Groups of 30 male A/J mice, six to eight weeks old, received a diet containing 0 or 0.75% BHA for two weeks (average intake, 187 mg) prior to intraperitoneal injection of 1000 mg/kg bw urethane and were then maintained on basal diet for a further four months. The average number of lung tumours per mouse, but not the percentage of mice with lung tumours, was significantly reduced in the group receiving BHA plus urethane (Witschi, 1981).

Groups of female inbred Swiss albino mice, ten weeks of age, were mated and administered 500 μg DMBA on day 17 of pregnancy. One group was also given 10 mg BHA twice a day by oral intubation from day 15 of gestation until three days after delivery. In the first generation of offspring (F_1), 22/31 of the progeny of DMBA-treated dams developed tumours compared to 9/38 progeny of dams treated with DMBA and BHA. Tumours were mainly lung adenomas, mammary tumours, ovarian tumours, malignant lymphomas, salivary-gland tumours, preputial-gland tumours, skin papillomas and subcutaneous sarcomas. In the F_2 generation, obtained by mating F_1 females with males from untreated dams, the tumour incidence in animals derived from the dams that received DMBA plus BHA was also lower than that in animals derived from dams that received DMBA alone (Rao, 1982).

Groups of female CF-1 mice, five weeks of age, were fed NIH-O7 diet (composed of natural foodstuffs) alone or containing 0.03, 0.1, 0.3 or 0.6% BHA. At seven weeks of age, the groups were given 15 mg/kg bw MAM acetate intraperitoneally four times over 11 days (low dose) or eight times over 22 days (high dose). Two weeks after the last administration of MAM acetate, feeding of BHA was discontinued. The experiment was terminated at 38 weeks from the start of exposure to MAM acetate. The incidences of colon tumours were 25% in the group given the low dose of MAM acetate alone, and, in the groups given MAM acetate and BHA, the incidences were 19% at 0.03%, 16% at 0.1%, 6% at 0.3% and 5% at 0.6% BHA. Similarly, the incidence of lung tumours was reduced from 26% to 3% with the highest dose of BHA. The incidences of colon and lung tumours were greater with the high dose of MAM acetate, and inhibition was less profound but still evident. BHA was also given at 0.6% in AIN-76 diet (semipurified diet; containing 20% casein, 0.3% DL-methionine, 52% corn starch, 13% dextrose, 5% Alphacel, 5% corn oil, 3.5% mineral mix, 1% revised vitamin mix and 0.2% choline bitartrate); inhibition of colon and lung carcinogenesis was also seen (Reddy et al., 1983a). In another experiment, BHA was fed from two weeks prior to MAM acetate administration until termination of the study at 38 weeks after the last carcinogen exposure. Again, BHA inhibited both colon and lung carcinogenesis when given in either NIH-07 or AIN-76 diet (Reddy & Maeura, 1984).

Rat: Two groups of 34 and 18 female Sprague-Dawley rats, seven weeks of age, were administered a single dose of 12 mg/ml DMBA in olive oil by oral intubation; one group was treated 1 h previously with 200 mg BHA. At 25 weeks of age, the incidences of mammary tumours were 80% in rats treated with DMBA alone and 39% in the BHA-pretreated group (Wattenberg, 1972).

Two groups of 30 and 20 albino rats [sex and strain unspecified], 40 days of age, were fed diets containing 33% bracken fern alone or in conjunction with 0.5% BHA, or 0.5% BHA alone for one year. BHA reduced the incidence of intestinal tumours from 100% to 75% and that of bladder tumours from 73% to 60%. BHA alone did not induce tumours (Pamukcu et al., 1977).

Groups of 30 female Sprague-Dawley rats, 50 days old, were administered a single intragastric dose of 10 mg DMBA and were fed diets containing either 20% corn oil, 18% coconut oil and 2% linoleic acid or 2% linoleic acid together with 0.3% BHA. No difference in mammary tumour incidence at six months was observed in any group compared to a control group that received the single dose of DMBA only (King & McCay, 1983).

Groups of 25 female Sprague-Dawley rats, 50 days old, were administered a single intragastric dose of 8 mg DMBA and were fed diets containing 0.25 or 0.5% BHA from two weeks before until one week after DMBA treatment. Both dose levels of BHA inhibited mammary carcinogenesis induced by DMBA treatment (McCormick et al., 1984).

Groups of 25 male Fischer 344 rats, weighing 80-100 g, were fed 10 mg/kg bw ciprofibrate alone or in conjunction with 0.5% BHA in the diet. After 60 weeks, 22/25 rats exposed to ciprofibrate alone had liver tumours >5 mm in diameter, whereas only 12/25 rats treated with ciprofibrate plus BHA had tumours of that size (Rao et al., 1984).

3.2 Other relevant biological data

(a) Experimental systems

The biological effects of BHA have been reviewed (WHO, 1974; International Programme for Chemical Safety, 1983). Unless otherwise indicated, neither the purity nor the isomer composition was specified in the studies considered by the Working Group.

Toxic effects

The oral LD_{50} of BHA was 2000 mg/kg bw in mice and 2200 mg/kg bw in rats (Lehman et al., 1951). The intraperitoneal LD_{50} in male Sprague-Dawley rats was 881 mg/kg bw (Takahashi et al., 1985).

(i) Gastrointestinal tract

Male and female Wistar Han/BGA rats were fed diets containing 2% BHA (purity, 99.5% 3-BHA) for up to four weeks. After one week, the epithelium of the forestomach displayed superficial necrosis, ulceration, mild hyperplasia and hyperkeratosis. Discontinuation of exposure resulted in recovery by week 4. After two weeks of feeding, the forestomach mucosa was markedly hyperplastic and hyperkeratotic; four weeks after exposure to BHA was discontinued, these changes had diminished in severity. After four weeks of feeding, the hyperplasia and hyperkeratosis were more advanced; four weeks after discontinuation of this exposure, mild hyperplasia persisted. Administration by gavage of 1 g/kg bw BHA per day for up to 32 days produced similar changes (Altmann et al., 1985).

Feeding of food-grade BHA at concentrations of 0.5-2% for nine days to weanling male Fischer 344 rats induced proliferation of the squamous epithelium of the forestomach, resulting in thickening of the mucosa. After 27 days of exposure, the changes were more severe and involved a greater area of the forestomach (Nera et al., 1984).

BHA fed at levels of 0.5% and 2% in the diet to Fischer 344 rats for 104 weeks increased the incidence of hyperplasia of the forestomach in a dose-dependent manner (Ito et al., 1983a).

Male Syrian golden hamsters were fed 1% 2- or 3-BHA or crude BHA (<98% 3-BHA) for one to four weeks. The incidence of severe hyperplasia in the forestomach was high in animals given 3-BHA or crude BHA for two weeks or more, but was similar to that in controls in those given 2-BHA (Ito *et al.*, 1984).

Pregnant Danish Landrace swine were fed diets containing up to 3.7% BHA for 16 weeks. No treatment-related lesion of the forestomach or glandular stomach was observed (Olsen, 1983).

Female cynomolgus monkeys were administered 125 or 500 mg/kg bw food-grade BHA by gavage in corn oil on five days per week for 17 weeks. The high dose was reduced to 250 mg/kg bw after 20 days because of toxicity. No treatment-related lesion was observed, but there was a 1.9-fold increase in the mitotic index of the epithelium of the distal oesophagus in BHA-exposed animals (Iverson *et al.*, 1985).

(ii) *Other*

In New Zealand white rabbits, five daily intragastric doses of 1 g BHA caused a ten-fold increase in sodium excretion and a 20% increase in potassium excretion in the urine. The serum potassium fell progressively with exposure. The adrenal cortex showed decreased fat staining of the zona glomerulosa and there was increased excretion of aldosterone in the urine, associated with the sodium and potassium loss (Denz & Llaurado, 1957).

Administration of 500 mg/kg bw BHA by gastric intubation to rhesus monkeys daily for four weeks resulted in an increase in liver weight; this effect was not seen with 50 mg/kg bw. Ultrastructurally, the high dose also produced pronounced proliferation of the hepatic smooth endoplasmic reticulum. No consistent change in serum cholesterol was found (Allen & Engblom, 1972).

BHA was fed at 0.5-2.0% in the diet for six weeks to male Fischer 344 rats which had undergone partial hepatectomy. The development of preneoplastic lesions of the liver induced by *N*-nitrosodiethylamine (200 mg/kg bw) was inhibited in a dose-dependent manner (Thamavit *et al.*, 1985).

A/J mice fed 0.75% BHA in the diet for eight weeks showed no change in proliferation of lung cells (Witschi & Doherty, 1984).

After intraperitoneal administration of >384 mg/kg bw per day BHA, intracranial haemorrhages were observed in dead rats and lung haemorrhages and epistasis in survivors (Takahashi *et al.*, 1985). Such changes were not observed after dietary administration (Takahashi & Hiraga, 1978).

Groups of Fischer 344 rats of both sexes were maintained on diets containing 0, 0.5 or 2.0% BHA for 104 weeks and then on basal diets until week 112. A significant decrease in brain weight was observed in treated males, and increases in the relative weights of salivary glands and hearts were seen in females (Ito *et al.*, 1983a).

Groups of four weanling dogs were fed BHA at 0, 5, 50 and 250 mg/kg bw for 15 months. Most animals fed the highest dose had liver-cell degeneration with diffuse granulocytic infiltration, normal lobular structure and no excessive connective tissue proliferation (Wilder *et al.*, 1960).

BHA was fed to groups of three beagle dogs at dose levels of 0, 0.3, 3, 30 and 100 mg/kg bw for one year. All animals survived; no pathological lesion was seen, and there was no demonstrable storage of BHA (Hodge *et al.*, 1964).

Effects on reproduction and prenatal toxicity

The effects of BHA on reproduction and prenatal toxicity have been reviewed (WHO, 1974; Branen, 1975; International Programme on Chemical Safety, 1983; Cosmetic Ingredient Review Expert Panel, 1984).

In ICI-SPF mice administered 500 mg/kg bw per day BHA in arachis oil by gavage for seven weeks before conception and until day 18 of gestation, maternal mortality was 25%. No significant sign of embryotoxicity or teratogenicity was reported (Clegg, 1965). [The Working Group noted that there was a high percentage of abortions in the treated group, which was not commented upon by the author.]

Groups of one Tuck albino and six Carworth SPF rats were administered a single dose of 1000 mg/kg bw BHA in arachis oil by oral intubation on day 9, 11 or 13 of gestation; some skeletal malformations were reported, which were considered to be spontaneous. [The Working Group noted the small number of animals per group and the use of one dose only.] No abnormality was reported in the offspring of groups of five and three Tuck albino rats administered 750 mg/kg bw per day BHA on days 1-20 of gestation or for 70 days before conception and throughout gestation (Clegg, 1965). [The Working Group noted the choice of a dose level that produced pronounced maternal toxicity and lethality, the small numbers used and the use of one dose only.]

Male and female Sprague-Dawley rats were fed a diet which already contained 0.005% BHA (but no butylated hydroxytoluene) supplemented with 0.125, 0.25 or 0.5% BHA for at least 14 days before mating; the treatment of females continued throughout gestation and lactation. In addition, the offspring were fed the BHA diets until at least 90 days of age. The high dose impaired the growth of offspring, slightly increased postnatal mortality, and produced marginal effects in a battery of behavioural tests. There was no sign of maternal toxicity (Vorhees *et al.*, 1981). [The Working Group noted that no cross-fostering was performed to differentiate between pre- and postnatal effects or between parentally transmitted and direct effects on the offspring.]

In 12 litters of Walter Reed-Carworth rats fed a total dose of 0.5 g BHA in the diet throughout gestation, no increase in resorption rate or malformations was reported (Telford *et al.*, 1962).

Groups of 13-18 pregnant New Zealand SPF rabbits received 50, 200 or 400 mg/kg bw food-grade BHA by gavage on days 7-18 of gestation. No treatment-related effect was observed in dams or offspring (Hansen & Meyer, 1978).

Groups of 9-13 female Danish Landrace pigs were fed diets containing 50, 200 or 400 mg/kg bw food-grade BHA per day from artificial insemination to day 110 of gestation, at which time the foetuses were removed by caesarean section. Body-weight gain was lower in dams fed 400 mg/kg bw, but no other sign of maternal toxicity, embryotoxicity or teratogenicity was reported (Hansen *et al.*, 1982).

After mating with untreated males, six female rhesus monkeys were fed BHA at a level that ensured a daily intake of 50 mg/kg bw (in a diet that also contained the same level of butylated hydroxytoluene) for two years. No maternal toxicity was seen and they produced normal progeny (Allen, 1976).

Absorption, distribution, excretion and metabolism

(i) *Pharmacokinetics*

In male and female Sprague-Dawley rats, BHA was absorbed rapidly after oral administration and metabolized. The main metabolites were 4-*O*-conjugates: the *O*-sulphate and the *O*-glucuronide (Astill *et al.*, 1960). [No data on absorption *via* the skin were available to the Working Group.]

After administration of a single oral dose of 1000 mg BHA to New Zealand white rabbits, 46% of the dose was excreted in the urine as glucuronides, 9% as ethereal sulphates and 6% as free phenols. Excretion of glucuronides was inversely dose dependent: 60% was recovered as glucuronides after a dose of 500 mg and 84% after 250 mg. Recovery of BHA as glucuronide after repeated dosing (three or four doses) was lower than that after a single dose (Dacre *et al.*, 1956).

Male mongrel dogs excreted 60% of an oral dose of 350 mg/kg bw BHA unchanged in the faeces within three days, and the remainder in the urine largely as sulphate conjugates of BHA, *tert*-butylhydroquinone and unidentified phenol. A small amount of glucuronide was also found in the urine (Astill *et al.*, 1962). Wilder *et al.* (1960) also found higher ratios of BHA sulphates to glucuronates in the urine of dogs.

BHA can be oxidized by tissue peroxidases to a derivative that can bind to DNA (Rahimtula, 1983).

(ii) *Effects on enzymes*

BHA binds to cytochrome P450 *in vitro* and inhibits a variety of enzyme activities (Yang *et al.*, 1974).

Addition of BHA to female CF-1 mouse liver and large intestine preparations *in vitro* inhibited NAD^+ (nicotinamide adenine dinucleotide)-dependent alcohol dehydrogenase activity (Wattenberg & Sparnins, 1979).

BHA has been reported to enhance glutathione *S*-transferase activities in rat and mouse liver and other tissues (Benson *et al.*, 1978, 1979). When 3-BHA and 2-BHA were fed to A/HeJ mice for two weeks at a dietary concentration of 0.5%, either singly or as mixtures of the isomers in different ratios, cytosolic glutathione *S*-transferase in the liver was induced to a higher level by 3-BHA than by 2-BHA, whereas in the forestomach the induction characteristics of the isomers were reversed. Sulfhydryl levels in these tissues followed the same trend. Significant synergistic effects of the two isomers were observed in the forestomach, but not in the liver. The epoxide hydrolase activity of isolated liver microsomes from the treated mice was enhanced by 3-BHA, but only marginally by 2-BHA (Lam *et al.*, 1981).

Feeding of BHA to female CF-1 mice at 0.03, 0.1, 0.3 and 0.6% in the diet for ten weeks produced a dose-related increase in glutathione transferase activity in cytosols from liver, small intestine and colon. The maximal increase in liver and small intestine was seven to eight fold, whereas that in colon was only two fold (Reddy & Maeura, 1984).

Administration of BHA at 0.5% in the diet to A/HeJ mice for two weeks increased cytochrome P450 levels 1.5 times, but did not alter arylhydrocarbon hydroxylase activity (Speier & Wattenberg, 1975). Microsomal preparations from the livers of female CF-1 mice fed diets containing 0.03, 0.1, 0.3 or 0.6% BHA showed a marked increase in the levels of cytochrome P450 and b_5, when compared to controls (Reddy et al., 1982).

Administration to rhesus monkeys of 50 or 500 mg/kg bw BHA daily for four weeks by oral intubation produced an elevation of hepatic nitroanisole demethylase activity by two weeks; at four weeks, this level was greater with the high dose but returned to normal with the low dose. No change in cytochrome P450 levels occurred (Allen & Engblom, 1972). Food-grade BHA was administered by gavage to cynomolgus monkeys at 500 mg/kg bw daily, five times per week for 20 days, after which the dose was reduced to 250 mg/kg bw for a final 65 days. No significant change was produced in the activities of a variety of liver monooxygenase enzymes, with the exception of decreased ethoxyresorufin deethylase activity (Iverson et al., 1985).

(iii)   *Modulation of the toxicity of other chemicals by BHA*

As a consequence of its effects on enzyme systems and possible antioxidant properties, BHA modifies the toxicity of a variety of chemicals. Some examples are presented.

Groups of female Sprague-Dawley rats were given 30 mg 7,12-dimethylbenz[a]anthracene (DMBA) intragastrically either alone or 1 h after oral administration of 100 or 200 mg BHA. After 72 h, adrenal necrosis was seen in 29/30 rats given DMBA alone, in 7/10 given the low dose of BHA with DMBA and in 0/10 given the high dose (Wattenberg, 1972).

Feeding of 1% BHA for 30 days or gavage administration of 500 mg/kg bw per day for five days to 10-12 week old (C3H×101)F$_1$ hybrid mice reduced the 30-day lethality due to ethyl methanesulphonate (Cumming & Walton, 1973).

Groups of 90-130 female CF-1 mice were fed two different diets containing 0, 0.03, 0.1, 0.3 or 0.6% BHA. After two weeks, all but ten mice in each group were injected intraperitoneally with 20 mg/kg bw methylazoxymethanol (MAM) acetate and a second injection was given four days later. Mortality among MAM acetate-treated mice on control diets was 80% and 92%, whereas that in mice fed diets with BHA was inversely related to the amount of BHA, being 0 and 1% in the groups fed 0.6%. Feeding of 0.3 or 0.6% BHA also reduced or eliminated histopathological changes observed in the livers and other organs of the mice (Reddy et al., 1982).

When BHA was fed to ICR/Ha mice prior to administration of benzo[a]pyrene, the formation of DNA adducts in the forestomach and liver, but not in the lung, was reduced (Ioannou et al., 1982a).

Mutagenicity and other short-term tests

BHA was not mutagenic to *Salmonella typhimurium* TA1535, TA1537, TA1538, TA98 or TA100 when tested at up to 1000 μg/plate in the presence of a metabolic system (S9) from the liver of polychlorinated biphenyl-induced rats (Joner, 1977; Bonin & Baker, 1980). It also gave negative results in a preincubation assay (10^{-6}-10^{-4}M) in strains TA1535 and TA98 in the absence of a metabolic system (Rosin & Stich, 1979) [details not given].

BHA was not mutagenic to *S. typhimurium* TA98 or TA100 in a host-mediated assay in mice given 0.75% BHA in the diet for ten days prior to testing. No mutagenicity was seen in 24-h urine samples from these mice tested in the presence of Aroclor-induced rat-liver S9 (Batzinger *et al.*, 1978) [details not given].

Sex-linked recessive lethal mutations were not induced in *Drosophila melanogaster* fed 1% solutions of BHA for 24 h (Miyagi & Goodheart, 1976). Similarly, neither sex-linked recessive lethal mutations nor loss of ring X^B chromosome were observed when male *D. melanogaster* were injected with 0.2 μl solutions of 0.001% BHA (Prasad & Kamra, 1974). [The Working Group noted that the authors interpreted this result as positive.]

BHA (1-10 μM) did not induce 6-thioguanine-resistant mutants in cultured Chinese hamster ovary cells in the presence of Aroclor-induced or uninduced rat-liver S9 or microsomes (Tan *et al.*, 1982) nor in Chinese hamster V79 cells (0.1-0.3 mM) in the presence of rat or hamster hepatocytes (Rogers *et al.*, 1985).

Chromosomal aberrations were not induced in cultured Chinese hamster CHL cells by 0.03 mg/ml [1.7×10^{-4}M] BHA (Ishidate & Odashima (1977). BHA (10^{-6}-10^{-3}M) did not induce sister chromatid exchanges or chromosomal aberrations in cultured Chinese hamster DON cells (Abe & Sasaki, 1977). [The Working Group noted that the authors interpreted these results as positive.]

[The Working Group was aware of reports of experiments in which the intention was to study the modulating effects of BHA on the activity of carcinogens/mutagens and in which treatment with BHA alone served as a control. Most of these reports could not be used to evaluate the mutagenic or related effects of BHA alone.]

Almost all studies (see Table 2) on the modulating effects of BHA on the mutagenic and related effects of known carcinogens/mutagens have been directed toward determining its effect on the metabolism of the test chemicals. The methods employed for this purpose can be separated into five groups: studies of the effects of BHA on

(A) directly-acting chemicals — BHA and a test chemical were added directly to an in-vitro assay system;

(B) exogenous metabolic systems — BHA and a test chemical were added to an in-vitro system containing an exogenous metabolic system;

(C) in-vivo metabolic systems — a BHA-induced metabolic system was added to an in-vitro assay with a test chemical;

Table 2. Results from short-term tests: modification of the effects of carcinogens/mutagens by BHA[a]

Test	Test organism/assay	Study design[b] (Exogenous metabolic system[c])	Combination with carcinogen/mutagen	Reported result	Comments	References
PROKARYOTES						
DNA damage	*Bacillus subtilis* (*rec*+/*rec*−)	A	Sodium nitrite	Enhancement		Natake *et al.* (1979)
	Haemophilus influenzae (transformation Ery**R**)	A	Sodium nitrite	Enhancement		Thomas *et al.* (1979)
	Calf thymus DNA (binding)	B (3MC-R-Micr)	Benzo[*a*]pyrene	Reduction		Piekarski *et al.* (1979)
		B (sheep seminal vesical microsomes)	*para*-Phenetidine	Reduction		Andersson *et al.* (1984)
		B (PB-R-Micr)	Aflatoxin B$_1$	Reduction		Bhattacharya *et al.* (1984)
		C (BHA-M-Micr)	Benzo[*a*]pyrene	Reduction		Rahimtula *et al.* (1982)
		C (BHA-M-liver nuclei)	Benzo[*a*]pyrene	Reduction		Hennig *et al.* (1983)
		(BHA-M-Micr)	Benzo[*a*]pyrene	No effect		
	Calf thymus DNA (binding)	C (BHA-M-Micr)	*trans*-7,8-Dihydroxy-7,8-dihydrobenzo[*a*]-pyrene	Reduction		Dock *et al.* (1982)
	Isolated DNA (binding)	C (BHA-M-Micr)	Benzo[*a*]pyrene	No effect	Source of DNA not given	Ioannou *et al.* (1982b)
		B (M-Micr)	Aflatoxin B$_1$	Reduction		Rahimtula & Martin (1984)
	Calf thymus DNA (binding)	C (BHA-M-Micr)	Aflatoxin B$_1$	Enhancement		Rahimtula & Martin (1984)

Table 2 (contd)

Test	Test organism/assay	Study design[b] (Exogenous metabolic system[c])	Combination with carcinogen/mutagen	Reported result	Comments	References
Mutation	*Salmonella typhimurium* (his^-/his^+)	A	N-Acetoxy-2-acetyl-aminofluorene	No effect	Strain TA98	Rosin & Stich 1979
		A	N-Methyl-N'-nitro-N-nitrosoguanidine	No effect	Strain TA1535	Rosin & Stich (1979)
		A	Sodium nitrite	No effect	Strains TA1535 and TA98; figures not given	Natake *et al.* (1979)
		A	γ-radiation	No effect	Strain TA100	Ben-Hur *et al.* (1981)
		B (Liver-PMS)	Benzo[a]pyrene 1-Aminoanthracene 2-Aminoanthraquinone Proflavine dihydrochloride Homidium bromide	Reduction Reduction Reduction Reduction Reduction	Strains TA1538 and TA98 [species and inducer of metabolic system not stated]	McKee & Tometsko (1979)
		B (Aro-R-PMS)	Aflatoxin B_1	Enhancement	Strain TA100	Shelef & Chin (1980)
		B (β-Naphthoflavone-R-PMS, Aro-R-PMS)	Benzo[a]pyrene	Reduction	Strain TA98	Rahimtula *et al.* (1977); Calle & Sullivan (1982)
		B (β-Naphthoflavone-R-PMS)	Benzo[a]pyrene (BP) 6-MeBP 10-MeBP	Reduction Reduction Reduction	Strain TA98	Calle *et al.* (1978)
		B (preparation from sheep seminal vesicles incubated with arachidonic acid)	BP-7,8-diol	Reduction	Strain TA98	Marnett *et al.* (1978)
		B (Aro-R-PMS)	Quercetin	Reduction	Strain TA98 [The Working Group noted only a slight reduction]	Hatcher & Bryan (1985)

Table 2 (contd)

Test	Test organism/assay	Study design[b] (Exogenous metabolic system[c])	Combination with carcinogen/mutagen	Reported result	Comments	References
Mutation (contd)	Salmonella typhimurium (his^-/his^+) (contd)	B (Aro-R-PMS)	3,2'-Dimethyl-4-aminobiphenyl	Reduction	Strains TA98 and TA100	Reddy et al. (1983b)
		C (BHA-M-Micr)	Aflatoxin B_1	Enhancement	Strain TA98	Rahimtula & Martin (1984)
		E (Host-mediated assay)	Aflatoxin B_1	No effect	Strain TA98	Chang & Wei (1982)
		E (Host-mediated assay and E (urine) (Aro-R-PMS)	Metronidazole	Reduction	Strains TA98 and TA100	Batzinger et al. (1978)
			Benzo[a]pyrene	Reduction		
			IA-4N-oxide	Reduction		
			Metrifonate	Reduction		
			Praziquantel	Reduction		
			Diazepam	Reduction		
			Mebendazole	Reduction		
			Hycanthone	Reduction		
			Oxamniquine	No effect		
			4-Nitro-4'-isothio-cyanodiphenylamine	No effect		
		E (Urine) (BHA-M-CytP450, BHA-R-CytP450)	Benzo[a]pyrene	Reduction	Strains TA98 and TA100	Benson et al. (1978)
GREEN PLANTS						
Mutation	Hordeum vulgare (chlorophyll mutants)	D	Propane sultone	Enhancement	Treatment of seeds	Kaul & Tandon (1981)
Chromosomal effects	Hordeum vulgare (aberrations)	D	Propane sultone	Enhancement	Treatment of seeds	Tandon & Kaul (1979); Kaul & Tandon (1981)
	Allium cepa (aberrations)	D	X-rays	Enhancement	Treatment of seeds	Kaul (1979)

Table 2 (contd)

Test	Test organism/ assay	Study design[b] (Exogenous metabolic system[c])	Combination with carcinogen/mutagen	Reported result	Comments	References
INSECTS						
Mutation	Drosophila melanogaster (sex-linked recessive lethals)	D	γ-rays	Enhancement		Prasad & Kamra (1974)
Chromosomal effects	Drosophila melanogaster (loss of ring X^B chromosome)	D	γ-rays	No effect	[The Working Group noted the very low dose of 0.2 μl of 0.001% BHA used.]	Prasad & Kamra (1974)
MAMMALIAN CELLS IN VITRO						
DNA damage	Mouse embryo cells	D	Benzo[a]pyrene	Reduction		Piekarski et al. (1979); Sawicki et al. (1980)
	Human skin (primary culture)	D	Benzo[a]pyrene	Reduction		
	Human lymphocytes (binding to DNA)	D	Benzo[a]pyrene	No effect		
	NIH Swiss mouse epidermal cells in culture (binding to DNA)	D	7,12-Dimethylbenz-[a]anthracene	Reduction		Shoyab (1979)
	Guinea-pig leucocytes (binding to DNA)	D	N-Methylaminoazobenzene + 12-0-tetradecanoylphorbol 13-acetate	Reduction		Takanaka et al. (1982)
	Primary mouse embryo cells in culture (binding to DNA)	D	7,12-Dimethylbenz-[a]anthracene	Reduction only of syn bay region of dihydrodiol epoxy adducts		Sawicki & Dipple (1983)

Table 2 (contd)

Test	Test organism/assay	Study design[b] (Exogenous metabolic system[c])	Combination with carcinogen/mutagen	Reported result	Comments	References
Mutation	Chinese hamster V79 cells (ouabain resistance)	B (SHE) A	Benzo[a]pyrene N-Acetoxy-2-acetyl-aminofluorene	Reduction No effect		Katoh et al. (1980)
Chromosomal effects	Human lymphocytes (aberrations)	D	12-0-Tetradecanoyl-phorbol 13-acetate	Reduction		Emerit et al. (1983)
MAMMALIAN CELLS IN VIVO						
DNA damage	CD-1 mice (binding to DNA from skin)	D	Benzo[a]pyrene 7,12-Dimethylbenz[a]anthracene	Reduction Reduction		Slaga & Bracken (1977)
	NIH Swiss mice (binding to DNA in skin)	D	7,12-Dimethylbenz[a]anthracene	No effect		Dipple et al. (1984)
	Sprague-Dawley rats (O^6-methylguanine in DNA from colon)	D	1,2-Dimethylhydrazine	No effect		Bull et al. (1981)
	A/HeJ mice (binding to DNA from lung, liver and forestomach)	D	Benzo[a]pyrene	Reduction		Anderson et al. (1981); Ioannou et al. (1982a); Adrianenssens et al. (1983)
Chromosomal effects	C57BL/6J mice (aberrations in colonic cells)	D	1,2-Dimethyl-hydrazine	Reduction		Wargovich et al. (1983)

[a]This table comprises selected assays and references and is not intended to be complete review of the literature.

[b]Studies are designed to investigate the effects of BHA on: A, directly-acting chemicals; B, exogenous metabolic system; C, in-vivo metabolic system; D, test chemicals in test organisms; E, in-vivo metabolism of test chemicals; see text for explanations.

[c]3MC, 3-methylcholanthrene-induced; R, rat; Micr, microsomes; M, mouse; PB, phenobarbital-induced; BHA, BHA-induced; PMS, postmitochondrial supernatant; Aro, Aroclor-induced; CytP450, purified cytochrome P450; SHE, Syrian hamster embryo cells

(D)   test chemicals in test organisms — BHA was administered to test organisms *in vitro* (systems not requiring an exogenous metabolic system) or *in vivo*, prior to or simultaneously with a test chemical; and

(E)   in-vivo metabolism of test chemicals — BHA was administered *in vivo* prior to or simultaneously with a test chemical and a host-mediated or urine mutagenesis assay was performed.

(b)   Humans

Toxic effects

No data were available to the Working Group.

Effects on reproduction and prenatal toxicity

No data were available to the Working Group.

Absorption, distribution, excretion and metabolism

When male volunteers were given an oral dose of 50 mg BHA, 27-77% was excreted in the urine as the glucuronide and urinary metabolites, as measured by paper chromatography. Urinary excretion of BHA was maximal within 17 h and complete by 48 h (Astill *et al.*, 1962). When human volunteers were given a single oral dose of ^{14}C-labelled BHA (approximately 0.5 mg/kg bw), 60-70% of the radioactivity was excreted in the urine within two days and 80-86.5% by day 11 (Daniel *et al.*, 1967). Four male volunteers were given 30 mg BHA orally and ten days later they were given another 5 mg. Approximately 20% of either dose was excreted in the urine as glucuronide within the first 24 h. Almost no free BHA was present in urine (Castelli *et al.*, 1984).

Mutagenicity and chromosomal effects

No data were available to the Working Group.

3.3 Case reports and epidemiological studies of carcinogenicity to humans

No data were available to the Working Group.

4. Summary of Data Reported and Evaluation

4.1 Exposure data

Butylated hydroxyanisole (BHA) has been used since 1947 as an antioxidant in many foods, including edible fats and oils, meats, cereals, potato products, baked goods, nuts, snack foods, chewing-gum and beverages. It has also been used extensively in cosmetics, especially lipsticks and eye shadow. There is widespread human exposure to this compound by ingestion and skin application.

4.2 Experimental data

Butylated hydroxyanisole was tested for carcinogenicity in two experiments in rats and in two experiments in hamsters by administration in the diet, inducing benign and malignant tumours of the forestomach.

Butylated hydroxyanisole was studied in mice and rats for its ability to modify the carcinogenicity of selected chemical agents. When administered with known carcinogens, butylated hydroxyanisole either enhanced, inhibited or had no effect on carcinogenicity (see also the 'General Remarks on the Substances Considered', p. 38).

Butylated hydroxyanisole administered to rats at maternally toxic and occasionally lethal doses during, or before, during and after, gestation induced slight embryotoxicity but no definite indication of teratogenicity. No effect was seen in rabbits, pigs or rhesus monkeys.

In rats, feeding of butylated hydroxyanisole in the diet caused superficial necrosis, ulceration and hyperplasia of the squamous epithelium of the forestomach. Induction of forestomach hyperplasia also occurs in hamsters. Administration of butylated hydroxyanisole by gavage to monkeys was associated with an elevated mitotic index in the squamous epithelium of the distal oesophagus.

Butylated hydroxyanisole was not mutagenic to *Salmonella typhimurium*, *Drosophila melanogaster* or to Chinese hamster cells *in vitro*. It did not cause chromosomal effects in *D. melanogaster* or in cultured Chinese hamster cells.

When tested in combination with other chemicals (usually known mutagens or carcinogens), butylated hydroxyanisole often modified their DNA damaging, mutagenic and clastogenic activities. In most studies, butylated hydroxyanisole reduced the activity of indirectly-acting mutagens/carcinogens.

4.3 Human data

No data were available to evaluate the carcinogenicity of butylated hydroxyanisole to humans.

4.4 Evaluation[1]

There is *sufficient evidence*[2] for the carcinogenicity of butylated hydroxyanisole to experimental animals.

No data were available on the carcinogenicity of butylated hydroxyanisole to humans.

---

[1]For definition of the italicized term, see Preamble, p. 18.
[2]In the absence of data on humans, it is reasonable, for practical purposes, to regard chemicals or exposures for which there is *sufficient evidence* of carcinogenicity in animals as if they presented a carcinogenic risk to humans.

Overall assessment of data from short-term tests: Butylated hydroxyanisole[a]

	Genetic activity			Cell transformation
	DNA damage	Mutation	Chromosomal effects	
Prokaryotes		−		
Fungi/Green plants				
Insects		−	−	
Mammalian cells (*in vitro*)		−	−	
Mammals (*in vivo*)				
Humans (*in vivo*)				
Degree of evidence in short-term tests for genetic activity: **No evidence**				Cell transformation: No data

[a]The groups into which the table is divided and the symbol used are defined on pp. 19-20 of the Preamble; the degrees of evidence are defined on pp. 20-21.

5. References

Abe, S. & Sasaki, M. (1977) Chromosome aberrations and sister chromatid exchanges in Chinese hamster cells exposed to various chemicals. *J. natl Cancer Inst.*, *58*, 1635-1641

Adriaenssens, P.I., White, C.M. & Anderson, M.W. (1983) Dose-response relationships for the binding of benzo(*a*)pyrene metabolites to DNA and protein in lung, liver, and forestomach of control and butylated hydroxyanisole-treated mice. *Cancer Res.*, *43*, 3712-3719

Allen, J.R. (1976) Long-term antioxidant exposure effects on female primates. *Arch. environ. Health*, *31*, 47-50

Allen, J.R. & Engblom, J.F. (1972) Ultrastructural and biochemical changes in the liver of monkeys given butylated hydroxytoluene and butylated hydroxytoluene. *Food Cosmet. Toxicol.*, *10*, 769-779

Altmann, H.-J., Wester, P.W., Matthiaschk, G., Grunow, W. & van der Heijden, C.A. (1985) Induction of early lesions in the forestomach of rats by 3-*tert*-butyl-4-hydroxyanisole (BHA). *Food Chem. Toxicol.*, *23*, 723-731

Anderson, M.W., Boroujerdi, M. & Wilson, A.G.E. (1981) Inhibition *in vivo* of the formation of adducts between metabolites of benzo(*a*)pyrene and DNA by butylated hydroxyanisole. *Cancer Res.*, *41*, 4309-4315

Andersson, B., Larsson, R., Rahimtula, A. & Moldéus, P. (1984) Prostaglandin synthase and horseradish peroxidase catalyzed DNA-binding of p-phenetidine. *Carcinogenesis*, 5, 161-165

Anon. (1983) Feast or famine: the future of chemicals in the food industry. *Chem. Purch.*, 19, 47-55

Astill, B.D., Fassett, D.W. & Roudabush, R.L. (1960) The metabolism of phenolic antioxidants. 2. The metabolism of butylated hydroxyanisole in the rat. *Biochem. J.*, 75, 543-551

Astill, B.D., Mills, J., Fassett, D.W., Roudabush, R.L. & Terhaar, C.J. (1962) Fate of butylated hydroxyanisole in man and dog. *J. agric. Food Chem.*, 10, 315-319

Batzinger, R.P., Ou, S.-Y. L. & Bueding, E. (1978) Antimutagenic effects of 2(3)-*tert*-butyl-4-hydroxyanisole and of antimicrobial agents. *Cancer Res.*, 38, 4478-4485

Ben-Hur, E., Green, M., Prager, A., Rosenthal, I. & Riklis, E. (1981) Differential protective effects of antioxidants against cell killing and mutagenesis of *Salmonella typhimurium* by γ radiation. *J. Radiat. Res.*, 22, 250-257

Benson, A.M., Batzinger, R.P., Ou, S.-Y.L., Bueding, E., Cha, Y.-N. & Talalay, P. (1978) Elevation of hepatic glutathione S-transferase activities and protection against mutagenic metabolites of benzo(a)pyrene by dietary antioxidants. *Cancer Res.*, 38, 4486-4495

Benson, A.M., Cha, Y.-N., Bueding, E., Heine, H.S. & Talalay, P. (1979) Elevation of extrahepatic glutathione S-transferase and epoxide hydratase activities by 2(3)-*tert*-butyl-4-hydroxyanisole. *Cancer Res.*, 39, 2971-2977

Berry, D.L., DiGiovanni, J., Juchau, M.R., Bracken, W.M., Gleason, G.L. & Slaga, T.J. (1978) Lack of tumor-promoting ability of certain environmental chemicals in a two-stage mouse skin tumorigenesis assay. *Res. Commun. chem. Pathol. Pharmacol.*, 20, 101-108

Bhattacharya, R.K., Firozi, P.F. & Aboobaker, V.S. (1984) Factors modulating the formation of DNA adduct by aflatoxin B₁ *in vitro*. *Carcinogenesis*, 5, 1359-1362

Bonin, A.M. & Baker, R.S.U. (1980) Mutagenicity testing of some approved food additives with the *Salmonella*/microsome assay. *Food Technol. Austr.*, 32, 608-611

Branen, A.L. (1975) Toxicology and biochemistry of butylated hydroxyanisole and butylated hydroxytoluene. *J. Am. Oil Chem. Soc.*, 52, 59-63

Bull, A.W., Burd, A.D. & Nigro, N.D. (1981) Effect of inhibitors of tumorigenesis on the formation of O^6-methylguanine in the colon of 1,2-dimethylhydrazine-treated rats. *Cancer Res.*, 41, 4938-3941

Calle, L.M. & Sullivan, P.D. (1982) Screening of antioxidants and other compounds for antimutagenic properties towards benzo[a]pyrene-induced mutagenicity in strain TA98 of *Salmonella typhimurium*. *Mutat. Res.*, 101, 99-114

Calle, L.M., Sullivan, P.D., Nettleman, M.D., Ocasio, I.J., Blazyk, J. & Jollick, J. (1978) Antioxidants and the mutagenicity of benzo(a)pyrene and some derivatives. *Biochem. biophys. Res. Commun.*, 85, 351-356

Castelli, M.G., Benfenati, E., Pastorelli, R., Salmona, M. & Fanelli, R. (1984) Kinetics of 3-*tert*-butyl-4-hydroxyanisole (BHA) in man. *Food Chem. Toxicol.*, *22*, 901-904

Chang, S.-C. & Wei, R.-D. (1982) In vivo mutagenicity of aflatoxin B_1 in rats. *J. Chin. biochem. Soc.*, *11*, 79-84

The Chemical Daily Co. (1980) *JCW Chemicals Guide*, Tokyo, p. 70

Chemical Dynamics Corp. (undated) *Butylated Hydroxyanisole: Material Safety Data Sheet* (*Product No. 15-1388-00*), South Plainfield, NJ

Clegg, D.J. (1965) Absence of teratogenic effect of butylated hydroxyanisole (BHA) and butylated hydroxytoluene (BHT) in rats and mice. *Food Cosmet. Toxicol.*, *3*, 387-403

Commission of the European Communities (1978) *Reports of the Scientific Committee for Food*, 5th Series, Brussels, pp. 13-25

Cosmetic Ingredient Review Expert Panel (1984) Final report on the safety assessment of butylated hydroxyanisole. *J. Am. Coll. Toxicol.*, *3*, 83-146

Cumming, R.B. & Walton, M.F. (1973) Modification of the acute toxicity of mutagenic and carcinogenic chemicals in the mouse by prefeeding with antioxidants. *Food Cosmet. Toxicol.*, *11*, 547-553

Dacre, J.C., Denz, F.A. & Kennedy, T.H. (1956) The metabolism of butylated hydroxy-anisole in the rabbit. *Biochem. J.*, *64*, 777-782

Daniel, J.W., Gage, J.C., Jones, D.I. & Stevens, M.A. (1967) Excretion of butylated hydroxytoluene (BHT) and butylated hydroxyanisole (BHA) by man. *Food Cosmet. Toxicol.*, *5*, 475-479

Denz, F.A. & Llaurado, J.G. (1957) Some effects of phenolic anti-oxidants on sodium and potassium balance in the rabbit. *Br. J. exp. Pathol.*, *38*, 515-524

Dilli, S. & Robards, K. (1977) Detection of the presence of BHA by a rapid spectrofluori-metric screening procedure. *Analyst*, *102*, 210-205

Dipple, A., Pigott, M.A., Bigger, C.A.H. & Blake, D.M. (1984) 7,12-Dimethylbenz[a]-anthracene-DNA binding in mouse skin: response of different mouse strains and effects of various modifiers of carcinogenesis. *Carcinogenesis*, *5*, 1087-1090

Dock, L., Rahimtula, A., Jernström, B. & Moldéus, P. (1982) Metabolism of (±)-*trans*-7,8-dihydroxy-7,8-dihydro-benzo[a]pyrene in mouse liver microsomes and the effect of 2(3)-*tert*-butyl-4-hydroxyanisole. *Carcinogenesis*, *3*, 697-701

Doeden, W.G., Bowers, R.H. & Ingala, A.C. (1979) Determination of BHA, BHT and TBHQ in edible fats and oils. *J. Am. Oil Chem. Soc.*, *56*, 12-14

Eastman Chemical Products, Inc. (1982) *Tenox^R Food-grade Antioxidants* (*Publ. No. ZG-109F*), Kingsport, TN

El-Rashidy, R. & Niazi, S. (1979) GLC determination of butylated hydroxyanisole in human plasma and urine. *J. pharm. Sci.*, *68*, 103-104

Emerit, I., Levy, A. & Cerutti, P. (1983) Suppression of tumor promoter phorbolmyristate acetate-induced chromosome breakage by antioxidants and inhibitors of arachidonic acid metabolism. *Mutat. Res.*, *110*, 327-335

Epstein, S.S., Joshi, S., Andrea, J., Forsyth, J. & Mantel, N. (1967) The null effect of antioxidants on the carcinogenicity of 3,4,9,10-dibenzpyrene to mice. *Life Sci.*, *6*, 225-233

Fazio, T., ed. (1984a) *Food additives: direct. Antioxidants.* In: Williams, S., ed., *Official Methods of Analysis of the Association of Official Analytical Chemists*, 14th ed., Arlington, VA, Association of Official Analytical Chemists, pp. 373-374

Fazio, T., ed. (1984b) *Food additives: direct. Antioxidants.* In: Williams, S., ed., *Official Methods of Analysis of the Association of Official Analytical Chemists*, 14th ed., Arlington, VA, Association of Official Analytical Chemists, pp. 374-375

Freydberg, N. & Gortner, W.A. (1982) *The Food Additives Book*, New York, Bantam Books, pp. 489-490

Gedeon, B.J., Chu, T. & Copeland, S. (1983) The identification of rubber compounding ingredients using thin layer chromatography. *Rubber Chem. Technol.*, *56*, 1080-1095

Giragosian, N.H. (1982) Food preservatives and antioxidants. *Chem. Purch.*, *18*, 27, 29-30, 33-34, 37

Hansen, E. & Meyer, O. (1978) A study of the teratogenicity of butylated hydroxyanisole on rabbits. *Toxicology*, *10*, 195-201

Hansen, E.V., Meyer, O. & Olsen, P. (1982) Study on toxicity of butylated hydroxyanisole (BHA) in pregnant gilts and their foetuses. *Toxicology*, *23*, 79-83

Hatcher, J.F. & Bryan, G.T. (1985) Factors affecting the mutagenic activity of quercetin for *Salmonella typhimurium* TA98: metal ions, antioxidants and pH. *Mutat. Res.*, *148*, 13-23

Hawley, G.G., ed. (1981) *The Condensed Chemical Dictionary*, 10th ed., New York, Van Nostrand Reinhold, p. 162

Hennig, E.E., Demkowicz-Dobrzański, K.K., Sawicki, J.T., Mojska, H. & Kujawa, M. (1983) Effect of dietary butylated hydroxyanisole on the mouse hepatic monooxygenase system of nuclear and microsomal fractions. *Carcinogenesis*, *4*, 1243-1246

Hirose, M., Masuda, A., Kurata, Y., Ikawa, E., Mera, Y. & Ito, N. (1986) Histological and autoradiographical studies on the forestomach of hamsters treated with 2-*tert*-butylated hydroxyanisole, 3-*tert*-butylated hydroxyanisole, crude butylated hydroxyanisole or butylated hydroxytoluene. *J. natl Cancer Inst.*, *76*, 143-149

Hodge, H.C., Fassett, D.W., Maynard, E.A., Downs, W.L. & Coye, R.D., Jr (1964) Chronic feeding studies of butylated hydroxyanisole in dogs. *Toxicol. appl. Pharmacol.*, *6*, 512-519

Hodge, H.C., Maynard, E.A., Downs, W.L., Ashton, J.K. & Salerno, L.L. (1966) Tests on mice for evaluating carcinogenicity. *Toxicol. appl. Pharmacol.*, *9*, 583-596

IARC (1977) *IARC Monographs on the Evaluation of the Carcinogenic Risk of Chemicals to Man*, Vol. 15, *Some Fumigants, the Herbicides 2,4-D and 2,4,5-T, Chlorinated Dibenzodioxins and Miscellaneous Industrial Chemicals*, Lyon, pp. 155-175

IARC (1982a) *IARC Monographs on the Evaluation of the Carcinogenic Risk of Chemicals to Humans*, Suppl. 4, *Chemicals, Industrial Processes and Industries Associated with Cancer in Humans (IARC Monographs Volumes 1 to 29)*, Lyon, pp. 50-51

IARC (1982b) *IARC Monographs on the Evaluation of the Carcinogenic Risk of Chemicals to Humans*, Suppl. 4, *Chemicals, Industrial Processes and Industries Associated with Cancer in Humans (IARC Monographs Volumes 1 to 29)*, Lyon, pp. 149-150

IARC (1982c) *IARC Monographs on the Evaluation of the Carcinogenic Risk of Chemicals to Humans*, Suppl. 4, *Chemicals, Industrial Processes and Industries Associated with Cancer in Humans (IARC Monographs Volumes 1 to 29)*, Lyon, pp. 115-116

ICIS Chemical Information System (1984) *Carbon-13 NMR Spectral Search System (CNMR)*, *Mass Spectral Search System* (MSSS), *Infrared Spectral Search System* (IRSS), *Information System for Hazardous Organics in Water* (ISHOW) and *Environmental Fate* (ENVIROFATE), Washington DC, Information Consultants, Inc.

Imaida, K., Fukushima, S., Shirai, T., Ohtani, M., Nakanishi, K. & Ito, N. (1983) Promoting activities of butylated hydroxyanisole and butylated hydroxytoluene on 2-stage urinary bladder carcinogenesis and inhibition of γ-glutamyl transpeptidase-positive foci development in the liver of rats. *Carcinogenesis*, *4*, 895-899

Imaida, K., Fukushima, S., Shirai, T., Masui, T., Ogiso, T. & Ito, N. (1984) Promoting activities of butylated hydroxyanisole, butylated hydroxytoluene, and sodium L-ascorbate on forestomach and urinary bladder carcinogenesis initiated with methyl-nitrosourea in F344 male rats. *Gann*, *75*, 769-775

International Life Sciences Institute (1984) *Butylated Hydroxyanisole (BHA). A Monograph*, Washington DC

International Programme on Chemical Safety (1983) *Toxicological Evaluation of Certain Food Additives and Food Contaminants (WHO Food Add. Ser. No. 18)*, Geneva, pp. 41-49

Ioannou, Y.M., Wilson, A.G.E. & Anderson, M.W. (1982a) Effect of butylated hydroxy-anisole, α-angelica lactone, and β-napthoflavone on benzo(α)pyrene: DNA adduct formation *in vivo* in the forestomach, lung, and liver of mice. *Cancer Res.*, *42*, 1199-1204

Ioannou, Y.M., Wilson, A.G.E. & Anderson, M.W. (1982b) Effect of butylated hydroxy-anisole on the metabolism of benzo[a]pyrene and the binding of metabolites to DNA, *in vitro* and *in vivo*, in the forestomach, lung and liver of mice. *Carcinogenesis*, *3*, 739-745

Isacoff, H. (1979) *Cosmetics*. In: Mark, H.F., Othmer, D.F., Overberger, C.G. & Seaborg, G.T., eds, *Kirk-Othmer Encyclopedia of Chemical Technology*, 3rd ed., Vol. 7, New York, John Wiley & Sons, pp. 143-176

Ishidate, M., Jr & Odashima, S. (1977) Chromosome tests with 134 compounds on Chinese hamster cells in vitro — a screening for chemical carcinogens. *Mutat. Res.*, *48*, 337-354

Isshiki, K., Tsumura, S. & Watanabe, T. (1980) Determination of preservatives, butylhydroxy-anisole and dibutylhydroxytoluene. *Agric. Biol. Chem.*, *44*, 1601-1607

Ito, N., Hagiwara, A., Shibata, M., Ogiso, T. & Fukushima, S. (1982) Induction of squamous cell carcinoma in the forestomach of F344 rats treated with butylated hydroxyanisole. *Gann*, *73*, 332-334

Ito, N., Fukushima, S., Hagiwara, A., Shibata, M. & Ogiso, T. (1983a) Carcinogenicity of butylated hydroxyanisole in F344 rats. *J. natl Cancer Inst.*, *70*, 343-352

Ito, N., Tsuda, H., Sakata, T., Hasegawa, R. & Tamano, S. (1983b) Inhibitory effect of butylated hydroxyanisole and ethoxyquin on the induction of neoplastic lesions in rat liver after an initial treatment with N-ethyl-N-hydroxyethylnitrosamine. *Gann*, *74*, 466-468

Ito, N., Fukushima, S., Imaida, K., Sakata, T. & Masui, T. (1983c) Induction of papilloma in the forestomach of hamsters by butylated hydroxyanisole. *Gann*, *74*, 459-461

Ito, N., Hirose, M., Kurata, Y., Ikawa, E., Mera, Y. & Fukushima, S. (1984) Induction of forestomach hyperplasia by crude butylated hydroxyanisole, a mixture of 3-*tert* and 2-*tert* isomers, in Syrian golden hamsters is due to 3-*tert*-butylated hydroxyanisole. *Gann*, *75*, 471-474

Ito, N., Fukushima, S. & Tsuda, H. (1985) Carcinogenicity and modification of the carcinogenic response by BHA, BHT, and other antioxidants. *Crit. Rev. Toxicol.*, *15*, 109-150

Ito, N., Fukushima, S., Tamano, S., Shibata, M. & Hagiwara, A. (1986) Dose-response study of forestomach carcinogenesis in F344 rats induced by butylated hydroxyanisole. *J. natl Cancer Inst.* (in press)

Iverson, F., Truelove, J., Nera, E., Wong, J., Lok, E. & Clayson, D.B. (1985) An 85-day study of butylated hydroxyanisole in the cynomolgus monkey. *Cancer Lett.*, *26*, 43-50

Joner, P.E. (1977) Butylhydroxyanisol (BHA), butylhydroxytoluene (BHT) and ethoxyquin (EMQ) tested for mutagenicity. *Acta vet. scand.*, *18*, 187-193

Jones, F.E., Komorowski, R.A. & Condon, R.E. (1984) The effects of ascorbic acid and butylated hydroxyanisole in the chemoprevention of 1,2-dimethylhydrazine-induced large bowel neoplasms. *J. surg. Oncol.*, *25*, 54-60

Kahl, R. (1984) Synthetic antioxidants: biochemical actions and interference with radiation, toxic compounds, chemical mutagens and chemical carcinogens. *Toxicology*, *33*, 185-228

Katoh, Y., Tanaka, M., Umezawa, K. & Takayama, S. (1980) Inhibition of mutagenesis in Chinese hamster V-79 cells by antioxidants. *Toxicol. Lett.*, *7*, 125-130

Kauffman, P. (1977) The separation of butylated hydroxyanisole isomers on Sephadex LH-20. *J. Chromatogr.*, *132*, 356-358

Kaul, B.L. (1979) Cytogenetic activity of some common antioxidants and their interaction with X-rays. *Mutat. Res.*, *67*, 239-247

Kaul, B.L. & Tandon, V. (1981) Modification of the mutagenic activity of propane sultone by some phenolic antioxidants. *Mutat. Res.*, *89*, 57-61

Keeley, D.E. (1980) *Ethers*. In: Mark, H.F., Othmer, D.F., Overberger, C.G. & Seaborg, G.T., eds, *Kirk-Othmer Encyclopedia of Chemical Technology*, 3rd ed., Vol. 9, New York, John Wiley & Sons, pp. 381-393

King, M.M. & McCay, P.B. (1983) Modulation of tumor incidence and possible mechanisms of inhibition of mammary carcinogenesis by dietary antioxidants. *Cancer Res., 43 (Suppl.)*, 2485s-2490s

King, P., Joseph, K.T. & Kissinger, P.T. (1980) Liquid chromatography with amperometric detection for determination of phenolic preservatives. *J. Assoc. off. anal. Chem., 63*, 137-142

Kline, D.A., Joe, F.L., Jr & Fazio, T. (1978) A rapid gas-liquid chromatographic method for the multidetermination of antioxidants in fats, oils, and dried food products. *Anal. Chem., 61*, 513-519

Lam, L.K.T., Pai, R.P. & Wattenberg, L.W. (1979) Synthesis and chemical carcinogen inhibitory activity of 2-*tert*-butyl-4-hydroxyanisole. *J. med. Chem., 22*, 569-571

Lam, L.K.T., Sparnins, V.L., Hochalter, J.B. & Wattenberg, L.W. (1981) Effects of 2- and 3-*tert*-butyl-4-hydroxyanisole on glutathione *S*-transferase and epoxide hydrolase activities and sulfhydryl levels in liver and forestomach of mice. *Cancer Res., 41*, 3940-3943

Lehman, A.J., Fitzhugh, O.G., Nelson, A.A. & Woodard, G. (1951) The pharmacological evaluation of antioxidants. *Adv. Food Res., 3*, 197-208

Majors, R.E. & Johnson, E.L. (1978) High-performance exclusion chromatography of low-molecular-weight additives. *J. Chromatogr., 167*, 17-30

Marnett, L.J., Reed, G.A. & Dennison, D.J. (1978) Prostaglandin synthetase dependent activation of 7,8-dihydro-7,8-dihydroxy-benzo(a)pyrene to mutagenic derivatives. *Biochem. biophys. Res. Commun., 82*, 210-216

Masui, T., Shibata, M., Tamano, S., Ono, S. & Hirose, M. (1985) *Species differences with regard to sequential changes induced by butylated hydroxyanisole in the forestomach of rats, mice and hamsters* (Abstract No. 85). In: *Proceedings of the Japanese Cancer Association, 44th Annual Meeting*, Tokyo, Japanese Cancer Association, p. 48

Masui, T., Hirose, M., Imaida, K., Fukushima, S., Tamano, S. & Ito, N. (1986) Sequential changes of the forestomach of F344 rats, Syrian golden hamsters, and B6C3F$_1$ mice treated with butylated hydroxyanisole. *Jpn. J. Cancer Res., 77*, 1083-1090

McClusky, G.A., Kondrat, R.W. & Cooks, R.G. (1978) Direct mixture analysis by mass-analyzed ion kinetic energy spectrometry using negative chemical ionization. *J. Am. chem. Soc., 100*, 6045-6051

McCormick, D.L., Major, N. & Moon, R.C. (1984) Inhibition of 7,12-dimethyl-benz(*a*)anthracene-induced rat mammary carcinogenesis by concomitant or post-carcinogen antioxidant exposure. *Cancer Res., 44*, 2858-2863

McKee, R.H. & Tometsko, A.M. (1979) Inhibition of promutagen activation by the antioxidants butylated hydroxyanisole and butylated hydroxytoluene. *J. natl Cancer Inst., 63*, 473-477

McKone, H.T. (1976) Determination of butylated hydroxyanisole (BHA) in cooking oils. *J. chem. Educ.*, *53*, 800

Miyagi, M.P. & Goodheart, C.R. (1976) Effects of butylated hydroxyanisole in *Drosophila melanogaster*. *Mutat. Res.*, *40*, 37-42

Natake, M., Danno, G.-I., Maeda, T., Kawamura, K. & Kanazawa, K. (1979) Formation of DNA-damaging and mutagenic activity in the reaction systems containing nitrite and butylated hydroxyanisole, tryptophan, or cysteine. *J. nutr. Sci. Vitaminol.*, *25*, 317-332

National Research Council (1981) *BHA*. In: *Food Chemicals Codex*, 3rd ed., Washington DC, National Academy of Sciences, pp. 37-38

Nera, E.A., Lok, E., Iverson, F., Ormsby, E., Karpinski, K.F. & Clayson, D.B. (1984) Short-term pathological and proliferative effects of butylated hydroxyanisole and other phenolic antioxidants in the forestomach of Fischer 344 rats. *Toxicology*, *32*, 197-213

Olsen, P. (1983) The carcinogenic effect of butylated hydroxyanisole on the stratified epithelium of the stomach in rat versus pig. *Cancer Lett.*, *21*, 115-116

Page, B.D. (1979) High performance liquid chromatographic determination of nine phenolic antioxidants in oils, lards, and shortenings. *J. Assoc. off. anal. Chem.*, *62*, 1239-1246

Pamukcu, A.M., Yalçiner, S. & Bryan, G.T. (1977) Inhibition of carcinogenic effect of bracken fern (*Pteridium aquilinum*) by various chemicals. *Cancer*, *40*, 2450-2454

Pellerin, F., Delaveau, P., Dumitrescu, D. & Safta, F. (1982) Identification and titration of BHA and BHT in chewing-gum preparations (Fr.). *Ann. pharm. fr.*, *40*, 221-230

Piekarski, L., Sawicki, J., Kugaczewska, M., Potocki, L.J., Sankowski, A., Uszyński, H., Malunowicz, E., Wojciechowska, M., Kolodziejska, A. & Fox, C.H. (1979) Inhibitory effect of the antioxidant butylated hydroxyanisole on the activation of the carcinogen benzo(a)pyrene. *Neoplasma*, *26*, 139-144

Prasad, O.M. & Kamra, O.P. (1974) Radiosensitization of *Drosophila* sperm by commonly used food additives — butylated hydroxyanisole and butylated hydroxytoluene. *Int. J. Radiat. Biol.*, *25*, 67-72

Rahimtula, A. (1983) In vitro metabolism of 3-*t*-butyl-4-hydroxyanisole and its irreversible binding to proteins. *Chem.-biol. Interactions*, *45*, 125-135

Rahimtula, A.D. & Martin, M. (1984) Dietary administration of 2(3)-*t*-butyl-4-hydroxy-anisole elevates mouse liver microsome-mediated DNA binding and mutagenicity of aflatoxin B_1. *Chem.-biol. Interactions*, *48*, 207-220

Rahimtula, A.D., Zachariah, P.K. & O'Brien, P.J. (1977) The effects of antioxidants on the metabolism and mutagenicity of benzo[*a*]pyrene *in vitro*. *Biochem. J.*, *164*, 473-475

Rahimtula, A.D., Jernström, B., Dock, L. & Moldéus, P. (1982) Effects of dietary and in vitro 2(3)-t-butyl-4-hydroxyanisole and other phenols on hepatic enzyme activities in mice. *Br. J. Cancer*, *45*, 935-944

Rao, A.R. (1982) Inhibitory action of BHA on carcinogenesis in F_1 and F_2 descendants of mice exposed to DMBA during pregnancy. *Int. J. Cancer*, *30*, 121-124

Rao, M.S., Lalwani, N.D., Watanabe, T.K. & Reddy, J.K. (1984) Inhibitory effect of antioxidants ethoxyquin and 2(3)-*tert*-butyl-4-hydroxyanisole on hepatic tumorigenesis in rats fed ciprofibrate, a peroxisome proliferator. *Cancer Res.*, *44*, 1072-1076

Reddy, B.S. & Maeura, Y. (1984) Dose-response studies of the effect of dietary butylated hydroxyanisole on colon carcinogenesis induced by methylazoxymethanol acetate in female CF1 mice. *J. natl Cancer Inst.*, *72*, 1181-1187

Reddy, B.S., Furuya, K., Hanson, D., DiBellow, J. & Berke, B. (1982) Effect of dietary butylated hydroxyanisole on methylazoxymethanol acetate-induced toxicity in mice. *Food Chem. Toxicol.*, *20*, 853-859

Reddy, B.S., Maeura, Y. & Weisburger, J.H. (1983a) Effect of various levels of dietary butylated hydroxyanisole on methylazoxymethanol acetate-induced colon carcinogenesis in CF1 mice. *J. natl Cancer Inst.*, *71*, 1299-1305

Reddy, B.S., Sharma, C. & Mathews, L. (1983b) Effect of butylated hydroxytoluene and butylated hydroxyanisole on the mutagenicity of 3,2'-dimethyl-4-aminobiophenyl. *Nutr. Cancer*, *5*, 153-158

Rogers, C.G., Nayak, B.N. & Héroux-Metcalf, C. (1985) Lack of induction of sister chromatid exchanges and of mutation to 6-thioguanine resistance in V79 cells by butylated hydroxyanisole with and without activation by rat or hamster hepatocytes. *Cancer Lett.*, *27*, 61-69

Rosin, M.P. & Stich, H.F. (1979) Assessment of the use of the *Salmonella* mutagenesis assay to determine the influence of antioxidants on carcinogen-induced mutagenesis. *Int. J. Cancer*, *23*, 722-727

Sadtler Research Laboratories (1980) *The Sadtler Standard Spectra, Cumulative Index*, Philadelphia, PA

Sawicki, J.T. & Dipple, A. (1983) Effects of butylated hydroxyanisole and butylated hydroxytoluene on 7,12-dimethylbenz[*a*]anthracene-DNA adduct formation in mouse embryo cell cultures. *Cancer Lett.*, *20*, 165-171

Sawicki, J., Selkirk, J.K., Kugaczewska, M., Piekarski, L. & McLeod, M.C. (1980) Benzo(a)pyrene metabolism and metabolites binding to DNA in the presence of BHA. *Arch. Geschwulstforsch.*, *50*, 317-321

Senten, J.R., Waumans, J.M. & Clement, J.M. (1977) Gas-liquid chromatographic determination of butylated hydroxyanisole and butylated hydroxytoluene in edible oils. *J. Assoc. off. anal. Chem.*, *60*, 505-508

Shelef, L.A. & Chin, B. (1980) Effect of phenolic antioxidants on the mutagenicity of aflatoxin B_1. *Appl. environ. Microbiol.*, *40*, 1039-1043

Shirai, T., Fukushima, S., Ohshima, M., Masuda, A. & Ito, N. (1984) Effects of butylated hydroxyanisole, butylated hydroxytoluene, and NaCl on gastric carcinogenesis initiated with *N*-methyl-*N'*-nitro-*N*-nitrosoguanidine in F344 rats. *J. natl Cancer Inst.*, *72*, 1189-1198

Shirai, T., Ikawa, E., Hirose, M., Thamavit, W. & Ito, N. (1985) Modification by five antioxidants of 1,2-dimethylhydrazine-initiated colon carcinogenesis in F344 rats. *Carcinogenesis*, *6*, 637-639

Shoyab, M. (1979) Evidence for translational control of the binding of 7,12-dimethylbenz-[*a*]anthracene to DNA of murine epidermal cell in culture. *Chem.-biol. Interactions*, *25*, 289-301

Slaga, T.J. & Bracken, W.M. (1977) The effects of antioxidants on skin tumor initiation and aryl hydrocarbon hydroxylase. *Cancer Res.*, *37*, 1631-1635

Speier, J.L. & Wattenberg, L.W. (1975) Alterations in microsomal metabolism of benzo[*a*]pyrene in mice fed butylated hydroxyanisole. *J. natl Cancer Inst.*, *55*, 469-472

Stoner, G.D., Shimkin, M.B., Kniazeff, A.J., Weisburger, J.H., Weisburger, E.K. & Gori, G.B. (1973) Test for carcinogenicity of food additives and chemotherapeutic agents by the pulmonary tumor response in strain A mice. *Cancer Res.*, *33*, 3069-3085

Takahashi, O. & Hiraga, K. (1978) The relationship between hemorrhage induced by butylated hydroxytoluene and its antioxidant properties or structural characteristics. *Toxicol. appl. Pharmacol.*, *46*, 811-814

Takahashi, O., Sakamoto, Y. & Hiraga, K. (1985) Lung hemorrhagic toxicity of butylated hydroxyanisole in the rat. *Toxicol. Lett.*, *27*, 15-25

Takanaka, K., O'Brien, P.J., Tsuruta, Y. & Rahimtula, A.D. (1982) Tumor promoter stimulated irreversible binding of *N*-methylaminoazobenzene to polymorphonuclear leukocyte DNA. *Cancer Lett.*, *15*, 311-315

Tan, E.-L., Schenley, R.L. & Hsie, A.W. (1982) Microsome-mediated cytotoxicity to CHO cells. *Mutat. Res.*, *103*, 359-365

Tandon, V. & Kaul, B.L. (1979) Influence of some phenolic antioxidants on radiomimetic activity of propane sultone. *Indian J. exp. Biol.*, *17*, 713-714

Telford, I.R., Woodruff, C.S. & Linford, R.H. (1962) Fetal resorption in the rat as influenced by certain antioxidants. *Am. J. Anat.*, *110*, 29-36

Thamavit, W., Tatematsu, M., Ogiso, T., Mera, Y., Tsuda, H. & Ito, N. (1985) Dose-dependent effects of butylated hydroxyanisole, butylated hydroxytoluene and ethoxyquin in induction of foci of rat liver cells containing the placental form of glutathione-*S*-transferase. *Cancer Lett.*, *27*, 295-303

Thomas, H.F., Hartman, P.E., Mudryj, M. & Brown, D.L. (1979) Nitrous acid mutagenesis of duplex DNA as a three-component system. *Mutat. Res.*, *61*, 129-151

Tsuda, H., Sakata, T., Shirai, T., Kurata, Y., Tamano, S. & Ito, N. (1984) Modification of *N*-methyl-*N*-nitrosourea initiated carcinogenesis in the rat by subsequent treatment with antioxidants, phenobarbital and ethinyl estradiol. *Cancer Lett.*, *24*, 19-27

US Department of Agriculture (1984) Animals and animal products. *US Code fed. Regul.*, *Title 9*, Parts 318.7, 381.147, pp. 209, 407

US Food and Drug Administration (1983a) *Butylated hydroxytoluene (BHT): Method II.* In: Warner, C., Modderman, J., Fazio, T., Beroza, M., Schwartzman, G. & Fominaya, K., eds, *Food Additives Analytical Manual*, Vol. 1, Arlington, VA, Association of Official Analytical Chemists, pp. 62-76

US Food and Drug Administration (1983b) *Butylated hydroxytoluene (BHT): Method I.* In: Warner, C., Modderman, J., Fazio, T., Beroza, M., Schwartzman, G. & Fominaya, K., eds, *Food Additives Analytical Manual*, Vol. 1, Arlington, VA, Association of Official Analytical Chemists, pp. 52-61

US Food and Drug Administration (1984a) Food and drugs. *US Code fed. Regul., Title 21,* Part 182.3169, p. 380

US Food and Drug Administration (1984b) Food and drugs. *US Code fed. Regul., Title 21,* Part 172.110, pp. 25-26

US Food and Drug Administration (1984c) Food and drugs. *US Code fed. Regul., Title 21,* Part 172.615, p. 58

US Food and Drug Administration (1984d) Food and drugs. *US Code fed. Regul., Title 21,* Part 172.515, p. 54

US Food and Drug Administration (1984e) Food and drugs. *US Code fed. Regul., Title 21,* Part 173.340, p. 119

US Food and Drug Administration (1984f) Food and drugs. *US Code fed. Regul., Title 21,* Part 181.24, p. 365

US Food and Drug Administration (1984g) Food and drugs. *US Code fed. Regul., Title 21,* Part 178.3570, p. 319

US Food and Drug Administration (1984h) Food and drugs. *US Code fed. Regul., Title 21,* Part 175.105, p. 125

Verma, K.K., Tripathi, R.P., Bajaj, I., Prakash, O. & Parihar, D.B. (1970) Studies on the synthesis of butylated hydroxyanisole. *J. Chromatogr., 52,* 507-511

Vorhees, C.V., Butcher, R.E., Brunner, R.L., Wootten, V. & Sobotka, T.J. (1981) Developmental neurobehavioral toxicity of butylated hydroxyanisole (BHA) in rats. *Neurobehav. Toxicol. Teratol., 3,* 321-329

Wang, J. & Freiha, B.A. (1983) Preconcentration and differential pulse voltammetry of butylated hydroxyanisole at a carbon paste electrode. *Anal. chim. Acta, 154,* 87-94

Wang, J. & Luo, D.-B. (1984) Competition studies on voltammetric measurements based on extractive accumulation into carbon paste electrodes. *J. electroanal. Chem., 179,* 251-261

Wargovich, M.J., Goldberg, M.T., Newmark, H.L. & Bruce, W.R. (1983) Nuclear aberrations as a short-term test for genotoxicity to the colon: evaluation of nineteen agents in mice. *J. natl Cancer Inst., 71,* 133-137

Wattenberg, L.W. (1972) Inhibition of carcinogenic and toxic effects of polycyclic hydrocarbons by phenolic antioxidants and ethoxyquin. *J. natl Cancer Inst., 48,* 1425-1430

Wattenberg, L.W. (1973) Inhibition of chemical carcinogen-induced pulmonary neoplasia by butylated hydroxyanisole. *J. natl Cancer Inst.*, *50*, 1541-1544

Wattenberg, L.W. & Sparnins, V.L. (1979) Inhibitory effects of butylated hydroxyanisole on methylazoxymethanol acetate-induced neoplasia of the large intestine and nicotinamide adenine dinucleotide-dependent alcohol dehydrogenase activity in mice. *J. natl Cancer Inst.*, *63*, 219-222

Wattenberg, L.W., Jerina, D.M., Lam, L.K.T. & Yagi, H. (1979) Neoplastic effects of oral administration of (±)-*trans*-7,8-dihydroxy-7,8-dihydrobenzo[*a*]pyrene and their inhibition by butylated hydroxyanisole. *J. natl Cancer Inst.*, *62*, 1103-1106

Wattenberg, L.W., Coccia, J.B. & Lam, L.K.T. (1980) Inhibitory effects of phenolic compounds on benzo(*a*)pyrene-induced neoplasia. *Cancer Res.*, *40*, 2820-2823

WHO (1974) *Toxicological Evaluation of Some Food Additives Including Anticaking Agents, Antimicrobials, Antioxidants, Emulsifiers and Thickening Agents* (*WHO Food Add. Ser. No. 5*), Geneva, pp. 148-155

WHO (1983) *Evaluation of Certain Food Additives and Food Contaminants* (*Tech. Rep. Ser. No. 696*), Geneva, pp. 13-14

Wilder, O.H.M., Ostby, P.C. & Gregory, B.R. (1960) Effect of feeding butylated hydroxyanisole to dogs. *J. agric. Food Chem.*, *8*, 504-506

Windholz, M., ed. (1983) *The Merck Index*, 10th Ed., Rahway, NJ, Merck & Co., p. 215

Witschi, H.P. (1981) Enhancement of tumor formation in mouse lung by dietary butylated hydroxytoluene. *Toxicology*, *21*, 95-104

Witschi, H. & Doherty, D.G. (1984) Butylated hydroxyanisole and lung tumor development in A/J mice. *Fundam. appl. Toxicol.*, *4*, 795-801

Witschi, H.P., Hakkinen, P.J. & Kehrer, J.P. (1981) Modification of lung tumor development in A/J mice. *Toxicology*, *21*, 37-45

Wyatt, D.M. (1981) Simultaneous analysis of BHA, TBHQ, BHT and propyl gallate by gas chromatography as extracted from refined vegetable oil. *J. Am. Oil Chem. Soc.*, *58*, 917-920

Yang, C.S., Strickhart, F.S. & Woo, G.K. (1974) Inhibition of the mono-oxygenase system by butylated hydroxyanisole and butylated hydroxytoluene. *Life Sci.*, *15*, 1497-1505

BUTYLATED HYDROXYTOLUENE (BHT)

1. Chemical and Physical Data

1.1 Synonyms and trade names

Chem. Abstr. Services Reg. No.: 128-37-0

Chem. Abstr. Name: 2,6-Bis(1,1-dimethylethyl)-4-methylphenol

IUPAC Systematic Name: 2,6-Di-*tert*-butyl-*para*-cresol

Synonyms: Butylhydroxytoluene; DBPC; dibutylated hydroxytoluene; di-*tert*-butyl-*para*-cresol; *ortho,ortho'*-di-*tert*-butyl-*para*-cresol; 1,3-di-*tert*-butyl-2-hydroxy-5-methylbenzene; 3,5-di-*tert*-butyl-4-hydroxytoluene; 3,5-di-*tert*-butyl-4-methylphenol; EEC No. 321; 4-methyl-2,6-di-*tert*-butylphenol; NCI-CO3598

Trade Names: Advastab 401; Agidol; Alkofen BP; Antioxidant 4; Antioxidant 29; Antioxidant 30; Antioxidant DBPC; Antioxidant 4K; Antioxidant KB; Buks; CAO-1; CAO-3; Catalin CAO-3; Chemanox 11; Dalpac; Deenax; Dibunol; Impruvol; Ionol; Ionole; Kerabit; Nocrac 200; Nonox TBC; Parabar 441; Paranox 441; Stavox; Sumilizer BHT; Sustane BHT; Swanox BHT; Tenamene 3; Tenox BHT: Topanol; Toxolan P; Vanlube PC; Vanlube PCX; Vianol; Vulkanox KB

1.2 Structural and molecular formulae and molecular weight

$C_{15}H_{24}O$
Mol. wt: 220.36

1.3 Chemical and physical properties of the pure substance

(*a*)   *Description*: White, crystalline solid (Hawley, 1981; Windholz, 1983; Sax, 1984)

(b)   *Boiling-point*: 265°C (Windholz, 1983; Sax, 1984; Weast, 1985); 136°C at 10 mm
      Hg (Weast, 1985)

(c)   *Melting-point*: 71°C (Weast, 1985)

(d)   *Density*: d_4^{20} 1.048 (Hawley, 1981; Windholz, 1983; Sax, 1984)

(e)   *Spectroscopy data*: Ultraviolet (Sadtler Research Laboratories, 1980 [9777[a]]),
      infrared (Sadtler Research Laboratories, 1980; prism [283, 540], grating [18002]),
      proton nuclear magnetic resonance (Sadtler Research Laboratories, 1980 [526]),
      C-13 nuclear magnetic resonance (Sadtler Research Laboratories, 1980 [4642];
      ICIS Chemical Information System, 1984 [CNMR]), fluorescence (Sadtler Research
      Laboratories, 1973 [22]) and mass spectral data (Grasselli & Ritchey, 1975; ICIS
      Chemical Information System, 1984 [MSSS]) have been reported.

(f)   *Solubility*: Very slightly soluble in water (0.4 mg/l at 20°C) (Verschueren, 1983);
      soluble in most aliphatic and aromatic hydrocarbon solvents, ketones, alcohols,
      linseed oil, food oils and fats (Grasselli & Ritchey, 1975; Hawley, 1981; Windholz,
      1983)

(g)   *Volatility*: Vapour pressure, 0.0075 mm Hg (Biesterfeld US, Inc., 1972), 0.01 mm
      Hg at 20°C (Uniroyal Chemical Co., 1984); relative vapour density (air = 1), 7.6
      (Verschueren, 1983; Sax, 1984; Uniroyal Chemical Co., 1984)

(h)   *Stability*: Flash-point, 126.6°C (open-cup) (Sax, 1984)

(i)   *Octanol/water partition coefficient (P)*: log P, 5.80 [ISHOW]; log P, 4.17
      [ENVIROFATE] (ICIS Chemical Information System, 1984)

(j)   *Conversion factor*: mg/m³ = 9.01 × ppm[b]

1.4 Technical products and impurities

The Food Chemical Codex (National Research Council, 1981) and the Joint FAO/WHO
Expert Committee on Food Additives (Food and Agricultural Organization, 1983) specify
that food-grade BHT assay at not less than 99.0% w/w of pure BHT, with a solidification
point not lower than 69.2°C. Maximum levels of arsenic (see IARC, 1982) and heavy metals
(as lead) are set at 3 and 10 mg/kg, respectively. Food-grade BHT is available in crystalline
form or as a fine powder (Sherwin-Williams, 1982; Koppers Co., Inc., undated).

---

[a]Spectrum number in Sadtler compilation

[b]Calculated from: mg/m³ = (molecular weight/24.45) × ppm, assuming standard temperature (25°C) and pressure (760 mm Hg)

Technical-grade BHT is available in crystalline or flake forms, or in molten form in bulk quantities. The crystalline/flake substance generally contains 98% w/w minimum active ingredient and has a solidification point not lower than 68.7-68.8°C. Molten BHT may be 78-84% pure, have a maximum of 0.5% water and a solidification point of approximately 56°C (Sherwin-Williams, 1982; Koppers Co., Inc., undated).

2. Production, Use, Occurrence and Analysis

2.1 Production and use

(a) Production

BHT is produced commercially by the alkylation of *para*-cresol with isobutylene. A US patent for this process was received in 1947 (Windholz, 1983).

US production of technical-grade BHT decreased from 5.4 million kg in 1977 to 3.6 million kg in 1983; US production of food-grade BHT was 4.9 million kg in 1977, but was not reported in 1983 (US International Trade Commission, 1978, 1984). US consumption of BHT was estimated at 3.5 million kg in 1981 (Anon., 1983). US demand has increased recently, due to growth in the rubber and plastics industries; demand was 8.2 million kg in 1983 and approximately 9 million kg in 1984. US capacity in 1984 was estimated at 12.3 million kg, provided by three primary producers (Anon., 1984).

BHT is also produced by several western European manufacturers, with three production/processing plants identified in the Federal Republic of Germany, two each in France, the Netherlands and the UK and one in Spain.

Fifteen companies in Japan reportedly produce BHT.

(b) Use

BHT is used as an antioxidant to help preserve and stabilize the flavour, colour, freshness and nutritive value of foods and animal feed products. It can improve the stability of pharmaceuticals, fat-soluble vitamins, cosmetics, petroleum-based lubricant and transformer oils, and gasoline and diesel fuels. The service life of rubber, elastomers and plastics is increased by the addition of BHT (Sherwin-Williams, 1982). In the USA, less than 5% is used in food or feed (Table 1).

Food products, food packaging and feed additives: BHT is reported to have been used in foods in the USA since 1949 (Federation of American Societies for Experimental Biology, 1973). It was found to be an effective antioxidant for animal fats in 1954 (Babich, 1982). The National Research Council (1972) of the US National Academy of Sciences as well as the Bureau of Foods (1973) reported that BHT was used in fats and oils, jams and jellies, sweet sauces, nut products, milk products, meat products, breakfast cereals, snack foods, hard and soft sweets, baked goods, confectionery frosting, gelatin puddings, frozen dairy products, gravies, alcoholic and nonalcoholic beverages, chewing-gum, soups, processed vegetables and fruit. The use of BHT in foods has decreased in recent years.

Table 1. Use of BHT in the USA[a]

Use	Percent
Plastics antioxidant	48
Rubber antioxidant	38
Petroleum additive	9
Other (including food additive)	5

[a]From Anon. (1984)

BHT is used as an antioxidant and stabilizer in paper and plastic food packaging materials. It is also used as an antioxidant for animal feeds to inhibit the development of rancidity in grain-seed oils and meals, and to preserve fat-soluble vitamins, particularly vitamins A and E (Sherwin-Williams, 1982).

Plastics: The largest current use of BHT is as a plastics antioxidant to prevent oxidation and free-radical formation, which alter the molecular structure of plastic materials, thereby diminishing their performance properties and shortening the serviceable life of the product (Sherwin-Williams, 1982). Although phenolic antioxidants are used in a number of plastics, such as polyurethanes, polyesters and polyvinyls, 70% of the BHT volume intended for use in plastics goes into polyolefins (Anon., 1983).

Rubber and synthetic elastomers: BHT was originally developed as an antioxidant for rubber and petroleum, and was patented for this application in 1947 (Babich, 1982). It is added at concentrations of 0.5-2.0% to natural rubber and to synthetic elastomer polymers such as ethylene-propylene-diene terpolymers, nitriles, styrene-butadiene rubber, butyl rubber, polyisoprene and neoprene to provide resistance to weathering and cracking and to maintain elasticity (Sherwin-Williams, 1982).

Petroleum products: BHT is used as an antioxidant in gasoline to prevent the formation during cracking of gums which clog fuel lines and cause mechanical failure. It is usually found in low concentrations in gasoline (0.001-0.008%), turbine oils (0.1%-1.0%) and insulating oils (0.2-0.3%), but at up to 2.0% in engine oils (Sherwin-Williams, 1982).

Miscellaneous uses: BHT is reportedly used in a wide variety of cosmetic products. Companies participating in a US Food and Drug Administration-sponsored cosmetic registration programme in 1981 indicated that BHT was used in 42 different product categories and in 668 of 20 578 cosmetic formulations. Of the formulations in which the concentration of BHT was reported, the majority (91%) had levels ≤0.1%; only one product category in the survey, eye-shadow products, contained as much as 1-5% BHT. Of the cosmetics reported in the survey, eye-shadow formulations represented the greatest use (128 products), followed by lipstick (79 products) (US Food and Drug Administration, 1981).

BHT has been used as a stabilizer for pyrethrin and vinyl phosphate insecticides and for synthetic detergents. It is sometimes present in asphalt floor tiles at concentrations of 0.1%

(Sherwin-Williams, 1982) and is used as an antiskinning agent in paints and inks (Windholz, 1983). It may also be present as an inhibitor in composite dental materials at concentrations of 0.006% or less (Paffenbarger & Rupp, 1979).

(c) Regulatory status and guidelines

Approximately 40 countries reportedly permit the use of BHT as a direct or indirect food additive (International Life Sciences Institute, 1984).

BHT was approved for use as a food additive by the US Food and Drug Administration prior to 1958 and was therefore classified as GRAS (Generally Recognized as Safe) under the 1958 Food Additives Amendment to the Food, Drug and Cosmetic Act. Food products regulated by this Act could contain a combined total of up to 0.02% BHT and butylated hydroxyanisole (see monograph p. 123), based on the fat content of the food. Foods covered by the Meat Inspection Act and the Poultry Inspection Act were permitted to contain no more than 0.01% of an individual antioxidant and 0.02% combined total (Babich, 1982).

Some restrictions on the uses of BHT in foods were proposed subsequently; current US regulations permit its use in certain potato products, rice, margarine, breakfast cereals, chewing-gum and certain meat products at specified levels ranging from 0.001-0.1% and in food packaging materials (US Food and Drug Administration, 1977; Babich, 1982; US Department of Agriculture, 1984; US Food and Drug Administration, 1984).

The Commission of the European Communities (1978) recommended a temporary acceptable daily intake (ADI) of 30 mg/adult in 1978 for BHT or BHT combined with butylated hydroxyanisole. The Joint FAO/WHO Expert Committee on Food Additives has set a temporary ADI of 0-0.5 mg/kg bw for BHT or combined BHT, butylated hydroxyanisole and tert-butylhydroquinone (WHO, 1983).

The American Conference of Governmental Industrial Hygienists (1984) recommends that occupational exposure to airborne BHT not exceed 10 mg/m³ as an eight-hour time-weighted average (TWA) or 20 mg/m³ in any 15-min period. These levels have been adopted in Finland (Työsuojeluhallitus, 1981). In Australia, Belgium, the Netherlands and Switzerland, the TWA for BHT is also set at 10 mg/m³ (International Labour Office, 1980).

2.2 Occurrence

(a) Natural occurrence

BHT is not known to occur as a natural product.

(b) Occupational exposure

In a purification and bagging plant for BHT, concentrations of 4.2-10.5 mg/m³ BHT vapour and aerosol were measured; the highest concentration was 619 mg/m³ in the area above a slop tank. After engineering and ventilation modifications, the exposure levels ranged from 1.6-2.6 mg/m³, and the highest area concentration measured was 15.4 mg/m³, which occurred during cleaning operations (Gilles & Lucas, 1975; Grote & Kupel, 1978).

(c)   Food

Concentrations of 6-31 mg/kg BHT have been measured in cereals and flour mixes, up to 292 mg/kg in wax wrappers from cereals (Kline et al., 1978), up to 82 mg/kg in oils and vegetable fats (Kline et al., 1978; Page, 1979), up to 216 mg/kg in five of eight chewing-gum samples and up to 530 mg/kg in basic gum (Pellerin et al., 1982).

The concentration of BHT in foods in the UK in the 1960s was estimated not to exceed 1 mg/kg of diet (Gilbert & Martin, 1967); some estimates of US per-caput daily intake ranged as high as 13.7 mg (0.2 mg/kg bw) (Federation of American Societies for Experimental Biology, 1973).

(d)   Human tissue levels

In a study reported in 1970, the BHT content of fat extracted from human subcutaneous adipose tissue at random post-mortems was determined by colour reaction after solvent extraction and steam distillation. Levels averaged 0.23 ± 0.15 mg/kg among 11 UK residents and 1.30 ± 0.82 mg/kg among 12 US residents (Collings & Sharratt, 1970). A level of 1.30 mg/kg corresponds to a tissue concentration of about 5 μM, at which modulation of prostaglandin synthesis occurs in vitro (Kahl, 1984).

2.3 Analysis

Analytical methods for determining quantities of antioxidants, including BHT, present in matrices are based on separation of the phenol by extraction, distillation, precipitation and chromatography, and quantitative measurement by colorimetric, ultraviolet, infrared and various other techniques (Stuckey, 1972). Examples of these methods as applied to various matrices are given in Table 2.

There is an analytical method of the US National Institute for Occupational Safety and Health for the determination of BHT in air by gas chromatography/flame-ionization detection (Taylor, 1977), a method of the International Union for Pure and Applied Chemistry—Food and Drug Administration (FDA)—Association of Official Analytical Chemists (AOAC) for the determination of BHT in oils and lard by liquid chromatography/ultra-violet detection (US Food and Drug Administration, 1983a; Fazio, 1984a), an FDA-AOAC method (vacuum sublimation/gas chromatography) for BHT in lard (US Food and Drug Administration, 1983b) and an AOAC method (gas chromatography/flame-ionization detection) for BHT in cereals (Fazio, 1984b).

3. Biological Data Relevant to the Evaluation of Carcinogenic Risk to Humans

3.1 Carcinogenicity studies in animals

Several reviews discuss carcinogenicity studies on BHT in experimental animals (WHO, 1974; Babich, 1982; International Programme on Chemical Safety, 1983; Malkinson, 1983; WHO, 1983; Kahl, 1984; Ito et al., 1985).

Table 2. Methods for the analysis of BHT

Sample matrix	Sample preparation	Assay procedure[a]	Reference
Air	Adsorb on silica gel; desorb on methanol-carbon disulphide	GC/FID	Taylor (1977); Grote & Kupel (1978)
Water	Extract into organic solvent; react with stable cation	SP	Clement & Gould (1980)
	Reverse phase	LC/ECD	Armentrout et al. (1979)
	Extract with dichloromethane	GC/MS	Jungclaus et al. (1976)
	Dilute with acetonitrile; reverse-phase elution	HPLC	Chao & Suatoni (1982)
Oils and lard	Dilute with hexane; extract with acetonitrile	LC/UV	US Food and Drug Administration (1983a); Fazio (1984a)
Lard	Sublime under vacuum	GC	US Food and Drug Administration (1983b)
Edible oils; cottonseed oil	Extract with acetonitrile	GC/FID	Senten et al. (1977); Wyatt (1981)
Edible fats and oils	Dilute with chloroform or tetrahydrofuran; filter	GPC/UV	Doeden et al. (1979); Majors & Johnson (1978)
Fats and mixed feeds	Solvent extraction	LC/PMD	Rékasi & Örsi (1976)
Cereals	Extract with carbon disulphide	GC/FID	Fazio (1984b)
Miscellaneous foods	Steam distill; extract with dichloromethane	GC	Isshiki et al. (1980)
Fats, oils and dried food products	Oil trap precolumn; inject diluted samples directly	GC	Kline et al. (1978)
Chewing-gum	Extract with hexane, alkaline dimethyl sulphoxide	HPLC	Pellerin et al. (1982)
Fuels	Direct injection	GC/MS	Bartl & Schaaff (1982)
Transformer oils	Dilute with hexane; elute with acetonitrile	LC/ECD (differential pulse voltammetry)	Foley & Kimmerle (1979)
Rubber	Extract with acetone	TLC	Gedeon et al. (1983)
Polymers	Dissolve in acetone or tetrachloro-ethylene; elute with tetrahydrofuran or tetrachloroethylene	GPC	Čoupek et al. (1972); Mirabella et al. (1976)
Volatiles released from polymers into the air		GC/MS	Kiselev et al. (1983)
Plastics	Extract with acetonitrile	LC/MS	Vargo & Olson (1985)

Table 2 (contd)

Sample matrix	Sample preparation	Assay procedure[a]	Reference
Polyethylene	Dissolve in toluene; heat; extract with solvent	GC/FID	Denning & Marshall (1972)
	Dissolve in decalin	HPLC	Schabron & Fenska (1980)
Adipose tissue	Extract serially with petroleum ether, benzene-petroleum and water-methanol; steam distill	Colorimetric (di-*ortho*-anisidine)	Collings & Sharratt (1970)

[a]Abbreviations: GC, gas chromatography; FID, flame-ionization detection; SP, spectrophotometric detection; LC, liquid chromatography; ECD, electrochemical detection; MS, mass spectrometry; HPLC, high-performance liquid chromatography; UV, ultraviolet detection; GPC, gel-permeation chromatography; PMD, photometric detection; TLC, thin-layer chromatography

[The Working Group noted that several studies are available in which BHT-treated animals were used as control groups for studies on the modulating effects of this chemical on the actions of carcinogens and in which the effect of BHT was examined for a shorter period than the standard two years (Wattenberg, 1972; Ulland et al., 1973; Witschi et al., 1977; Clapp et al., 1979; Witschi & Lock, 1979; Witschi, 1981; Imaida et al., 1983; Tatsuta et al., 1983; Williams et al., 1983; Witschi & Morse, 1983; Imaida et al., 1984; Shirai et al., 1984). These studies could not be used to evaluate the carcinogenicity of BHT alone, but some of them are considered in section 3.1(c).]

(a) Oral administration

Mouse: Groups of approximately 50 male BALB/c mice, eight weeks of age, were fed a diet containing 0 or 0.75% BHT [purity unspecified] for life. About 66% of mice in each group were killed 12 months after the start of the experiment and the rest at 18 months. At 12 months, no difference was found in the incidence of lung tumours or reticulum-cell sarcomas between the 19 surviving BHT-treated and the 50 surviving control animals. At 18 months, 11 BHT-treated and 25 control mice were still alive; BHT treatment was associated with a higher incidence of lung tumours (in 7/11 animals, 64% *versus* 6/25, 24%; $p < 0.025$) and a lower incidence of reticulum-cell sarcomas (1/8, 12.5% *versus* 14/25, 56%; $p < 0.05$) (Clapp et al., 1974). [The Working Group noted the small number of animals used.]

Groups of 100 male and 50 female BALB/c mice, eight weeks old, were fed a diet containing 0 or 0.75% BHT [purity unspecified] for 18 months, at which time all animals were sacrificed. No difference was observed in the incidence of lung tumours or reticulum-cell sarcomas between treated and control mice. No liver tumour, thymic lymphoma, myeloid leukaemia or tumour of the forestomach was seen in BHT-treated mice. At the end of the experiment, $>90\%$ of animals in all groups were still alive (Clapp *et al.*, 1978).

Groups of 50 male and 50 female B6C3F$_1$ mice, six weeks old, were fed diets containing 0.3 (low dose) or 0.6% (high dose) BHT (99.9% pure; purity confirmed by gas chromatography) for 107 or 108 weeks, at which time the experiment was terminated. A control group of 20 males and 20 females was used. Survival at termination of the experiment was $>82\%$ in the BHT-treated groups and $>60\%$ in controls. A statistically significant increase in the incidence of alveolar/bronchiolar adenomas or adenocarcinomas was observed in low-dose ($p = 0.009$) but not in high-dose females (1/20 control, 16/46 low-dose and 7/50 high-dose); no such increase was observed in males (7/20 control, 21/50 low-dose and 17/49 high-dose). No other change in the incidence of neoplasms was reported (National Cancer Institute, 1979).

Groups of 51 or 52 male or female B6C3F$_1$ mice, six weeks old, were fed diets containing 0.02, 0.1 or 0.5% food-additive grade BHT [purity unspecified] for 96 weeks and were maintained on basal diet for a further eight weeks, at which time the experiment was terminated. A control group of 50 mice of each sex was fed basal diet alone for 104 weeks. Survival at termination of the experiment was $>60\%$ in all groups. Tumours were found in a variety of tissues in both control and BHT-treated groups. The differences in the incidence of neoplasms between control and BHT-treated groups were not statistically significant (Shirai *et al.*, 1982).

Rat: In an early experiment, groups of 15 male and 15 female Wistar rats [age unspecified] were fed diets containing 0, 0.2, 0.5, 0.8 or 1% BHT ('melting point of 68.5°C; corresponds to a mole purity of 97.8%') in 1% lard for two years. Six to nine female rats and eight to 11 male rats in each of the treated groups survived for two years and were examined grossly. Sections taken for microscopic examination were reported to demonstrate malignant neoplasms in four control and five treated females and in two control and one treated male; the author concluded that there was no treatment-related tumour (Deichmann *et al.*, 1955). [The Working Group noted the inadequate reporting of data and the small numbers of animals used.]

Groups of 50 male and 50 female Fischer 344 rats, six weeks of age, were fed diets containing 0.3 or 0.6% BHT (99.9% pure; purity confirmed by gas chromatography) for 105 weeks. Control groups of 20 males and 20 females received the basal diet only. At termination of the experiment, 65% control and $>72\%$ BHT-treated rats were still alive. In males, interstitial-cell tumours of the testes and pheochromocytomas of the adrenal gland were the most frequently observed neoplasms. In females, there were fibroadenomas of the mammary gland and endometrial stromal polyps of the uterus. The incidences of tumours reported were similar in control and treated groups (National Cancer Institute, 1979).

Groups of 57 male and 57 female Wistar rats, seven weeks of age, were fed diets containing 0.25 or 1.0% BHT [purity unspecified] for 104 weeks. A control group of 36 male and 36 female rats was fed basal diet only. Survival at the time of appearance of the first tumour (69 weeks) was $>70\%$ in all groups, and that at the end of the experiment was $>40\%$. A statistically significantly increased incidence of pituitary adenomas was observed in low-dose ($p < 0.05$) but not in high-dose treated females (0/32 control, 6/46 low-dose, 3/51 high-dose). The authors concluded that the tumours observed did not seem to be induced by BHT treatment (Hirose *et al.*, 1981).

Groups of 60, 40, 40 or 60 Wistar SPF rats of each sex, seven weeks of age, were fed diets containing food-grade BHT (purity, >99.5%) to give doses of 0, 25, 100 or 500 mg/kg bw for 13 weeks, after which time the males and females within each group were mated. Females were maintained on treatment throughout pregnancy and nursing. Groups of 100, 80, 80 and 100 offspring of each sex (F_1) were continued on the same treatment, except that the high-dose level was reduced to 250 mg/kg bw due to renal toxicity in animals of the parental generation. The experiment was terminated when the progeny were 141-144 weeks of age. Survival at that time was 44% in treated males and 39% in treated females in the high-dose F_1 group, as compared to 16% in control males and 17% in control females. F_1 males and females in the high-dose groups were reported to have increased incidences of adenomas and carcinomas of the liver as compared to controls. Liver tumours were reported only in rats more than 115 weeks old; no liver tumour occurred prior to that time. In males, one adenoma and one carcinoma occurred in controls; one adenoma and no carcinoma at 25 mg/kg bw; five adenomas and one carcinoma at 100 mg/kg bw; and 18 adenomas, eight carcinomas and one haemangioendotheliosarcoma at 250 mg/kg bw. In females, the respective numbers were two and 0 in controls; three and 0 at 25 mg/kg bw; six and 0 at 100 mg/kg bw; and 12 and two at 250 mg/kg bw (Olsen *et al.*, 1983, 1986). [The Working Group noted that, due to large differences in survival between treatment and control groups, it is difficult to draw conclusions about the significance of the observed incidences of liver lesions in the treated groups.]

Dog: A group of six adult mongrel dogs [sex unspecified] was fed a daily diet of ground meat containing 0.0025, 0.005 or 0.01% BHT (purity, 97.8%) for 260 days over one year (estimated intake: 4538, 6058, 12 237, 13 210, 16 636 and 24 411 mg/kg bw BHT). All animals survived the study period, and no tumour was found by gross or histological examination (Deichmann *et al.*, 1955). [The Working Group noted the apparent absence of a control group and the short period of observation.]

(b) *Intraperitoneal administration*

Mouse: In a screening assay based on the production of lung tumours in A/He mice, groups of 15 males and 15 females, six to eight weeks of age, were given thrice-weekly intraperitoneal injections (0.1 ml/dose) of BHT [purity unspecified] in tricaprylin or tricaprylin alone for eight weeks (total doses, 1.2 or 6.0 g/kg bw), and were sacrificed after 24 weeks on study. All BHT-treated mice (except for two high-dose males) survived the entire test period. No difference was observed in the incidence or number of tumours/mouse between BHT-treated and control animals: controls: incidence, 20-28%; number of tumours/mouse, 0.20-0.24; BHT-treated: incidence, 20-27% (3/13 in high-dose males, 3/15 in high-dose females, 3/15 in low-dose males and 4/15 in low-dose females); number of tumours/mouse, 0.20-0.31 (Stoner *et al.*, 1973).

(c)   *Administration with known carcinogens*

(i)   *Sequential exposures*

Mouse: Groups of male Swiss-Webster or A/J mice [number unspecified], six weeks of age, were given a single intraperitoneal injection of 1 mg/g bw urethane or saline; one week later some groups received weekly injections of 250 mg/kg bw BHT. At week 13, the incidences of lung tumours in Swiss-Webster mice were 93% in those receiving urethane and BHT treatment and 71% in those receiving urethane treatment only. The incidence of lung tumours in A/J mice at week 10 was 100% in those receiving urethane and BHT treatment and 83% in those receiving urethane treatment only. No lung tumour was observed in Swiss-Webster mice treated with BHT alone (Witschi *et al.*, 1977). [These findings were confirmed and extended in subsequent studies (Witschi & Lock, 1979; Witschi, 1981; Witschi *et al.*, 1981; Witschi & Morse, 1983).]

Administration of 800 mg/kg BHT either two or 26 days after administration of urethane did not affect lung tumorigenicity in CFLP mice (Bojan *et al.*, 1978).

Groups of 30 female CD-1 mice, six to eight weeks of age, received a single topical application of 200 nmol 7,12-dimethylbenz[*a*]anthracene (DMBA) on a shaven area of back skin; one group subsequently received twice weekly applications of 1 mg BHT on the same area for 30 weeks. The incidence of skin papillomas was 6% in mice receiving DMBA plus BHT compared with 0% in those receiving DMBA only. The difference was not statistically significant. No tumour was observed in a further group receiving treatment with BHT only (Berry *et al.*, 1978).

Groups of five different strains of mice received a single intraperitoneal injection of 1000 mg/kg bw urethane followed one week later by six weekly intraperitoneal injections of 200 mg/kg bw BHT. The number of lung tumours per mouse in animals receiving urethane plus BHT was enhanced over that in mice receiving urethane alone in all strains except strain 129 (2.2 as compared to 2.0/mouse), as follows (urethane alone *versus* urethane plus BHT): A, 30.2 *versus* 42.2/mouse; SWR, 26.2 *versus* 36.0/mouse; BALB/cBy, 2.4 *versus* 8.4/mouse; and RIIIS, 1.3 *versus* 2.7/mouse (Malkinson & Beer, 1984).

Rat: Groups of 120 male Sprague-Dawley rats, 22 days of age, were fed 0.02% 2-acetylaminofluorene in the diet for 18 days; one week later, a group was fed 0.5% BHT in the diet for 407 days. The incidence of liver tumours was 7% in the group treated with 2-acetylaminofluorene only, compared to 26% in that treated with 2-acetylaminofluorene and BHT (Peraino *et al.*, 1977).

When 0.66% BHT was administered in the diet after ten weekly subcutaneous injections of 7.4 mg/kg bw azoxymethane to male Fischer 344 rats, the overall incidence of gastro-intestinal and ear-duct tumours was not affected but the multiplicity of gastrointestinal tumours was increased: 1.7 after azoxymethane plus BHT *versus* 1.4 after azoxymethane alone (Weisburger *et al.*, 1977).

Groups of 25-26 male Fischer 344 rats, six weeks old, were given 0.01 or 0.05% *N*-nitrosobutyl-*N*-(4-hydroxybutyl)amine in the drinking-water for four weeks and were subsequently fed on basal diet or diet containing 1% BHT for 32 weeks. Administration of BHT after the low dose of nitrosamine induced an increase in the incidence of urinary bladder hyperplasia over that seen with the nitrosamine alone ($p < 0.05$). Administration of BHT after the high dose of nitrosamine increased the incidences of bladder hyperplasia, papillomas ($p < 0.05$) and carcinomas over that with the nitrosamine alone ($p < 0.05$): bladder carcinomas occurred in 5/26 animals receiving nitrosamine alone and in 13/24 animals receiving nitrosamine plus BHT. No bladder lesion was observed in a group of animals receiving BHT only (Imaida et al., 1983).

Groups of 12-14 male Fischer 344 rats, seven weeks of age, were fed a diet containing 0.02% 2-acetylaminofluorene for eight weeks. Two weeks later, animals were fed either basal diet or basal diet containing 0.03, 0.1, 0.3 or 0.6% BHT for 22 weeks. The incidences of liver neoplasms were 21% in the group receiving 2-acetylaminofluorene only and 33%, 25%, 50% and 67% in the groups also receiving BHT. Only the highest concentration produced a significant increase in liver carcinogenesis induced by 2-acetylaminofluorene (Maeura & Williams, 1984).

Groups of 10 or 25 female Sprague-Dawley rats, 50 days old, were given an intragastric dose of 8 mg DMBA and were fed diets containing 0.25 or 0.5% BHT beginning one week after DMBA exposure. BHT treatment was reported to inhibit mammary carcinogenesis (McCormick et al., 1984).

Two groups of 20 male Fischer 344 rats, six weeks of age, were given a single dose of 150 mg/kg bw N-methyl-N'-nitro-N-nitrosoguanidine by intragastric intubation. One week later, one group was fed a diet containing 1.0% BHT for 51 weeks. BHT treatment did not affect the incidence of stomach tumours (Shirai et al., 1984).

Groups of 30 male Fischer 344 rats, seven weeks old, received twice-weekly intraperitoneal injections of 20 mg/kg bw N-methyl-N-nitrosourea (MNU) in citrate buffer or citrate buffer alone (controls) for four weeks, followed by a basal diet containing 0 or 1% BHT for 32 weeks; all animals were killed at 36 weeks. The first tumour-bearing animal died at week 24. MNU alone produced 6/22 adenomas and 1/22 adenocarcinoma of the thyroid; in combination with BHT, MNU treatment resulted in 11/17 adenomas of the thyroid ($p < 0.05$) and 0/17 adenocarcinomas. BHT treatment alone produced no tumour of the thyroid. MNU or BHT alone failed to cause papillomas or carcinomas of the urinary bladder; however, when MNU treatment was followed by BHT, 9/15 rats developed papillomas ($p < 0.001$) and 4/15 developed carcinomas ($p < 0.05$) of the urinary bladder. MNU alone produced papillomas (8/22) but no squamous-cell carcinoma of the forestomach; when MNU was followed by BHT, the incidence of neither papillomas (7/17) nor squamous-cell carcinomas (1/17) of the forestomach was augmented. BHT alone produced no tumour of the forestomach (Imaida et al., 1984).

Groups of 20 male Fischer 344 rats, six weeks old, were given 20 mg/kg bw 1,2-dimethylhydrazine (DMH) in 0.9% saline or saline alone by subcutaneous injection once a week for four weeks. One week after the last treatment with DMH, two groups were fed basal diet containing 0 or 1.0% BHT for 36 weeks. At the end of this period, the animals in the group treated only with DMH (controls) had 5/18 adenomas and 7/18 adenocarcinomas of the colon; animals treated with DMH and BHT had 4/19 adenomas and 9/19 adenocarcinomas of the colon. Differences between the control and treated groups were not significant (Shirai *et al.*, 1985).

(ii)   *Prior or concomitant exposure*

Mouse: Groups of 19-20 female Ha/ICR mice, nine to ten weeks of age, were fed diets containing 0.03% benzo[*a*]pyrene alone or with 1.0% BHT for 28 days, after which they were maintained on basal diet until 28-40 weeks of age. The incidences of forestomach tumours were 68% in animals fed benzo[*a*]pyrene only and 50% in those fed benzo[*a*]pyrene plus BHT. Groups of nine to 12 female A/HeJ mice, nine to ten weeks of age, were fed diets containing 0.1% benzo[*a*]pyrene alone or 0.1% benzo[*a*]pyrene plus 0.5% BHT for two weeks. When 21 weeks old, the incidences of forestomach tumours were 100% in the group receiving benzo[*a*]pyrene alone and 22% in that fed benzo[*a*]pyrene plus BHT (Wattenberg, 1972).

Groups of 30-40 male BALB/c mice, eight weeks of age, were fed diets containing 0.75% BHT for 16 months either alone or concomitantly with 0.004% N-nitrosodiethylamine in the drinking-water for seven weeks starting when the mice were 11 weeks old. In mice killed at 12 months of age, the incidence of lung tumours was 45% in those given the nitrosamine alone and 35% in those given nitrosamine plus BHT. At 18 months of age, the incidence was 100% in both groups (Clapp *et al.*, 1974).

A group of 30 female Charles River CD-1 mice, seven to nine weeks of age, received a single topical application of 1 mg BHT 5 min before a single application of 2.56 μg DMBA on an area of shaved back skin, followed one week later by twice-weekly promoting applications of 10 μg 12-*O*-tetradecanoylphorbol 13-acetate (TPA) for 20 weeks. A second group of 30 mice received three applications of 1 mg BHT 6 h before, 5 min before and 6 h after DMBA treatment, followed one week later by the same TPA treatment. Another group received DMBA and TPA treatment only. At 28 weeks, the incidences of skin papillomas were 57%, 35% and 82% in the three groups, respectively (Slaga & Bracken, 1977).

Groups of male Swiss-Webster mice, six weeks old, were given a single intraperitoneal injection of 300 mg/kg bw BHT 1 h or one to seven days before intraperitoneal injection of 1 mg/g bw urethane. No effect on lung tumour incidence was observed compared to mice receiving urethane treatment only (Witschi *et al.*, 1977). [These findings were confirmed in subsequent studies (Witschi & Lock, 1979; Witschi, 1981).]

Groups of 100 male and 50 female BALB/c mice, eight weeks of age, were fed diets containing 0.75% BHT either alone or concomitantly with 0.004% N-nitrosodiethylamine in the drinking-water for seven weeks starting when the mice were 11 weeks of age. In female mice followed for up to 18 months of age, the incidence of squamous-cell carcinomas of the forestomach was 100% after nitrosamine alone and 77% in those given nitrosamine plus BHT. The incidence of forestomach tumours in males and the incidences of nitrosamine-induced lung tumours in mice of each sex were not affected by BHT (Clapp *et al.*, 1978).

Groups of female CFLP mice, 30-35 days of age, were given a single intraperitoneal injection of 1000 mg/kg bw urethane. When 400 or 800 mg/kg bw BHT were administered for one to eight days [route unspecified] six or seven days before administration of urethane, the multiplicity of lung tumours was increased: in mice given 800 mg/kg BHT six days before urethane, there were 2.46 tumours/mouse *versus* 1.06 in mice given only urethane, while in mice given 400 or 800 mg/kg BHT seven days before urethane, there were 2.21 and 2.89, respectively, *versus* 1.36 (Bojan *et al.*, 1978).

Groups of 35-38 male and 27-28 female BALB/c mice, eight weeks of age, were fed 0.75% BHT continuously; one group received 10 weekly subcutaneous injections of 20 mg/kg bw DMH beginning at 11 weeks of age. At termination of the experiment, ten months after the first injection of DMH, the incidence of colon neoplasms in males given DMH was 75% and that in the group fed DMH plus BHT was 34%. No reduction occurred in female mice (Clapp *et al.*, 1979).

Rat: A group of 34 female Sprague-Dawley rats, seven weeks of age, received a single dose of 12 mg DMBA by oral intubation; one group of 18 rats was treated 1 h previously with 200 mg BHT. At 25 weeks of age, the incidence of mammary tumours was 80% in rats treated with DMBA only and 28% in those pretreated with BHT (Wattenberg, 1972).

Groups of 10-20 male and 10-20 female Charles River CD rats, six weeks old, were fed standard diet or a diet containing 0.66% BHT together with 0.0223% 2-acetylaminofluorene (AAF) for 24 weeks (males) or 32 weeks (females). At 37 weeks, 7/10 (70%) males given AAF and 4/20 (20%) males given AAF plus BHT had liver tumours; of the females, 2/10 (20%) given AAF and 6/20 (33%) of those given AAF plus BHT had mammary adenocarcinomas. In similar experiments with *N*-hydroxy-2-acetylaminofluorene, 60% of males had liver tumours, reduced to 15% by the addition of BHT, and 70% of females had mammary tumours, reduced to 35% by BHT. Similar data were obtained in male Fischer 344 rats with lower levels of carcinogens and BHT (Ulland *et al.*, 1973).

Groups of 25-50 male Fischer 344 rats, six weeks of age, were given weekly subcutaneous injections of 7.4 mg/kg bw azoxymethane for ten weeks; one group was fed a diet containing 0.66% BHT starting two weeks before azoxymethane treatment and ending at the end of azoxymethane exposure. Another group received the BHT diet for 12 weeks after the end of azoxymethane administration. At 40 weeks of study, 87% of rats given azoxymethane alone had tumours of either the gastrointestinal tract or ear duct. With concurrent administration of BHT, the overall tumour incidence was decreased to 58%; the number of gastrointestinal tumours per animal was 1.0 in animals given azoxymethane plus BHT *versus* 1.4 in those given azoxymethane alone, and the incidence of ear-duct tumours was 24% *versus* 52%, respectively (Weisburger *et al.*, 1977).

One group of ten male Sprague-Dawley rats was given weekly doses of 30 mg/kg bw DMH by stomach tube for the first nine weeks of the study (total, ten doses) and one group of ten males was given DMH and fed a diet containing 0.66% BHT. At 23 weeks, the incidence of rats with colon tumours and the multiplicity of tumours were the same in the two groups (Barbolt & Abraham, 1979).

Groups of 30 female Sprague-Dawley rats, three weeks of age, were fed one of three experimental diets differing in level or type of fat; each of the diets was fed with or without 0.7% BHT. At 50 days of age, some groups were given 10 mg DMBA by stomach tube.

Animals were monitored for development of mammary tumours up to 180 days of age. The average numbers of tumours/rat were: 2% linoleic acid diet, 2.20; the same plus BHT, 1.77; 20% corn oil diet, 3.25; the same plus BHT, 2.33; 18% coconut oil plus 2% linoleic acid diet, 2.39; the same plus BHT, 1.77 (King et al., 1979).

Groups of 27 or 42 young (110-140 g bw) male Sprague-Dawley rats were fed a basal diet containing 0.05% 3'-methyl-4-dimethylaminoazobenzene with or without 0.5% BHT for nine weeks, when the experiment was terminated. The incidences of hepatocellular carcinomas were 38/42 in rats fed the carcinogen alone and 3/27 in those fed carcinogen plus BHT (Daoud & Griffin, 1980).

Groups of 16 female Sprague-Dawley rats (per cage), three weeks of age, were fed diets containing 0.3% BHT; at 50 days of age, some groups received either 50 mg/kg bw MNU intravenously or 10 mg DMBA intragastrically alone or with the BHT diet. By 27 weeks, rats given DMBA only developed a 100% incidence of mammary tumours, whereas those also given BHT had only a 54% incidence; with MNU there was no difference in mammary tumour incidence (King et al., 1981).

Groups of 56 or 41 male Fischer 344 rats, 11 weeks old, were fed diets containing 0.02% AAF either alone or with 0.6% BHT for 25 weeks, when the experiment was terminated. At that time, the incidences of hepatocellular carcinomas were 17/56 in the group receiving AAF only and 2/41 in the group receiving AAF plus BHT. In the latter group, 17 animals had bladder papillomas and three had carcinomas, whereas no such neoplasm occurred in the group receiving AAF only (Williams et al., 1983). In a subsequent study, it was reported that proportional inhibition of liver carcinogenesis was seen with 0.03, 0.1, 0.3 and 0.6% BHT. Bladder tumours occurred in the group receiving 0.03% BHT plus AAF, and the incidence increased with the concentration of BHT in the diet (Maeura et al., 1984).

Groups of 21-60 female Sprague-Dawley rats, 50 days old, were given a single dose of 5 or 15 mg DMBA by intragastric intubation either alone or together with a NIH-07, cereal-based diet containing 0.03, 0.1, 0.3 or 0.6% BHT beginning 14 days before DMBA administration and continuing for 14 days after. The cumulative incidence of mammary tumours, adenocarcinomas and fibroadenomas was determined 160 days after DMBA administration. After 5 mg DMBA, all four doses of BHT inhibited mammary tumour development; inhibition was approximately 50% in animals receiving 0.6% BHT. With 15 mg DMBA, only the high dose of BHT inhibited mammary carcinogenesis significantly. BHT also inhibited the induction of adrenocortical nodules. When 0.6% BHT was fed in AIN-76A (semipurified, deficient in vitamin K) diet to rats given either 5 or 15 mg DMBA, inhibition of carcinogenicity with the low dose was marginal and there was no inhibition with the high dose (Cohen et al., 1984).

Groups of 25 female Sprague-Dawley rats, 50 days old, were given a single intragastric dose of 8 mg DMBA, and diets containing 0.25 or 0.5% BHT were fed beginning two weeks before DMBA exposure and continuing until one week after. BHT treatment inhibited mammary carcinogenesis: DMBA alone, 88%; DMBA plus 0.25% BHT, 68%; DMBA plus 0.5% BHT, 52% (McCormick et al., 1984).

3.2 Other relevant biological data

(a) *Experimental systems*

The biological effects of BHT have been reviewed (WHO, 1974; Babich, 1982; International Programme on Chemical Safety, 1983; Malkinson, 1983).

Toxic effects

The oral LD_{50} of BHT in rats was reported to be 890 mg/kg bw (Bär *et al.*, 1977), 1700-1970 mg/kg bw (albino Wistar rats) (Deichmann *et al.*, 1955) and 2450 mg/kg bw (Karplyuk, 1959). Approximate lethal doses were 940-2100 mg/kg bw in cats, 2100-3200 mg/kg bw in New Zealand rabbits and 10 700 mg/kg bw in guinea-pigs (Deichmann *et al.*, 1955).

(i) *Lung*

The pulmonary toxicity attributed to BHT has been summarized recently (Kehrer & Kacew, 1985).

Intraperitoneal injection of 400 mg/kg bw BHT in corn oil to male Swiss Webster mice produced perivascular oedema and necrosis of type 1 alveolar cells within three days. This was followed by division of type 2 cells, which repopulated the alveolar wall (Adamson *et al.*, 1977), accounting for the proliferation of pulmonary cells reported by Marino and Mitchell (1972). Feeding of 0.75% BHT in the diet to A/J mice resulted in a significant increase in the proliferation of sessile alveolar lung cells (Witschi & Doherty, 1984).

BHT-induced lung damage is associated with increases in lung weight, DNA synthesis (Witschi & Saheb, 1974), RNA and protein synthesis (Saheb & Witschi, 1975), cyclic guanosine monophosphate content (Kuo *et al.*, 1978) and protein phosphorylation (Malkinson, 1979). The metabolism of BHT to a lung-toxic species appears to be mediated by a cytochrome-P450 system (Kehrer & Kacew, 1985). Mice of the ddY strain, aged seven weeks, responded to an intraperitoneal injection of 400 mg/kg bw BHT with a significant reduction in the glutathione content of the lung but not of the liver or kidney (Masuda & Nakayama, 1984). BHT binds to mouse lung tissue to a greater extent than to liver or kidney tissue; and more is bound in mouse tissues than in rat (Kehrer & Witschi, 1980).

After intraperitoneal injection of BALB/c mice, six to eight weeks old, with 400 mg/kg bw BHT, a very slight increase in collagen fibres was seen occasionally in the interstitium of the alveolar walls one year after exposure (Haschek *et al.*, 1982). In a chronic bioassay of BHT in rats, focal alveolar histiocytosis occurred in the lungs of 5% of control males and 11% of control females. In rats fed diets containing 0.3 or 0.6% BHT, histiocytosis occurred in 8% and 14% of males and in 25% and 43% of females, respectively (National Cancer Institute, 1979).

(ii) *Other*

Weanling male Norway hooded rats were fed diets containing 0.001, 0.1 or 0.5% BHT and 0, 10 or 20% lard for five weeks. An approximately 40% increase in serum cholesterol levels occurred only in those fed the highest levels of BHT and lard. Serum phospholipid levels were also increased (Day *et al.*, 1959). Other studies have also revealed elevation of serum cholesterol by BHT in Norway hooded (Johnson & Hewgill, 1961) and Sprague-Dawley rats (Frawley *et al.*, 1965). Intragastric administration of 500 mg/kg bw BHT to rhesus monkeys for four weeks did not alter serum cholesterol levels (Allen & Engblom, 1972).

Feeding of a diet containing 0.1% BHT to Norway hooded rats for seven weeks reduced the weight gain of males on a 20% lard diet but not that of males or females fed 10% lard. Liver weight was significantly increased (Brown *et al.*, 1959).

Feeding of 1% BHT to albino Wistar rats for 24 months increased the weights of the brain and liver (Deichmann *et al.*, 1955). Increased liver weight after feeding of BHT has been reported in numerous publications (e.g., Johnson & Hewgill, 1961).

Feeding of female Alderley-Park-SPF Wistar rats diets containing 0.01, 0.1, 1.0 or 5.0% BHT for up to 28 days produced a dose-related increase in the activity of liver aminopyrine demethylase. Ultrastructurally, smooth endoplasmic reticulum in hepatocytes was increased proportionally to dose, as determined using a differential point-counting technique. After discontinuation of BHT, the content of smooth endoplasmic reticulum returned to normal within 10-20 days (Botham *et al.*, 1970). Similar changes in smooth endoplasmic reticulum were reported by Lane and Lieber (1967).

Administration of 50 or 500 mg/kg bw BHT by gastric intubation to rhesus monkeys for four weeks produced no increase in liver weight or liver DNA, RNA or protein content. The hepatocytes of monkeys given the high dose showed moderate proliferation of smooth endoplasmic reticulum (Allen & Engblom, 1972).

Effects on reproduction and prenatal toxicity

The effects of BHT on reproduction and prenatal toxicity have been reviewed (WHO, 1974; Babich, 1982; International Programme on Chemical Safety, 1983).

Groups of four male and 24 female outbred albino mice were fed a diet containing 0.1 or 0.5% BHT and 10% or 20% lard from weaning for lifespan. They were allowed to mate and produce offspring for approximately 18 months. The number of live-born progeny was reduced by about 10% in the high-dose group, but no other sign of toxicity was observed in the parents or offspring. In particular, no case of anophthalmia was observed in the 7765 offspring (Johnson, 1965).

Evans No. 1 mice were administered 750 mg/kg bw BHT in arachis oil per day by gavage throughout gestation (five dams), or before and throughout gestation (seven dams). Normal litters were produced. Administration of a single dose of 1000 mg/kg bw BHT in arachis oil to groups of two female Evans No. 1 mice throughout gestation resulted in no embryo-toxicity and only one case of microphthalmia. Groups of nine to 20 ICI-SPF mice were given 250, 300 or 500 mg/kg bw BHT per day for seven weeks before conception and throughout gestation. With 250 mg/kg bw there was 33% maternal mortality; all ten survivors produced normal offspring. Maternal survival was very low at the higher dosages (Clegg, 1965). [The Working Group noted the small number of animals used, the poor selection of doses and the poor reporting of the study.]

Walter Reed-Carworth rats fed 0.5% BHT on days 1-22 of gestation produced 11 litters; no abnormal foetus was observed and there was no increase in resorption rates (Telford *et al.*, 1962). Groups of 11 rats [strain unspecified] were fed 0.0125, 0.0625, 0.313 or 1.55% BHT in the diet throughout gestation. Maternal weight loss and death of all foetuses were observed in the group fed 1.55% BHT; animals fed lower concentrations produced normal litters (Ames *et al.*, 1956). In the offspring of groups consisting of one Tuck albino and six Carworth SPF rats receiving a single dose of 1000 mg/kg bw BHT in arachis oil on day 9, 11 or 13 of gestation, no significant embryotoxic or teratogenic effect was reported. [The Working Group noted the occurrence of skeletal anomalies that were not commented upon by the author.] No abnormality was observed in the offspring of Tuck albino rats receiving 750 mg/kg bw per day throughout gestation, in offspring of Tuck and Benger hooded rats receiving the same dose for ten weeks before and throughout gestation, or in the offspring of Benger hooded and Porton SPF albino rats receiving 500 mg/kg bw BHT per day during seven weeks before and throughout gestation (Clegg, 1965). [The Working Group noted the small number of animals per group, the inadequate selection of doses and the poor reporting of results.]

In long-term feeding experiments with BHT, groups of 24 or 16 male and female Norway hooded rats received 0.1% BHT with 10% hydrogenated coconut oil for two years or 0.1 or 0.5% BHT with 10 or 20% lard for six months. Reproduction was impaired compared with controls, and three of the 30 litters contained anophthalmic offspring (Brown *et al.*, 1959). [The Working Group noted that data on the distribution of anophthalmic offspring among the different treatment groups were not given.]

Groups of male and female Wistar SPF rats were fed 0 or 500 mg/kg bw BHT per day in the diet for 13 weeks before conception and throughout gestation and lactation. In the treated group, a reduction in weight gain was reported for the parent generation before and during gestation. Number of offspring, birth weight and length of gestation were similar in the two groups. Independently of prenatal exposure, offspring nursed by treated dams (cross-fostering) had reduced weight gain, and several developmental parameters were adversely affected during the lactation period. These effects were attributed to a maternal influence (Meyer & Hansen, 1980). [The Working Group did not find the evidence for delayed development convincing.] In a similar experiment, groups of male and female Sprague-Dawley albino rats were fed 0.03, 0.1 or 0.3% BHT in a 20% fat diet until second and third generations had been bred. A reduction in growth rate of 10-20% and a 20% increase in serum cholesterol levels were observed in parents and offspring treated with 0.3%. No adverse reaction was reported in the groups fed 0.03 or 0.1% (Frawley *et al.*, 1965). Groups of male and female Sprague-Dawley rats were fed 0.125, 0.25 or 0.5% BHT in the diet (also containing 0.005% butylated hydroxyanisole) for at least two weeks before mating; treatment of females was continued throughout gestation and lactation. A reduction in maternal and offspring weight gain was observed with the high dose, and a dose-dependent increase in offspring mortality was seen with the high and medium doses. No effect on behavioural development was detected after weaning (Vorhees *et al.*, 1981). [The Working Group noted that no cross-fostering was performed to differentiate between parentally transmitted effects and those occurring postnatally.]

It was reported in an abstract that ^{14}C-BHT administered to rats on day 10 of gestation crossed the placenta and reached a maximum concentration in the foetus between 1 and 2 h after the injection [route unspecified], which then declined rapidly (Shipp, 1973).

Absorption, distribution, excretion and metabolism

(i) *Pharmacokinetics*

After a single oral dose of 1 mg ^{14}C-BHT to Alderley-Park-SPF albino Wistar rats, 24% and 37% was excreted in the urine and 42% and 35% in faeces in males and females, respectively (Daniel & Gage, 1965). In BALB/c mice, 40% of an intragastric dose was taken up by the tissues within 30 min by males, whereas only 10% was absorbed in females (Daugherty *et al.*, 1980).

In male and female BALB/c mice, a single intragastric dose was widely distributed to various tissues within 30 min, primarily to the small intestine, squamous stomach, liver and kidney; lung showed no greater accumulation than most other tissues (Daugherty *et al.*, 1980). Similar findings were reported by Matsuo *et al.* (1984).

In BALB/c mice, approximately 75% of a single oral dose was excreted in the urine during the first 24 h; this was followed by a slower phase during which an additional 10% was excreted over the next four days. The total amount found in the faeces was less than 1% (Daugherty *et al.*, 1980). Female rats have greater urinary excretion of BHT than male rats (Daniel & Gage, 1965; Tye *et al.*, 1965), whereas male BALB/c mice excreted BHT more rapidly than females (Daugherty *et al.*, 1980).

Enterohepatic circulation of BHT has been reported in rats (Daniel & Gage, 1965; Ladomery *et al.*, 1967a). Feeding of a diet containing 0.5% BHT to male and female rats for up to 50 days resulted in average levels of 30 and 45 mg/kg in fat and 1 and 3 mg/kg in liver in males and females, respectively. On cessation of treatment, the level in fat fell, with a half-life of seven to ten days (Daniel & Gage, 1965).

The metabolism of BHT in rats has been studied extensively. The predominant metabolic pathway involves oxidation of the 4-methyl group (Wright *et al.*, 1965; Daniel *et al.*, 1968). The major metabolites are 3,5-di-*tert*-butyl-4-hydroxybenzoic acid, both free and as a glucuronide, and *S*-(3,5-di-*tert*-butyl-4-hydroxybenzyl)-*N*-acetylcysteine, with minor amounts of 3,5-di-*tert*-butyl-4-hydroxybenzyl alcohol, 3,5-di-*tert*-butyl-4-hydroxy-benzaldehyde and 1,2-bis(3,5-di-*tert*-butyl-4-hydroxyphenyl)ethane (Daniel *et al.*, 1968; Branen, 1975). Moreover, BHT-quinone methide (2,6-di-*tert*-butyl-4-methylene-2,5-cyclo-hexadienone), a reactive metabolite, has been identified in the liver (Takahashi & Hiraga, 1979) and bile (Tajima *et al.*, 1981) of rats.

The concentration of glutathione in rat liver and in mouse lung decreased to about 50% and 80%, respectively, of the control values 4-12 h after intraperitoneal administration of 400 mg/kg bw to rats and 3000 mg/kg bw BHT to mice (Tajima *et al.*, 1984, 1985). It has been demonstrated recently that BHT is converted to *S*-(3,5-di-*tert*-butyl-4-hydroxybenzyl)-glutathione (BHT-glutathione) by rat-liver microsomes in the presence of NADPH, molecular oxygen and glutathione. Cytochrome P450 inhibitors, such as SKF-525A, metyrapone and carbon monoxide, significantly inhibit BHT-glutathione formation, suggesting that BHT is converted by cytochrome P450 monooxygenases to a chemically reactive metabolite — possibly BHT-quinone methide, which forms BHT-glutathione by nonenzymatic conjugation with glutathione (Tajima et al., 1985). Previous studies with ^{14}C-BHT showed that it is bound irreversibly to liver, lung and kidney macromolecules in both mice (Kehrer & Witschi, 1980) and rats (Nakagawa et al., 1979a) following administration in vivo. Furthermore, irreversible binding of BHT metabolites to rat lung and liver microsomes in vitro has been reported, which could be prevented by the addition of thiol compounds such as glutathione and cysteine (Nakagawa et al., 1979b).

The major metabolites of BHT in rat urine are (Fig. 1): 3,5-di-tert-4-hydroxybenzoic acid (BHT-acid; III), both free (9% of the dose) and as a glucuronide (15%), and S-(3,5-di-tert-butyl-4-hydroxybenzyl)-N-acetylcysteine (V; [amount unspecified]). The ester glucuronide and mercapturic acid were major metabolites in rat bile, while free BHT-acid was the main component in the faeces (Daniel et al., 1968). In addition, 1,2-bis(3,5-di-tert-butyl-4-hydroxyphenyl)ethane has been identified in rat bile (Ladomery et al., 1967b).

Fig. 1. Metabolism of BHT in rats and humans[a]

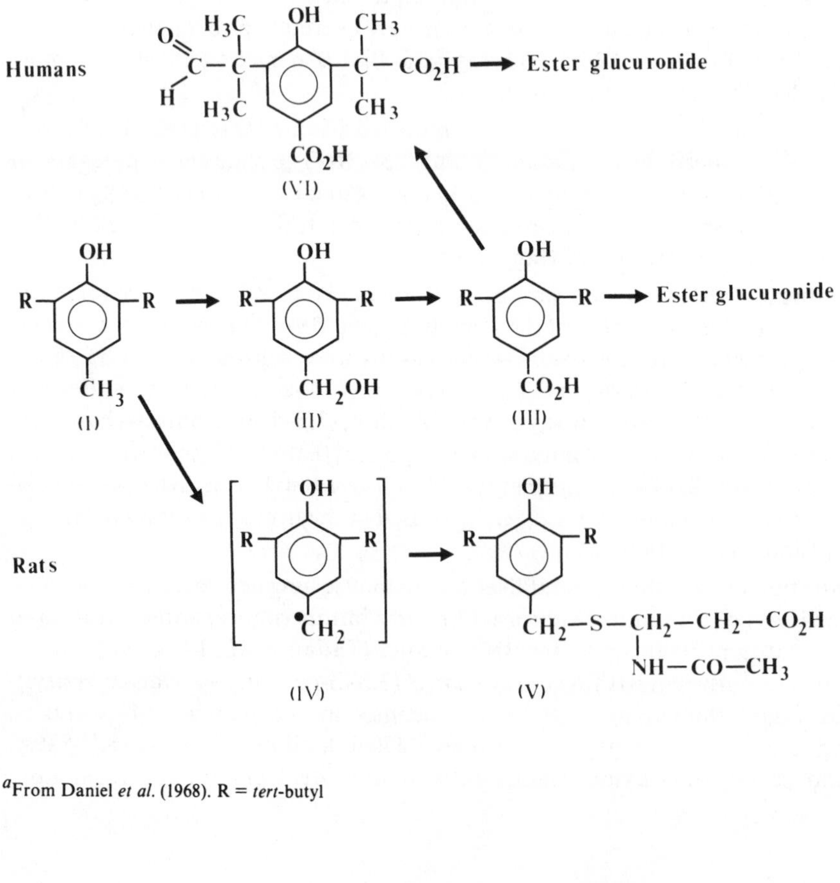

[a]From Daniel et al. (1968). R = tert-butyl

Metabolites produced in mice are similar to those produced in rats, except that the major biotransformation in mice was by oxidation of *tert*-methyl groups (Matsuo *et al.*, 1984).

In rabbits, orally administered BHT was metabolized to 2,6-di-*tert*-butyl-4-hydroxy-methylphenol, 3,5-di-*tert*-butyl-4-hydroxybenzoic acid and 4,4′-ethylenebis(2,6-di-*tert*-butylphenol). The urinary metabolites comprised 38% of the administered dose as glucuronides, 17% as sulphates and 7% as free phenols. Unchanged BHT was isolated from the faeces but not the urine (Akagi & Aoki, 1962).

(ii)   *Effects on enzymes*

As a consequence of the increases in the amounts of smooth endoplasmic reticulum (Lane & Lieber, 1967; Botham *et al.*, 1970) and of cytochrome P450 in the liver (Kawano *et al.*, 1980), many associated enzyme activities are increased.These include aminopyrine demethylase (Gilbert & Goldberg, 1965; Botham *et al.*, 1970), biphenyl 4-hydroxylase (Creaven *et al.*, 1966), epoxide hydratase (Kahl & Wulff, 1979) and *para*-nitroanisole-*O*-demethylase (Allen & Engblom, 1972; Halladay *et al.*, 1980), some of which are also increased in extrahepatic tissues. Other enzyme activities increased by BHT treatment include plasma esterase (Tyndall *et al.*, 1975), liver glutathione transferase (Awasthi *et al.*, 1983) and liver γ-glutamyl transpeptidase (Furukawa *et al.*, 1984).

BHT binds to cytochrome P450 *in vitro* (Yang et al., 1974).

(iii)   *Modulation of the toxicity of BHT by other chemicals*

Male BALB/c mice, 20-30 g, were given a single intraperitoneal injection of 400 mg/kg bw BHT either alone or with intraperitoneal administration of the enzyme inhibitors SKF-525A (up to 50 mg/kg bw) or piperonyl butoxide (up to 800 mg/kg bw). Incorporation of radioactive thymidine into pulmonary DNA, as evidence of regeneration following injury, was greatly reduced by the enzyme inhibitors, indicating a protective effect (Kehrer & Witschi, 1980).

Mice of the ddY strain, seven weeks of age, were given a single intraperitoneal injection of 400 mg/kg bw BHT either alone or following intraperitoneal administration of the enzyme inhibitors diethyldithiocarbamate (up to 300 mg/kg bw) or carbon disulphide (up to 100 mg/kg bw). Measurement of lung weight three and six days after exposure, as evidence of pulmonary injury, showed that the enzyme inhibitors abolished the BHT-induced increase in weight (Masuda & Nakayama, 1984).

The pulmonary toxicity of BHT in male ddY mice was assessed by measurement of wet lung weight in relationship to body weight. When mice were killed four days after an intraperitoneal injection of 270 or 400 mg/kg bw BHT, a 30-50% increase in relative lung weight was observed. Later exposure to diethyl maleate, a glutathione-depleting agent, or exposure to buthionine sulphoximine, an inhibitor of glutathione biosynthesis, enhanced the effects of BHT by approximately three fold (Mizutani *et al.*, 1984).

Several agents including oxygen (Haschek *et al.*, 1982), X-radiation (Haschek *et al.*, 1980) and prednisolone (Hakkinen *et al.*, 1983) have been found to enhance greatly for at least one year the development of pulmonary fibrosis in mice exposed to a single toxic intraperitoneal dose of 300 or 400 mg/kg bw BHT.

(iv) *Modulation of the toxicity of other chemicals by BHT*

As a consequence of its effects on enzyme systems and possible antioxidant properties, BHT modifies the toxicity of a variety of chemicals. Some examples are presented.

Feeding of 0.75% BHT to $(C3H\times101)F_1$ hybrid mice, 10-12 weeks old, reduced the 30-day mortality caused by a single intraperitoneal injection of various chemicals (ethyl-, methyl- [females only], *n*-propyl- and isopropyl methanesulphonate, ethylene dibromide, *N*-nitrosodiethylamine and cyclophosphamide) (Cumming & Walton, 1973).

Groups of seven-week-old female Sprague-Dawley rats were given 30 mg 7,12-dimethylbenz[*a*]anthracene (DMBA) intragastrically either alone or 1 h after oral administration of 200 mg BHT. Adrenal necrosis was seen 72 h later in 29/30 rats given DMBA only and in 0/10 rats given DMBA plus BHT (Wattenberg, 1972).

Mutagenicity and other short-term tests

BHT (10 mg/disc) gave negative results in the *Bacillus subtilus rec*$^{+/-}$ assay (Kinae *et al.*, 1981). It was not mutagenic to *Salmonella typhimurium* TA1535, TA1537, TA1538, TA98 or TA100 when tested at up to 1000 μg/plate in the presence of a metabolic system (S9) from the liver of rats uninduced or induced with polychlorinated biphenyls (Joner, 1977; Bruce & Heddle, 1979; Bonin & Baker, 1980; Kinae *et al.*, 1981).

Chromosomal aberrations were not induced in seeds of *Crepis capillaris* soaked in a solution of 10 μg/ml BHT (Alekperov *et al.*, 1975).

BHT did not induce sex-linked recessive lethal mutations, translocations or loss of X^B chromosome in *Drosophila melanogaster* when males were injected with 0.2 μl of solutions of 0.001% (Kamra, 1973; Prasad & Kamra, 1974). [The Working Group noted that the authors interpreted these results as positive.]. Sex-linked recessive lethal mutations and translocations were not observed in *D. melanogaster* when males were injected with 0.4 μl of a 0.05% solution or fed 0.2% BHT for seven days (Mazar Barnett & Muñoz, 1980). Similarly, Sankaranayanan (1983) observed no sex-linked recessive lethal mutation, chromosomal translocation or dominant lethal mutation when male or female *D. melanogaster* were raised in a medium containing 0.05% BHT.

BHT (tested at 1, 5 and 10 μg/ml) was reported to induce 8-azaguanine-resistant mutants with low survival in Chinese hamster V79 cells in the presence of S9 from uninduced mice (Paschin & Bahitova, 1984). In the absence of S9, concentrations of up to 0.075 mg/ml BHT did not induce polyploidy or chromosomal aberrations in cultured Chinese hamster lung cells [details not given] (Ishidate *et al.*, 1980).

Following oral administration of 5 mg ^{14}C-BHT to rats, radioactivity was bound to liver DNA (Nakagawa *et al.*, 1980). [The Working Group noted that the effect was small and that the adducts were not identified.]

Dominant lethal mutations were not induced when male ICR/Ha Swiss mice were given a single intraperitoneal injection of 250-2000 mg/kg bw BHT and mated for eight successive weeks (Epstein *et al.*, 1972).

When doses of up to 1000 mg/kg bw BHT were administered intraperitoneally to C57BL/6 × C3H/He mice for five successive days, no increase in micronuclei in bone marrow was observed in mice sacrificed on day 5 (4 h after the last injection), while sperm abnormalities were observed in animals sacrificed on day 40 (Bruce & Heddle, 1979).

[The Working Group was aware of reports of experiments in which the intention was to study the modulating effects of BHT on the activity of carcinogens/mutagens and in which treatment with BHT alone served as a control. Most of these reports could not be used to evaluate the mutagenic or related effects of BHT alone.]

Almost all studies (see Table 3) on the modulating effects of BHT on the mutagenic and related effects of known carcinogens/mutagens have been directed toward determining its effect on the metabolism of the test chemicals. The methods employed for this purpose can be separated into four groups: studies on the effects of BHT on

(A)   directly-acting chemicals — BHT and a test chemical were added directly to an in-vitro assay system;

(B)   exogenous metabolic system — BHT and a test chemical were added to an in-vitro assay system containing an exogenous metabolic system;

(C)   in-vivo metabolic system — a BHT-induced metabolic system was added to an in-vitro assay with a test chemical; and

(D)   test chemicals in test organisms — BHT was administered to test organisms *in vitro* (systems not requiring an exogenous metabolic system) or *in vivo*, prior to or simultaneously with a test chemical.

(b)   *Humans*

Toxic effects

No data were available to the Working Group.

Effects on reproduction and prenatal toxicity

No data were available to the Working Group.

Absorption, distribution, excretion and metabolism

When two male volunteers were administered a single oral dose of 40 mg ^{14}C-labelled BHT, about 50% of the radioactivity appeared in the urine within 24 h, and a total of 75% was excreted in the urine by the end of the observation period (Daniel *et al.*, 1967). Most was excreted as the glucuronide of a metabolite in which the 4-methyl group and one *tert*-butyl methyl group were oxidized to carboxyl groups and another *tert*-butyl methyl group was oxidized probably to an aldehyde. Free and conjugated BHT-acid (III, Fig. 1) were minor urinary components, and the mercapturic acid (V) was virtually absent (Daniel *et al.*, 1968).

Mutagenicity and chromosomal effects

No data were available to the Working Group.

Table 3. Results from short-term tests: modification of the effects of carcinogens/mutagens by BHT[a]

Test	Test organism/ assay	Study design[b] (Exogenous metabolic system[c])	Combination with carcinogen/mutagen	Reported result	Comments	References
PROKARYOTES						
DNA damage	Calf thymus DNA (binding)	C (BHT-PMS)	Aflatoxin B₁	No effect		Fukayama & Hsieh (1984)
		B (PB-R-Micr)	Aflatoxin B₁	Reduction		Bhattacharya et al. (1984)
	Exogenous DNA (binding)	B (rabbit, sheep seminal vesical Micr, bladder, liver and kidney Micr)	2-Amino-4-(5-nitro-2-furyl)thiazole	Reduction		Mattammal et al. (1981, 1982)
	Calf thymus DNA (binding)	B (PB/3MC-rabbit-Cyt-P450 and PB/3MC-rabbit-Micr)	(-)trans-7,8-Dihydro-xy-7,8-dihydrobenzo-[a]pyrene	No effect		Belvedere et al. (1980)
	Haemophilus influenzae (transformation Ery^R)	A	Sodium nitrite	Enhancement		Thomas et al. (1979)
Mutation	Salmonella typhimurium (his⁻/his⁺)	A	γ-radiation	No effect	Strain TA100	Ben-Hur et al. (1981)
		A	Methyl methane sulphonate	No effect	Strains TA98, TA100, TA1537 and TA1538	McKee & Tometsko (1979)
			2,4-Dinitro-1-fluoro-benzene	No effect		
			2,4-Dinitrophenyl hydrazine	No effect		
			9-Aminoacridine	No effect		
		B (liver-PMS)	Benzo[a]pyrene	Reduction	Strains TA1538 and TA98 [species and inducer of metabolic system not stated]	McKee & Tometsko (1979)
			1-Aminoanthracene	Reduction		
			2-Aminoanthraquinone	Reduction		
			Proflavine dihydrochloride	Reduction		
			Homidium bromide	Reduction		
		B (Aro-R-PMS)	Aflatoxin B₁	Enhancement	Strains TA98 and TA100	Shelef & Chin (1980)

Table 3 (contd)

Test	Test organism/assay	Study design[b] (Exogenous metabolic system[c])	Combination with carcinogen/mutagen	Reported result	Comments	References
		B (β-Naphthoflavone-R-PMS)	Benzo[a]pyrene (BP) 6-Methyl-BP 10-Methyl-BP	Reduction Reduction Reduction	Strain TA98	Calle et al. (1978); Calle & Sullivan (1982)
		B (Aro-R-PMS)	3,2'-Dimethyl-4-aminobiphenyl	Reduction	Strains TA98 and TA100	Reddy et al. (1983a,b)
		C (BHT-R-PMS)	3,2'-Dimethyl-4-aminobiphenyl	Reduction	Strains TA98 and TA100	Reddy et al. (1983a,b)
		B (3MC-R or M liver nuclei prep.)	N-Hydroxy-2-acetyl-aminofluorene	Reduction	Strain TA1538	Sakai et al. (1978)
		B (Aro-R-PMS)	Quinoline	Reduction	Strain TA100	Hollstein et al. (1978)
		C (BHT-R-PMS)	Aflatoxin B_1	Reduction	Strain TA98	Fukayama & Hsieh (1984)
		C (BHT-R-PMS)	Benzo[a]pyrene 2-Aminofluorene 2-Acetylaminofluorene	No effect Enhancement Enhancement	Strain TA98; 0.5% BHT in diet for 6 days; rats fed a diet with unsaturated or hydrogenated fats	Ponder & Green (1985)
GREEN PLANTS						
Mutation	Hordeum vulgare (chlorophyll mutants)	D (seeds)	Propane sultone	Enhancement	Treatment of seeds	Kaul & Tandon (1981)
Chromosomal effects	Hordeum vulgare (aberrations)	D (seeds)	Propane sultone	Enhancement	Treatment of seeds	Tandon & Kaul (1979); Kaul & Tandon (1981)
	Allium cepa (aberrations)	D (seeds)	X-rays	Enhancement	Treatment of seeds	Kaul (1979)
	Crepis capillaris L. (aberrations)	D	γ-rays Ethyleneimine	Reduction Reduction	Treatment of seeds	Alekperov et al. (1975, 1976)

Table 3 (contd)

Test	Test organism/assay	Study design[b] (Exogenous metabolic system[c])	Combination with carcinogen/mutagen	Reported result	Comments	References
INSECTS						
Mutation	*Drosophila melanogaster* (sex-linked recessive lethals)	D	γ-rays	Enhancement	[The Working Group noted the very low dose of 0.2 μl of 0.001% BHT used.]	Prasad & Kamra (1974)
		D	Ethyl methane-sulphonate	Reduction		Ives & Demick (1974)
		D	X-rays	Reduction		Mazar Barnett & Muñoz (1980)
		D	X-rays	Reduction	Reduction in spermatids but not in autosomal recessive lethals	Sankaranarayanan (1983)
			Diepoxybutane	Reduction		
			N-Nitrosodiethylamine	Reduction		
		D	Ethyl methanesulphonate	Enhancement		Mazar Barnett & Muñoz (1983)
			Diethyl sulphate	Enhancement		
Chromosomal effects	*Drosophila melanogaster* (translocations)	D	γ-rays	Enhancement	[The Working Group noted the very low dose of 0.2 μl of 0.001% BHT used.]	Kamra (1973)
		D	X-rays	No effect		Ives & Demick (1974)
	Drosophila melanogaster (chromosome loss; loss of ring X[B] chromosome)	D	γ-rays	No effect	[The Working Group noted the very low dose of 0.2 μl of 0.001% BHT) used.]	Prasad & Kamra (1974)

Table 3 (contd)

Test	Test organism/ assay	Study design[b] (Exogenous metabolic system[c])	Combination with carcinogen/mutagen	Reported result	Comments	References
	Drosophila melanogaster (translocation, dominant lethals)	D	X-rays	No effect		Mazar Barnett & Muñoz (1980)
	Drosophila melanogaster (X chromosome loss, dominant lethals)	D	X-rays	No effect		Sankaranarayanan (1983)
	Drosophila melanogaster (translocations)	D	X-rays	Reduction	Reduction in spermatids only	Sankaranarayanan (1983)
MAMMALIAN CELLS *IN VITRO*						
DNA damage	Chinese hamster V79 (unscheduled DNA synthesis)	A	Ultraviolet light (254 nm); *N*-acetoxy-2-acetylaminofluorene	No effect		Goodman *et al.* (1976)
	Human bronchial cells (binding to DNA)	D	Benzo[*a*]pyrene	Reduction		Harris *et al.* (1976)
	Human lymphocytes (unscheduled DNA synthesis)	D	Ultraviolet light (254 nm)	Reduction		Daugherty *et al.* (1978)
	NIH Swiss mouse epidermal cells in culture (binding to DNA)	D	7,12-Dimethylbenz[*a*]-anthracene	Reduction		Shoyab (1979)
	Human colonic tissues, primary culture (binding to DNA)	D	1,2-Dimethylhydra-zine	Reduction		Autrup *et al.* (1980)

Table 3 (contd)

Test	Test organism/ assay	Study design[b] (Exogenous metabolic system[c])	Combination with carcinogen/mutagen	Reported result	Comments	References
	Human skin fibroblasts (unscheduled DNA synthesis)	B	Aflatoxin B₁ N-Nitrosodimethyl-amine	Reduction Reduction		Wei et al. (1981)
	NIH Swiss mouse embryo cell culture (binding to DNA)	D	7,12-Dimethylbenz-[a]anthracene	No effect		Sawicki & Dipple (1983)
Mutation	Chinese hamster V79 (ouabain resistance)	B (SHE)	Benzo[a]pyrene	Reduction		Katoh et al. (1980)
	Chinese hamster V79 (8-azaguanine resistance)	B (M-PMS)	Benzo[a]pyrene	Reduction		Paschin & Bahitova (1984)
Chromosomal effects	Human lymphocytes (aberrations)	D	7,12-Dimethylbenz-[a]anthracene	Reduction	[The Working Group noted the high number of aberrations in the negative control.]	Shamberger et al. (1973)
		D	12-O-Tetradecanoyl-phorbol 13-acetate	Reduction		Emerit et al. (1983)
MAMMALIAN CELLS IN VIVO						
DNA damage	Sprague-Dawley rat (binding to liver DNA)	D	2-Acetylaminofluorene	Reduction		Goodman et al. (1976)
	CD-1 mice (binding to DNA from skin)	D	Benzo[a]pyrene 7,12-Dimethylbenz-[a]anthracene	Reduction Reduction		Slaga & Bracken (1977)
	Sprague-Dawley rat (O⁶-methylguanine in DNA from colon)	D	1,2-Dimethylhydrazine	No effect		Bull et al. (1981)

Table 3 (contd)

Test	Test organism/assay	Study design[b] (Exogenous metabolic system[c])	Combination with carcinogen/mutagen	Reported result	Comments	References
	CD rat (binding to liver DNA)	D	N-2-Acetylamino-fluorene (AAF) N-OH-N-2-AAF	Reduction		Grantham et al. (1973)
	NIH Swiss mouse (binding to DNA in skin)	D	7,12-Dimethylbenz[a]-anthracene	No effect		Dipple et al. (1984)
	BALB/c mouse (binding to DNA in stomach and liver)	D	N-Nitrosodiethylamine	Reduction		Daugherty (1984)
	Sprague-Dawley rat, lactating females (binding to liver nuclear DNA)	D	Aflatoxin B$_1$	Reduction		Fukayama et al. (1984)
CELL TRANSFORMATION	C3H/10T1/2 mouse embryo fibroblasts, clone 8 (morphological transformation)	D	3-Methylcholanthrene	Enhancement		Djurhuus & Lillehaug (1982)

[a]This table comprises selected assays and references and is not intended to be a complete review of the literature.

[b]Studies are designed to investigate the effects of BHT on: A, directly-acting chemicals; B, exogenous metabolic system; C, in-vivo metabolic system; D, test chemicals in test organisms; see text for explanations.

[c]BHT, BHT-induced; PMS, postmitochondrial supernatant; PB, phenobarbital-induced; R, rat; Micr, microsomes; CytP450, purified cytochrome P450; Aro, Aroclor-induced; 3MC, 3-methylcholanthrene-induced; M, mouse; SHE, Syrian hamster embryo cells

3.3 Case reports and epidemiological studies of carcinogenicity to humans

No data were available to the Working Group.

4. Summary of Data Reported and Evaluation

4.1 Exposure data

Butylated hydroxytoluene (BHT) has been used since 1947 as a common antioxidant in rubber and petroleum products and, more recently, in plastics. It has been used since 1949 as an antioxidant in many fat-containing foods, in edible fats and oils and in cosmetics. There is thus widespread human exposure to this compound.

4.2 Experimental data

Butylated hydroxytoluene was tested for carcinogenicity in mice and rats by oral administration in the diet. In one study in mice, there was no difference in tumour incidence among treated and control groups. Another study in mice showed an increased incidence of pulmonary tumours in females at the lower but not at the higher dose level. In another study in mice using one dose level and a small number of animals, the number of mice with lung tumours was increased by feeding of butylated hydroxytoluene; this finding was not confirmed in a further study by the same investigator using a larger number of animals. In one study in rats, no increase in tumour incidence was seen. An increased incidence of pituitary adenomas was observed in female rats at the lower but not at the higher dose level in another study. In one further experiment in rats, liver tumours were observed; however, this study could not be evaluated because of differential survival among control and treated groups.

Butylated hydroxytoluene was studied in mice and rats for its ability to modify the carcinogenicity of selected chemical agents. When administered with known carcinogens, butylated hydroxytoluene either enhanced, inhibited or had no effect on carcinogenicity (see also the 'General Remarks on the Substances Considered', p. 38).

No adequate data were available to evaluate the reproductive effects or prenatal toxicity of butylated hydroxytoluene to experimental animals.

In mice, a single intraperitoneal dose or feeding of butylated hydroxytoluene can cause pulmonary alveolar cell necrosis and proliferation. Butylated hydroxytoluene also induces proliferation of smooth endoplasmic reticulum in rat-liver cells, leading to hepatomegaly.

Butylated hydroxytoluene did not induce DNA damage in *Bacillus subtilis* or mutation in *Salmonella typhimurium*. It did not induce chromosomal aberrations in plants or mutation or chromosomal aberrations in *Drosophila melanogaster*. In one study, it was reported to be mutagenic to cultured Chinese hamster cells in the presence of an exogenous metabolic system. Binding of butylated hydroxytoluene to the DNA of liver of rats treated *in vivo* has been reported. It did not induce micronuclei in bone marrow or dominant lethal mutations in mice. It induced sperm abnormalities in mice.

When tested in combination with other chemicals (usually, known mutagens or carcinogens), butylated hydroxytoluene often modified the DNA-damaging, mutagenic and clastogenic activities. In most studies, butylated hydroxytoluene reduced the activity of indirectly-acting mutagens or carcinogens.

Overall assessment of data from short-term tests: Butylated hydroxytoluene[a]

	Genetic activity			Cell transformation
	DNA damage	Mutation	Chromosomal effects	
Prokaryotes	−	−		
Fungi/Green plants			−	
Insects		−	−	
Mammalian cells (*in vitro*)		?		
Mammals (*in vivo*)	?		−	
Humans (*in vivo*)				
Degree of evidence in short-term tests for genetic activity: **Inadequate**				Cell transformation: No data

[a]The groups into which the table is divided and the symbols used are defined on pp. 19-20 of the Preamble; the degrees of evidence are defined on pp. 20-21.

4.3 Human data

No data were available to evaluate the carcinogenicity of butylated hydroxytoluene to humans.

4.4 Evaluation[1]

There is *limited evidence* for the carcinogenicity of butylated hydroxytoluene in experimental animals.

No evaluation could be made of the carcinogenicity of butylated hydroxytoluene to humans.

---

[1]For definition of the italicized term, see Preamble, p. 18.

5. References

Adamson, I.Y.R., Bowden, D.H., Cote, M.G. & Witschi, H. (1977) Lung injury induced by butylated hydroxytoluene. Cytodynamic and biochemical studies in mice. *Lab. Invest.*, *36*, 26-32

Akagi, M. & Aoki, I. (1962) Studies on food additives. VI. Metabolism of 2,6-di-*tert*-butyl-*p*-cresol (BHT) in a rabbit. (1) Determination and paper chromatography of a metabolite. *Chem. pharm. Bull.*, *10*, 101-105

Alekperov, U.K., Abutalybov, M.G. & Bagirova, A.D. (1975) Ionol modification of natural and induced chromosome aberrations in *Crepis capillaris* L. (Wallr.). *Dokl. biol. Sci.*, *220*, 31-32

Alekperov, U.K., Abutalybov, M.G. & Bagirova, A.D. (1976) Studies on the mechanism of the action of antimutagens. I. Specific modification by ionol of aberrations induced by different factors. *Genetica*, *12*, 41-46

Allen, J.R. & Engblom, J.F. (1972) Ultrastructural and biochemical changes in the liver of monkeys given butylated hydroxytoluene and butylated hydroxyanisole. *Food Cosmet. Toxicol.*, *10*, 769-779

American Conference of Governmental Industrial Hygienists (1984) *Threshold Limit Values for Chemical Substances and Physical Agents in the Work Environment and Biological Exposure Indices with Intended Changes for 1984-85*, Cincinnati, OH, p. 18

Ames, S.R., Ludwig, M.I., Swanson, W.J. & Harris, P.L. (1956) Effects of DPPD, methylene blue, BHT, and hydroxyquinone on reproductive process in the rat. *Proc. Soc. exp. Biol. Med.*, *93*, 39-42

Anon. (1983) Uniroyal gives antioxidants a big vote of confidence as US recovery takes hold. *Chem. Mark. Rep.*, *224*, 4, 18

Anon. (1984) Chemical profile: BHT. *Chem. Mark. Rep.*, *226*, 54

Armentrout, D.N., McLean, J.D. & Long, M.W. (1979) Trace determination of phenolic compounds in water by reversed phase liquid chromatography with electrochemical detection using a carbon-polyethylene tubular anode. *Anal. Chem.*, *51*, 1039-1045

Autrup, H., Harris, C.C., Schwartz, R.D., Trump, B.F. & Smith, L. (1980) Metabolism of 1,2-dimethylhydrazine by cultured human colon. *Carcinogenesis*, *1*, 375-380

Awasthi, Y.C., Partridge, C.A. & Dao, D.D. (1983) Effect of butylated hydroxytoluene on glutathione *S*-transferase and glutathione peroxidase activities in rat liver. *Biochem. Pharmacol.*, *32*, 1197-1200

Babich, H. (1982) Butylated hydroxytoluene (BHT): A review. *Environ. Res.*, *29*, 1-29

Bär, V., Erdélyi, V., Foris, G., Pollak, Z. & Eckhardt, S. (1977) Biopharmacological investigation of 6,6'-methylene-bis/2,2,4-trimethyl-1,2-dihydroquinoline (MTDQ) a radical binding antioxidant of secondary amine type. *Neoplasma*, *24*, 253-258

Barbolt, T.A. & Abraham, R. (1979) Lack of effect of butylated hydroxytoluene on dimethylhydrazine-induced colon carcinogenesis in rats. *Experientia*, *35*, 257-258

Bartl, P. & Schaaff, A. (1982) Direct determination of antioxidants in aviation turbine fuels by gas chromatography/mass spectrometry. *Fresenius Z. anal. Chem.*, *310*, 250-251

Belvedere, G. Miller, H., Vatsis, K.P., Coon, M.J. & Gelboin, H.V. (1980) Hydroxylation of benzo[*a*]pyrene and binding of (-)*trans*-7,8-dihydroxy-7,8-dihydrobenzo[*a*]pyrene metabolites to deoxyribonucleic acid catalyzed by purified forms of rabbit liver microsomal cytochrome P-450. *Biochem. Pharmacol.*, *29*, 1693-1702

Ben-Hur, E., Green, M., Prager, A., Rosenthal, I. & Riklis, E. (1981) Differential protective effects of antioxidants against cell killing and mutagenesis of *Salmonella typhimurium* by γ radiation. *J. Radiat. Res.*, *22*, 250-257

Berry, D.L., DiGiovanni, J., Juchau, M.R., Bracken, W.M., Gleason, G.L. & Slaga, T.J. (1978) Lack of a tumor-promoting ability of certain environmental chemicals in a two-stage mouse skin tumorigenesis assay. *Res. Commun. chem. Pathol. Pharmacol.*, *20*, 101-108

Bhattacharya, R.K., Firozi, P.F. & Aboobaker, V.S. (1984) Factors modulating the formation of DNA adduct by aflatoxin B_1 *in vitro*. *Carcinogenesis*, *5*, 1359-1362

Biesterfeld US, Inc. (1972) *Butylated Hydroxytoluene: Material Safety Data Sheet*, Avon, CT

Bojan, F., Nagy, A. & Herman, K. (1978) Effect of butylated hydroxytoluene and paraquat on urethan tumorigenesis in mouse lung. *Bull. environ. Contam. Toxicol.*, *20*, 573-576

Bonin, A.M. & Baker, R.S.U. (1980) Mutagenicity testing of some approved food additives with the *Salmonella*/microsome assay. *Food Technol. Aust.*, *32*, 608-611

Botham, C.M., Conning, D.M., Hayes, J., Litchfield, M.H. & McElligott, T.F. (1970) Effects of butylated hydroxytoluene on the enzyme activity and ultrastructure of rat hepatocytes. *Food Cosmet. Toxicol.*, *8*, 1-8

Branen, A.L. (1975) Toxicology and biochemistry of butylated hydroxyanisole and butylated hydroxytoluene. *J. Am. Oil Chem. Soc.*, *52*, 59-63

Brown, W.D., Johnson, A.R. & O'Halloran, M.W. (1959) The effect of the level of dietary fat on the toxicity of phenolic antioxidants. *Aust. J. exp. Biol.*, *37*, 533-547

Bruce, W.R. & Heddle, J.A. (1979) The mutagenic activity of 61 agents as determined by the micronucleus, *Salmonella*, and sperm abnormality assays. *Can. J. Genet. Cytol.*, *21*, 319-333

Bull, A.W., Burd, A.D. & Nigro, N.D. (1981) Effect of inhibitors of tumorigenesis on the formation of O^6-methylguanine in the colon of 1,2-dimethylhydrazine-treated rats. *Cancer Res.*, *41*, 4938-4941

Bureau of Foods (1973) *Evaluation of the Health Aspects of Butylated Hydroxytoluene as a Food Ingredient (SCOGS-2)*, Washington DC, Food and Drug Administration, Department of Health, Education, and Welfare, pp. 2-3

Calle, L.M. & Sullivan, P.D. (1982) Screening of antioxidants and other compounds for antimutagenic properties towards benzo[*a*]pyrene-induced mutagenicity in strain TA98 of *Salmonella typhimurium*. *Mutat. Res.*, *101*, 99-114

Calle, L.M., Sullivan, P.D., Nettleman, M.D., Ocasio, I.J., Blazyk, J. & Jollick, J. (1978) Antioxidants and the mutagenicity of benzo(a)pyrene and some derivatives. *Biochem. biophys. Res. Commun.*, *85*, 351-356

Chao, G.K.-J. & Suatoni, J.C. (1982) Determination of phenolic compounds by HPLC. *J. chromatogr. Sci.*, *20*, 436-440

Clapp, N.K., Tyndall, R.L., Cumming, R.B. & Otten, J.A. (1974) Effects of butylated hydroxytoluene alone or with diethylnitrosamine in mice. *Food Cosmet. Toxicol.*, *12*, 367-371

Clapp, N.K., Tyndall, R.L., Satterfield, L.C., Klima, W.C. & Bowles, N.D. (1978) Selective sex-related modification of diethylnitrosamine-induced carcinogenesis in BALB/c mice by concomitant administration of butylated hydroxytoluene. *J. natl Cancer Inst.*, *61*, 177-182

Clapp, N.K., Bowles, N.D., Satterfield, L.C. & Klima, W.C. (1979) Selective protective effect of butylated hydroxytoluene against 1,2-dimethylhydrazine carcinogenesis in BALB/c mice. *J. natl Cancer Inst.*, *63*, 1081-1087

Clegg, D.J. (1965) Absence of teratogenic effect of butylated hydroxyanisole (BHA) and butylated hydroxytoluene (BHT) in rats and mice. *Food Cosmet. Toxicol.*, *3*, 387-403

Clement, N.R. & Gould, J.M. (1980) Quantitative detection of hydrophobic antioxidants such as butylatedhydroxytoluene and butylatedhydroxyanisole in picomole amounts. *Anal. Biochem.*, *101*, 299-304

Cohen, L.A., Polansky, M., Furuya, K., Reddy, M., Berke, B. & Weisburger, J.H. (1984) Inhibition of chemically induced mammary carcinogenesis in rats by short-term exposure to butylated hydroxytoluene (BHT): interrelationships among BHT concentration, carcinogen dose, and diet. *J. natl Cancer Inst.*, *72*, 165-174

Collings, A.J. & Sharratt, M. (1970) The BHT content of human adipose tissue. *Food Cosmet. Toxicol.*, *8*, 409-412

Commission of the European Communities (1978) *Reports of the Scientific Committee for Food*, 5th Series, Brussels, pp. 13-25

Čoupek, J., Pokorný, S., Protivová, J., Holčík, J., Karvaš, M. & Pospíšil, J. (1972) Antioxidants and stabilizers. XXXIII. Analysis of stabilizers of isotactic polypropylene: application of gel permeation chromatography. *J. Chromatogr.*, *65*, 279-286

Creaven, P.J., Davies, W.H. & Williams, R.T. (1966) The effect of butylated hydroxytoluene, butylated hydroxyanisole and octyl gallate upon liver weight and biphenyl 4-hydroxylase activity in the rat. *J. Pharm. Pharmacol.*, *18*, 485-489

Cumming, R.B. & Walton, M.F. (1973) Modification of the acute toxicity of mutagenic and carcinogenic chemicals in the mouse by prefeeding with antioxidants. *Food Cosmet. Toxicol.*, *11*, 547-553

Daniel, J.W. & Gage, J.C. (1965) The absorption and excretion of butylated hydroxytoluene (BHT) in the rat. *Food Cosmet. Toxicol.*, *3*, 405-415

Daniel, J.W., Gage, J.C., Jones, D.I. & Steven, M.A. (1967) Excretion of butylated hydroxytoluene (BHT) and butylated hydroxyanisole by man. *Food Cosmet. Toxicol.*, *5*, 475-479

Daniel, J.W., Gage, J.C. & Jones, D.I. (1968) The metabolism of 3,5-di-*tert*-butyl-4-hydroxytoluene in the rat and in man. *Biochem. J.*, *106*, 783-790

Daoud, A.H. & Griffin, A.C. (1980) Effect of retinoic acid, butylated hydroxytoluene, selenium and sorbic acid on azo-dye hepatocarcinogenesis. *Cancer Lett.*, *9*, 299-304

Daugherty, J.P. (1984) Mechanism of butylated hydroxytoluene-associated modification of diethylnitrosamine-induced squamous stomach carcinoma. *Food Chem. Toxicol.*, *22*, 951-961

Daugherty, J.P., Davis, S. & Yielding, K.L. (1978) Inhibition by butylated hydroxytoluene of excision repair synthesis and semiconservative DNA synthesis. *Biochem. biophys. Res. Commun.*, *80*, 963-969

Daugherty, J.P., Beach, L., Franks, H., Dean, A., Dees, J., Dees, R., Harmeson, P. & Mauldin, P. (1980) Tissue distribution and excretion of radioactivity in male and female mice after a single administration of [^{14}C]butylated hydroxytoluene. *Res. Commun. Subst. Abuse*, *1*, 99-110

Day, A.J., Johnson, A.R., O'Halloran, M.W. & Schwartz, C.J. (1959) The effect of the antioxidant butylated hydroxy toluene on serum lipid and glycoprotein levels in the rat. *Aust. J. exp. Biol.*, *37*, 295-305

Deichmann, W.B., Clemmer, J.J., Rakoczy, R. & Bianchine, J. (1955) Toxicity of ditertiarybutylmethylphenol. *Arch. ind. Health*, *11*, 93-101

Denning, J.A. & Marshall, J.A. (1972) The identification of antioxidants in polyethylene by gas chromatography. *Analyst*, *97*, 710-712

Dipple, A., Pigott, M.A., Bigger, C.A.H. & Blake, D.M. (1984) 7,12-Dimethylbenz[a]-anthracene-DNA binding in mouse skin: response of different mouse strains and effects of various modifiers of carcinogenesis. *Carcinogenesis*, *5*, 1087-1090

Djurhuus, R. & Lillehaug, J.R. (1982) Butylated hydroxytoluene: tumor-promoting activity in an *in vitro* two-stage carcinogenesis assay. *Bull. environ. Contam. Toxicol.*, *29*, 115-120

Doeden, W.G., Bowers, R.H. & Ingala, A.C. (1979) Determination of BHA, BHT, and TBHQ in edible fats and oils. *J. Am. Oil Chem. Soc.*, *56*, 12-14

Emerit, I., Levy, A. & Cerutti, P. (1983) Suppression of tumor promoter phorbolmyristate acetate-induced chromosome breakage by antioxidants and inhibitors of arachidonic acid metabolism. *Mutat. Res.*, *110*, 327-335

Epstein, S.S., Arnold, E., Andrea, J., Bass, W. & Bishop, Y. (1972) Detection of chemical mutagens by the dominant lethal assay in the mouse. *Toxicol. appl. Pharmacol.*, *23*, 288-325

Fazio, T. (1984a) *20. Food Additives: Direct. Antioxidants. Antioxidants in oils and fats.* In: Williams, S., ed., *Official Methods of Analysis of the Association of Official Analytical Chemists*, 14th ed., Arlington, VA, Association of Official Analytical Chemists, pp. 373-374

Fazio, T. (1984b) *20. Food Additives: Direct. Antioxidants. BHA and BHT in cereals.* In: Williams, S., ed., *Official Methods of Analysis of the Association of Official Analytical Chemists*, 14th ed., Arlington, VA, Association of Official Analytical Chemists, pp. 374-375

Federation of American Societies for Experimental Biology (1973) *SCOGS-2 Report Evaluation of the Health Aspects of Butylated Hydroxytoluene as a Food Ingredient*, Bethesda, MD, Life Sciences Research Office

Foley, L. & Kimmerle, F.M. (1979) Pulse voltammetric determination of butylated hydroxytoluene in transformer oils. *Anal. Chem., 51*, 818-822

Food and Agricultural Organization (1983) *Specifications for Identity and Purity (FAO Food and Nutrition Paper No. 28)*, Rome, pp. 11-12

Frawley, J.P., Kohn, F.E., Kay, J.H. & Calandra, J.C. (1965) Progress report on multigeneration reproduction studies in rats fed butylated hydroxytoluene (BHT). *Food Cosmet. Toxicol., 3*, 377-386

Fukayama, M.Y. & Hsieh, D.P.H. (1984) The effects of butylated hydroxytoluene on the in vitro metabolism, DNA-binding and mutagenicity of aflatoxin B_1 in the rat. *Food. Chem. Toxicol., 22*, 355-360

Fukayama, M.Y., Helferich, W.G. & Hsieh, D.P.H. (1984) Effect of butylated hydroxytoluene on the disposition of [^{14}C]aflatoxin B_1 in the rat. *Food Chem. Toxicol., 22*, 857-860

Furukawa, K., Maeura, Y., Furukawa, N.T. & Williams, G.M. (1984) Induction by butylated hydroxytoluene of rat liver γ-glutamyl transpeptidase activity in comparison to expression in carcinogen-induced altered lesions. *Chem.-biol. Interactions, 48*, 43-58

Gedeon, B.J., Chu, T. & Copeland, S. (1983) The identification of rubber compounding ingredients by using thin layer chromatography. *Rubber Chem. Technol., 56*, 1080-1095

Gilbert, D. & Goldberg, L. (1965) Liver response tests. III. Liver enlargement and stimulation of microsomal processing enzyme activity. *Food Cosmet. Toxicol., 3*, 417-432

Gilbert, D. & Martin, A.D. (1967) Food antioxidants in tissue culture. *Nature, 216*, 1254

Gilles, D. & Lucas, J.B. (1975) *Health Hazard Evaluation/Toxicity Determination Report 74-114-207, Koppers Company, Incorporated, Oil City, PA (PB 249 387)*, Rockville MD, National Institute for Occupational Safety and Health

Goodman, J.I., Trosko, J.E. & Yager, J.D., Jr (1976) Studies on the mechanism of inhibition of 2-acetylaminofluorene toxicity by butylated hydroxytoluene. *Chem.-biol. Interactions, 12*, 171-182

Grantham, P.H., Weisburger, J.H. & Weisburger, E.K. (1973) Effect of the antioxidant butylated hydroxytoluene (BHT) on the metabolism of the carcinogens N-2-fluorenylacetamide and N-hydroxy-N-2-fluorenylacetamide. *Food Cosmet. Toxicol.*, *11*, 209-217

Grasselli, J.G. & Ritchey, A.M., eds (1975) *CRC Atlas of Spectral Data and Physical Constants for Organic Compounds*, Vol. 2, Cleveland, OH, CRC Press, p. 279

Grote, A.A. & Kupel, R.E. (1978) Sampling and analysis of 2,6-di-*t*-butyl-*p*-cresol (DBPC). *Am. ind. Hyg. Assoc. J.*, *39*, 78-82

Hakkinen, P.J., Schmoyer, R.L. & Witschi, H.P. (1983) Potentiation of butylated-hydroxytoluene-induced acute lung damage by oxygen. Effects of prednisolone and indomethacin. *Am. Rev. resp. Dis.*, *128*, 648-651

Halladay, S.C., Ryerson, B.A., Smith, C.R., Brown, J.P. & Parkinson, T.M. (1980) Comparison of effects of dietary administration of butylated hydroxytoluene or a polymeric antioxidant on the hepatic and intestinal cytochrome P-450 mixed-function-oxygenase system of rats. *Food Cosmet. Toxicol.*, *18*, 569-574

Harris, C.C., Frank, A.L., van Haaften, C., Kaufman, D.G., Connor, R., Jackson, F., Barrett, L.A., McDowell, E.M. & Trump, B.F. (1976) Binding of [³H]benzo(*a*)pyrene to DNA in cultured human bronchus. *Cancer Res.*, *36*, 1011-1018

Haschek, W.M., Meyer, K.R., Ullrich, R.L. & Witschi, H.P. (1980) Potentiation of chemically induced lung fibrosis by thorax irradiation. *Int. J. Radiat. Oncol. Biol. Phys.*, *6*, 449-455

Haschek, W.M., Klein-Szanto, A.J.P., Last, J.A., Reiser, K.M. & Witschi, H. (1982) Long-term morphologic and biochemical features of experimentally induced lung fibrosis in the mouse. *Lab. Invest.*, *46*, 438-449

Hawley, G.G., ed. (1981) *The Condensed Chemical Dictionary*, 10th ed., New York, Van Nostrand Reinhold, p. 328

Hirose, M., Shibata, M., Hagiwara, A., Imaida, K. & Ito, N. (1981) Chronic toxicity of butylated hydroxytoluene in Wistar rats. *Food Cosmet. Toxicol.*, *19*, 147-151

Hollstein, M., Talcott, R. & Wei, E. (1978) Quinoline: conversion to a mutagen by human and rodent liver. *J. natl Cancer Inst.*, *60*, 405-410

IARC (1982) *IARC Monographs on the Evaluation of the Carcinogenic Risk of Chemicals to Humans*, Suppl. 4, *Chemicals, Industrial Processes and Industries Associated with Cancer in Humans, IARC Monographs, Volumes 1 to 29*, Lyon, pp. 50-51

ICIS Chemical Information System (1984) *Carbon-13 NMR Spectral Search System (CNMR), Mass Spectral Search System (MSSS), Infrared Spectral Search System (IRSS), Information System for Hazardous Organics in Water (ISHOW)*, and *Environmental Fate* (ENVIROFATE), Washington DC, Information Consultants

Imaida, K., Fukushima, S., Shirai, Y., Ohtani, M., Nakanishi, K. & Ito, N. (1983) Promoting activities of butylated hydroxyanisole and butylated hydroxytoluene on 2-stage urinary bladder carcinogenesis and inhibition of γ-glutamyl transpeptidase-positive foci development in the liver of rats. *Carcinogenesis*, *4*, 895-899

Imaida, K., Fukushima, S., Shirai, T., Masui, T., Ogiso, T. & Ito, N. (1984) Promoting activities of butylated hydroxyanisole, butylated hydroxytoluene and sodium L-ascorbate on forestomach and urinary bladder carcinogenesis initiated with methyl-nitrosourea in F344 male rats. *Gann, 75,* 769-775

International Labour Office (1980) *Occupational Exposure Limits for Airborne Toxic Substances, A Tabular Compilation of Values from Selected Countries,* 2nd (rev.) ed. (*Occupational Safety and Health Series No. 37*), Geneva, pp. 88-89

International Life Sciences Institute (1984) *Butylated Hydroxytoluene (BHT). A Monograph,* Washington DC

International Programme on Chemical Safety (1983) *Toxicological Evaluation of Certain Food Additives and Food Contaminants (WHO Food Add. Ser. No. 18*), Geneva, pp. 50-58

Ishidate, M., Jr, Yoshikawa, K. & Sofuni, T. (1980) A primary screening for mutagenicity of food additives in Japan. *Mutagens Toxicol., 3,* 82-90

Isshiki, K., Tsumura, S. & Watanabe, T. (1980) Determination of preservatives, butyl-hydroxyanisole and dibutylhydroxytoluene. *Agric. Biol. Chem., 44,* 1601-1607

Ito, N., Fukushima, S. & Tsuda, H. (1985) Carcinogenicity and modification of the carcinogenic response by BHA, BHT, and other antioxidants. *Crit. Rev. Toxicol., 15,* 109-150

Ives, P.T. & Demick, D.F. (1974) BHT modification of rates of induced mutagenesis. *Drosophila Inf. Serv., 51,* 133

Johnson, A.R. (1965) A re-examination of the possible teratogenic effects of butylated hydroxytoluene (BHT) and its effect on the reproductive capacity of the mouse. *Food Cosmet. Toxicol., 3,* 371-375

Johnson, A.R. & Hewgill, F.R. (1961) The effect of the antioxidants, butylated hydroxy anisole, butylated hydroxy toluene, and propyl gallate on growth, liver and serum lipids and serum sodium levels of the rat. *Aust. J. exp. Biol., 39,* 353-360

Joner, P.E. (1977) Butylhydroxyanisol (BHA), butylhydroxytoluene (BHT) and ethoxy-quin (EMQ) tested for mutagenicity. *Acta vet. scand., 18,* 187-193

Jungclaus, G.A., Games, L.M. & Hites, R.A. (1976) Identification of trace organic compounds in tire manufacturing plant wastewaters. *Anal. Chem., 48,* 1894-1896

Kahl, R. (1984) Synthetic antioxidants: biochemical actions and interference with radiation, toxic compounds, chemical mutagens and chemical carcinogens. *Toxicology, 33,* 185-228

Kahl, R. & Wulff, U. (1979) Induction of rat hepatic epoxide hydratase by dietary antioxidants. *Toxicol. appl. Pharmacol., 47,* 217-227

Kamra, O.P. (1973) Radiosensitizing property of butylated hydroxytoluene in *Drosophila* sperm. *Int. J. Radiat. Biol., 23,* 295-297

Karplyuk, I.A. (1959) Toxicologic characteristics of phenolic antioxidants of alimentary fats. (Russ). *Vop. Pitan., 18,* 24-29

Katoh, Y., Tanaka, M., Umezawa, K. & Takayama, S. (1980) Inhibition of mutagenesis in Chinese hamster V-79 cells by antioxidants. *Toxicol. Lett.*, *7*, 125-130

Kaul, B.L. (1979) Cytogenetic activity of some common antioxidants and their interaction with X-rays. *Mutat. Res.*, *67*, 239-247

Kaul, B.L. & Tandon, V. (1981) Modification of the mutagenic activity of propane sultone by some phenolic antioxidants. *Mutat. Res.*, *89*, 57-61

Kawano, S., Nakao, T. & Hiraga, K. (1980) Species and strain differences in the butylated hydroxytoluene (BHT)-producing induction of hepatic drug oxidation enzymes. *Jpn. J. Pharmacol.*, *30*, 861-870

Kehrer, J.P. & Kacew, S. (1985) Systemically applied chemicals that damage lung tissue. *Toxicology*, *35*, 251-293

Kehrer, J.P. & Witschi, H. (1980) Effects of drug metabolism inhibitors on butylated hydroxytoluene-induced pulmonary toxicity in mice. *Toxicol. appl. Pharmacol.*, *53*, 333-342

Kinae, N., Hashizume, T., Makita, T., Tomita, I., Kimura, I. & Kanamori, H. (1981) Studies on the toxicity of pulp and paper mill effluents — I. Mutagenicity of the sediment samples derived from kraft paper mills. *Water Res.*, *15*, 17-24

King, M.M., Bailey, D.M., Gibson, D.D., Pitha, J.V. & McCay, P.B. (1979) Incidence and growth of mammary tumors induced by 7,12-dimethylbenz[a]anthracene as related to the dietary content of fat and antioxidant. *J. natl Cancer Inst.*, *63*, 657-663

King, M.M., McCay, P.B. & Kosanke, S.D. (1981) Comparison of the effect of butylated hydroxytoluene on N-nitrosomethylurea and 7,12-dimethylbenz[a]anthracene-induced mammary tumors. *Cancer Lett.*, *14*, 219-226

Kiselev, A.V., Maltsev, V.V., Saada, B. & Valovoy, V.A. (1983) Gas chromatography-mass spectrometry of volatiles released from plastics used as building materials. *Chromatographia*, *17*, 539-544

Kline, D.A., Joe, F.L., Jr & Fazio, T. (1978) A rapid gas-liquid chromatographic method for the multidetermination of antioxidants in fats, oils, and dried food products. *J. Assoc. off. anal. Chem.*, *61*, 513-519

Koppers Co., Inc. (undated) *DBPC^R and BHT Antioxidants* (*Tech. Bull. OM-115-31*), Pittsburgh, PA

Kuo, J.F., Brackett, N.L., Stubbs, J.W., Shoji, M. & Helfman, D. (1978) Involvements of cyclic nucleotide systems in enlarged mice lungs produced by butylated hydroxytoluene. *Biochem. Pharmacol.*, *27*, 1671-1675

Ladomery, L.G., Ryan, A.J. & Wright, S.E. (1967a) The excretion of [^{14}C]butylated hydroxytoluene in the rat. *J. Pharm. Pharmacol.*, *19*, 383-387

Ladomery, L.G., Ryan, A.J. & Wright, S.E. (1967b) The biliary metabolites of butylated hydroxytoluene in the rat. *J. Pharm. Pharmacol.*, *19*, 388-394

Lane, B.P. & Lieber, C.S. (1967) Effects of butylated hydroxytoluene on the ultrastructure of rat hepatocytes. *Lab. Invest.*, *16*, 342-348

Maeura, Y. & Williams, G.M. (1984) Enhancing effect of butylated hydroxytoluene on the development of liver altered foci and neoplasms induced by *N*-2-fluorenylacetamide in rats. *Food Chem. Toxicol.*, *22*, 191-198

Maeura, Y., Weisburger, J.H. & Williams, G.M. (1984) Dose-dependent reduction of *N*-2-fluorenylacetamide-induced liver cancer and enhancement of bladder cancer in rats by butylated hydroxytoluene. *Cancer Res.*, *44*, 1604-1610

Majors, R.E. & Johnson, E.L. (1978) High-performance exclusion chromatography of low-molecular-weight additives. *J. Chromatogr.*, *167*, 17-30

Malkinson, A.M. (1979) Altered phosphorylation of lung proteins following administration of butylated hydroxytoluene (BHT) to mice. *Life Sci.*, *24*, 465-471

Malkinson, A.M. (1983) Review: putative mutagens and carcinogens in foods. III. Butylated hydroxytoluene (BHT). *Environ. Mutagenesis*, *5*, 353-362

Malkinson, A.M. & Beer, D.S. (1984) Pharmacologic and genetic studies on the modulatory effects of butylated hydroxytoluene on mouse lung adenoma formation. *J. natl Cancer Inst.*, *73*, 925-933

Marino, A.A. & Mitchell, J.T. (1972) Lung damage in mice following intraperitoneal injection of butylated hydroxytoluene. *Proc. Soc. exp. Biol. Med.*, *140*, 122-125

Masuda, Y. & Nakayama, N. (1984) Prevention of butylated hydroxytoluene-induced lung damage by diethyldithiocarbamate and carbon disulfide in mice. *Toxicol. appl. Pharmacol.*, *75*, 81-90

Matsuo, M., Mihara, K., Okuno, M., Ohkawa, H. & Miyamoto, J. (1984) Comparative metabolism of 3,5-di-*tert*-butyl-4-hydroxytoluene (BHT) in mice and rats. *Food chem. Toxicol.*, *22*, 345-354

Mattammal, M.B., Zenser, T.V. & Davis, B.B. (1981) Prostaglandin hydroperoxidase-mediated 2-amino-4-(5-nitro-2-furyl)[^{14}C]thiazole metabolism and nucleic acid binding. *Cancer Res.*, *41*, 4961-4966

Mattammal, M.B., Zenser, T.V. & Davis, B.B. (1982) Anaerobic metabolism and nuclear binding of the carcinogen 2-amino-4-(5-nitro-2-furyl)thiazole (ANFT). *Carcinogenesis*, *3*, 1339-1344

Mazar Barnett, B. & Muñoz, E.R. (1980) Modification of radiation-induced genetic damage in *Drosophila melanogaster* male germ cells by butylated hydroxytoluene. *Int. J. Radiat. Biol.*, *38*, 559-566

Mazar Barnett, B. & Muñoz, E.R. (1983) Recessive lethals induced by ethyl methane-sulfonate and diethyl sulfate in *Drosophila melanogaster* post-meiotic male cells pre-treated with butylated hydroxytoluene. *Mutat. Res.*, *110*, 49-57

McCormick, D.L., Major, N. & Moon, R.C. (1984) Inhibition of 7,12-dimethyl-benz(*a*)anthracene-induced rat mammary carcinogenesis by concomitant or postcarcinogen antioxidant exposure. *Cancer Res.*, *44*, 2858-2863

McKee, R.H. & Tometsko, A.M. (1979) Inhibition of promutagen activation by the antioxidants butylated hydroxyanisole and butylated hydroxytoluene. *J. natl Cancer Inst.*, *63*, 473-477

Meyer, O. & Hansen, E. (1980) Behavioural and developmental effects of butylated hydroxytoluene dosed to rats *in utero* and in the lactation period. *Toxicology, 16,* 247-258

Mirabella, F.M., Jr, Barrall, E.M., II & Johnson, J.F. (1976) A rapid technique for the qualitative analysis of polymers and additives using stop-and-go g.p.c. and i.r. *Polymer, 17,* 18-20

Mizutani, T., Nomura, H., Yamamoto, K. & Tajima, K. (1984) Modification of butylated hydroxytoluene-induced pulmonary toxicity in mice by diethyl maleate, buthionine sulfoximine, and cysteine. *Toxicol. Lett., 23,* 327-331

Nakagawa, Y., Hiraga, K. & Suga, T. (1979a) Biological fate of butylated hydroxytoluene (BHT); binding *in vivo* of BHT to macromolecules of rat liver. *Chem. pharm. Bull., 27,* 442-446

Nakagawa, Y., Hiraga, K. & Suga, T. (1979b) Biological fate of butylated hydroxytoluene (BHT); binding *in vitro* of BHT to liver microsomes. *Chem. pharm. Bull., 27,* 480-485

Nakagawa, Y., Hiraga, K. & Suga, T. (1980) Biological fate of butylated hydroxytoluene (BHT) — binding of BHT to nucleic acid *in vivo. Biochem. Pharmacol., 29,* 1304-1306

National Cancer Institute (1979) *Bioassay of Butylated Hydroxytoluene (BHT) for Possible Carcinogenicity (CAS No. 128-37-0)* (*Tech. Rep. Ser. No. 150*), Bethesda, MD

National Research Council (1972) *Subcommitte on Review of the GRAS List (Phase II). A Comprehensive Survey of Industry on the Use of Food Chemicals Generally Recognized as Safe (GRAS)* (*PB 221 949*), Washington DC, National Academy of Sciences

National Research Council (1981) *BHT.* In: *Food Chemicals Codex,* 3rd ed., Washington DC, National Academy of Sciences, p. 38

Olsen, P., Bille, N. & Meyer, O. (1983) Hepatocellular neoplasms in rats induced by butylated hydroxytoluene (BHT). *Acta pharmacol. toxicol., 53,* 433-434

Olsen, P., Meyer, O., Bille, N. & Würtzen, G. (1986) Carcinogenicity study on butylated hydroxytoluene (BHT) in Wistar rats exposed *in utero. Food chem. Toxicol., 24,* 1-12

Paffenbarger, G.C. & Rupp, N.W. (1979) *Dental materials.* In: Mark, H.F., Othmer, D.F., Overberger, C.G. & Seaborg, G.T., eds, *Kirk-Othmer Encyclopedia of Chemical Technology,* 3rd ed., Vol. 7, New York, John Wiley & Sons, pp. 461-521

Page, B.D. (1979) High-performance liquid chromatographic determination of nine phenolic antioxidants in oils, lards, and shortenings. *J. Assoc. off. anal. Chem., 62,* 1239-1246

Paschin, Y.V. & Bahitova, L.M. (1984) Inhibition of the mutagenicity of benzo[*a*]pyrene in the V79/HGPRT system by bioantioxidants. *Mutat. Res., 137,* 57-59

Pellerin, F., Delaveau, P., Dumitrescu, D. & Safta, F. (1982) Identification and titration of BHA and BHT in chewing-gum preparations (Fr.). *Ann. pharm. Fr., 40,* 221-230

Peraino, C., Fry, R.J.M., Staffeldt, E. & Christopher, J.P. (1977) Enhancing effects of phenobarbitone and butylated hydroxytoluene on 2-acetylaminofluorene-induced hepatic tumorigenesis in the rat. *Food Cosmet. Toxicol., 15,* 93-96

Ponder, D.L. & Green, N.R. (1985) Effects of dietary fats and butylated hydroxytoluene on mutagen activation in rats. *Cancer Res.*, *45*, 558-560

Prasad, O. & Kamra, O.P. (1974) Radiosensitization of *Drosophila* sperm by commonly used food additives — butylated hydroxyanisole and butylated hydroxytoluene. *Int. J. Radiat. Biol.*, *25*, 67-72

Reddy, B.S., Sharma, C. & Mathews, L. (1983a) Effect of butylated hydroxytoluene and butylated hydroxyanisole on the mutagenicity of 3,2'-dimethyl-4-aminobiphenyl. *Nutr. Cancer*, *5*, 153-158

Reddy, B.S., Hanson, D., Mathews, L. & Sharma, C. (1983b) Effect of micronutrients, antioxidants and related compounds on the mutagenicity of 3,2'-dimethyl-4-aminobiphenyl, a colon and breast carcinogen. *Food chem. Toxicol.*, *21*, 129-132

Rékasi, T. & Orsi, F. (1976) Determination of butylhydroxytoluene in mixed feeds by a photometric method I (Hung.). *Elelmiszeroizsgalati Kozl*, *22*, 316-321

Sadtler Research Laboratories (1973) *Fluorescence Spectra*, Philadelphia, PA

Sadtler Research Laboratories (1980) *The Sadtler Standard Spectra, Cumulative Index*, Philadelphia, PA

Saheb, W. & Witschi, H. (1975) Lung growth in mice after a single dose of butylated hydroxytoluene. *Toxicol. appl. Pharmacol.*, *33*, 309-319

Sakai, S., Reinhold, C.E., Wirth, P.J. & Thorgeirsson, S.S. (1978) Mechanism of *in vitro* mutagenic activation and covalent binding of N-hydroxy-2-acetylaminofluorene in isolated liver cell nuclei from rat and mouse. *Cancer Res.*, *38*, 2058-2067

Sankaranarayanan, K. (1983) The effects of butylated hydroxytoluene on radiation and chemically-induced genetic damage in *Drosophila melanogaster*. *Mutat. Res.*, *108*, 203-223

Sawicki, J.T. & Dipple, A. (1983) Effects of butylated hydroxyanisole and butylated hydroxytoluene on 7,12-dimethylbenz[a]anthracene-DNA adduct formation in mouse embryo cell cultures. *Cancer Lett.*, *20*, 165-171

Sax, N.I. (1984) *Dangerous Properties of Industrial Materials*, 6th ed., New York, Van Nostrand Reinhold, pp. 426-427, 919

Schabron, J.F. & Fenska, L.E. (1980) Determination of BHT, Irganox 1076, and Irganox 1010 antioxidant additives in polyethylene by high performance liquid chromatography. *Anal. Chem.*, *52*, 1411-1415

Senten, J.R., Waumans, J.M. & Clement, J.M. (1977) Gas-liquid chromatographic determination of butylated hydroxyanisole and butylated hydroxytoluene in edible oils. *J. Assoc. off. anal. Chem.*, *60*, 505-508

Shamberger, R.J., Baughman, F.F., Kalchert, S.L., Willis, C.E. & Hoffman, G.C. (1973) Carcinogen-induced chromosomal breakage decreased by antioxidants. *Proc. natl Acad. Sci. USA*, *70*, 1461-1463

Shelef, L.A. & Chin, B. (1980) Effect of phenolic antioxidants on the mutagenicity of aflatoxin B_1. *Appl. environ. Microbiol.*, *40*, 1039-1043

Sherwin-Williams (1982) *BHT: The Versatile Antioxidant for Today ... and Tomorrow* (*Bull. AOX-12*), Cleveland, OH

Shipp, B.D. (1973) The ^{14}C-synthesis, distribution, placental transfer, and fetal radio-protective properties of 2,6-di-*tert*-butyl-p-cresol. *Diss. Abstr. int. B, 33*, 4565B-4566B

Shirai, T., Hagiwara, A., Kurata, Y., Shibata, M., Fukushima, S. & Ito, N. (1982) Lack of carcinogenicity of butylated hydroxytoluene on long-term administration to B6C3F$_1$ mice. *Food Chem. Toxicol., 20*, 861-865

Shirai, T., Fukushima, S., Ohshima, M., Masuda, A. & Ito, N. (1984) Effects of butylated hydroxyanisole, butylated hydroxytoluene and NaCl on gastric carcinogenesis initiated with *N*-methyl-*N'*-nitro-*N*-nitrosoguanidine in F344 rats. *J. natl Cancer Inst., 72*, 1189-1198

Shirai, T., Ikawa, E., Hirose, M., Thamavit, W. & Ito, N. (1985) Modification by five antioxidants of 1,2-dimethylhydrazine-initiated colon carcinogenesis in F344 rats. *Carcinogenesis, 6*, 637-639

Shoyab, M. (1979) Evidence for translational control of the binding of 7,12-dimethylbenz-[*a*]anthracene to DNA of murine epidermal cell in culture. *Chem.-biol. Interactions, 25*, 289-301

Slaga, T.J. & Bracken, W.M. (1977) The effects of antioxidants on skin tumor initiation and aryl hydrocarbon hydroxylase. *Cancer Res., 37*, 1631-1635

Stoner, G.D., Shimkin, M.B., Kniazeff, A.J., Weisburger, J.H., Weisburger, E.K. & Gori, G.B. (1973) Test for carcinogenicity of food additives and chemotherapeutic agents by the pulmonary tumor response in strain A mice. *Cancer Res., 33*, 3069-3085

Stuckey, B.N. (1972) *Antioxidants as food stabilizers*. In: Furia, T.E., ed., *Handbook of Food Additives*, 2nd ed., Cleveland, OH, CRC Press, pp. 185-223

Tajima, K., Yamamoto, K. & Mizutani, T. (1981) Biotransformation of butylated hydroxytoluene (BHT) to BHT-quinone methide in rats. *Chem. pharm. Bull., 29*, 3738-3741

Tajima, K., Yamamoto, K. & Mizutani, T. (1984) Metabolic activation and glutathione conjugation of butylated hydroxytoluene. *J. Pharm. Dyn., 7*, 5-89

Tajima, K., Yamamoto, K. & Mizutani, T. (1985) Formation of a glutathione conjugate from butylated hydroxytoluene by rat liver microsomes. *Biochem. Pharmacol., 34*, 2109-2114

Takahashi, O. & Hiraga, O. (1979) 2,6-Di-*tert*-butyl-4-methylene-2,5-cyclohexadienone: a hepatic metabolite of butylated hydroxytoluene in rats. *Food Cosmet. Toxicol., 17*, 451-454

Tandon, V. & Kaul, B.L. (1979) Influence of some phenolic antioxidants on radiomimetic activity of propane sultone. *Indian J. exp. Biol., 17*, 713-714

Tatsuta, M., Mikuni, T. & Taniguchi, H. (1983) Protective effect of butylated hydroxytoluene against induction of gastric cancer by *N*-methyl-*N'*-nitro-*N*-nitrosoguanidine in Wistar rats. *Int. J. Cancer, 32*, 253-254

Taylor, D.G. (1977) *NIOSH Manual of Analytical Methods*, 2nd ed., Vol. 1 (*DHEW (NIOSH) Publ. No. 77-157-A*), Washington DC, Government Printing Office, pp. 226-1 — 226-8

Telford, I.R., Woodruff, C.S. & Linford, R.H. (1962) Fetal resorption in the rat as influenced by certain antioxidants. *Am. J. Anat.*, *110*, 29-36

Thomas, H.F., Hartman, P.E., Mudryj, M. & Brown, D.L. (1979) Nitrous acid mutagenesis of duplex DNA as a three-component system. *Mutat. Res.*, *61*, 129-151

Tye, R., Engel, J.D. & Rapien, I. (1965) Disposition of butylated hydroxytoluene (BHT) in the rat. *Food Cosmet. Toxicol.*, *3*, 547-551

Tyndall, R.L., Colyer, S. & Clapp, N. (1975) Early alterations in plasma esterases with associated pathology following oral administration of diethylnitrosamine and butylated hydroxytoluene singly or in combination. *Int. J. Cancer*, *16*, 184-191

Työsuojeluhallitus (National Finnish Board of Occupational Safety and Health) (1981) *Airborne Contaminants in the Workplace* (*Saf. Bull. 3*) (Finn.), Tampere, p. 10

Ulland, B.M., Weisburger, J.H., Yamamoto, R.S. & Weisburger, E.K. (1973) Antioxidants and carcinogenesis: butylated hydroxytoluene, but not diphenyl-*p*-phenylenediamine, inhibits cancer induction by *N*-2-fluorenylacetamide and by *N*-hydroxy-*N*-2-fluorenylacetamide in rats. *Food Cosmet. Toxicol.*, *11*, 199-207

Uniroyal Chemical Co. (1984) *Naugard BHT: Material Safety Data Sheet*, Middlebury, CT

US Department of Agriculture (1984) Animals and animal products. *US Code fed. Regul.*, *Title 9*, Parts 318.7, 319.700, 381.147, pp. 208, 246-247, 407

US Food and Drug Administration (1977) Butylated hydroxytoluene. Use restrictions. *Fed. Regist.*, *42*, 27603-27609

US Food and Drug Administration (1981) *Number of Brand Name Products in Each Product Code, Cosmetic Product Formulation Data*, Washington DC, Division of Cosmetics Technology, pp. 33-34

US Food and Drug Administration (1983a) *Butylated hydroxytoluene (BHT): Method II*. In: Warner, C., Modderman, J., Fazio, T., Beroza, M., Schwartzman, G. & Fominaya, K., eds, *Food Additives Analytical Manual*, Vol. 1, Arlington, VA, Association of Official Analytical Chemists, pp. 62-76

US Food and Drug Administration (1983b) *Butylated hydroxytoluene (BHT): Method I*. In: Warner, C., Modderman, J., Fazio, T., Beroza, M., Schwartzman, G. & Fominaya, K., eds, *Food Additives Analytical Manual*, Vol. 1, Arlington, VA, Association of Official Analytical Chemists, pp. 52-61, 74-76

US Food and Drug Administration (1984) Food and drugs. *US Code fed. Regul.*, *Title 21*, Parts 172.115, 172.615, 173.340, 174.5, 175.105, 175.125, 175.300, 176.210, 177.2260, 177.2600, 178.3570, 181.24, 182.3173, pp. 26, 58, 119, 126, 138, 148, 193, 271, 285, 319, 365, 380

US International Trade Commission (1978) *Synthetic Organic Chemicals, US Production and Sales, 1977* (*USITC Publ. 920*), Washington DC, National Technical Information Service, p. 357

US International Trade Commission (1984) *Synthetic Organic Chemicals, US Production and Sales, 1983 (USITC Publ. 1588)*, Washington DC, National Technical Information Service, p. 255

Vargo, J.D. & Olson, K.L. (1985) Identification of antioxidant and ultraviolet light stabilizing additives in plastics by liquid chromatography/mass spectrometry. *Anal. Chem.*, *57*, 672-675

Verschueren, K. (1983) *Handbook of Environmental Data on Organic Chemicals*, 2nd ed., New York, Van Nostrand Reinhold, p. 467

Vorhees, C.V., Butcher, R.E., Brunner, R.L. & Sobotka, T.J. (1981) Developmental neurobehavioural toxicity of butylated hydroxytoluene in rats. *Food Cosmet. Toxicol.*, *19*, 153-162

Wattenberg, L.W. (1972) Inhibition of carcinogenic and toxic effects of polycyclic hydrocarbons by phenolic antioxidants and ethoxyquin. *J. natl Cancer Inst.*, *48*, 1425-1430

Weast, R.C., ed. (1985) *CRC Handbook of Chemistry and Physics*, 66th ed., Boca Raton, FL, CRC Press, p. C-410

Wei, L., Whiting, R.F. & Stich, H.F. (1981) *Inhibition of chemical mutagenesis: an application of chromosome aberration and DNA synthesis assays using cultured mammalian cells.* In: Stich, H.F. & San, R.H.C., eds, *Short-Term Tests for Chemical Carcinogenesis*, New York, Springer-Verlag, pp. 428-437

Weisburger, E.K., Evarts, R.P. & Wenk, M.L. (1977) Inhibitory effect of butylated hydroxytoluene (BHT) on intestinal carcinogenesis in rats by azoxymethane. *Food Cosmet. Toxicol.*, *15*, 139-141

WHO (1974) *Toxicological Evaluation of Some Food Additives Including Anticaking Agents, Antimicrobials, Antioxidants, Emulsifiers and Thickening Agents (WHO Food Add. Ser. No. 5)*, Geneva, pp. 156-169

WHO (1983) *Evaluation of Certain Food Additives and Contaminants (WHO Tech. Rep. Ser. No. 696)*, Geneva, pp. 14-15

Williams, G.M., Maeura, Y. & Weisburger, J.H. (1983) Simultaneous inhibition of liver carcinogenicity and enhancement of bladder carcinogenicity of *N*-2-fluorenylacetamide by butylated hydroxytoluene. *Cancer Lett.*, *19*, 55-60

Windholz, M., ed. (1983) *The Merck Index*, 10th ed., Rahway, NJ, Merck & Co., pp. 215-216

Witschi, H.P. (1981) Enhancement of tumor formation in mouse lung by dietary butylated hydroxytoluene. *Toxicology*, *21*, 95-104

Witschi, H.R. & Doherty, D.G. (1984) Butylated hydroxyanisole and lung tumor development in A/J mice. *Fundam. appl. Toxicol.*, *4*, 795-801

Witschi, H. & Lock, S. (1979) Enhancement of adenoma formation in mouse lung by butylated hydroxytoluene. *Toxicol. appl. Pharmacol.*, *50*, 391-400

Witschi, H.R. & Morse, C.C. (1983) Enhancement of lung tumor formation in mice by dietary butylated hydroxytoluene: dose-time relationships and cell kinetics. *J. natl Cancer Inst.*, *71*, 859-866

Witschi, H. & Saheb, W. (1974) Stimulation of DNA synthesis in mouse lung following intraperitoneal injection of butylated hydroxytoluene. *Proc. Soc. exp. Biol. Med.*, *147*, 690-693

Witschi, H., Williamson, D. & Lock, S. (1977) Enhancement of urethan tumorigenesis in mouse lung by butylated hydroxytoluene. *J. natl Cancer Inst.*, *58*, 301-305

Witschi, H.P., Hakkinen, P.J. & Kehrer, J.P. (1981) Modification of lung tumor development in A/J mice. *Toxicology*, *21*, 37-45

Wright, A.S., Akintonwa, D.A.A., Crowne, R.S. & Hathway, D.E. (1965) The metabolism of 2,6-di-*tert*-butyl-4-hydroxymethylphenol (Ionox 100) in the dog and rat. *Biochem. J.*, *97*, 303-310

Wyatt, D.M. (1981) Simultaneous analysis of BHA, TBHQ, BHT and propyl gallate by gas chromatography as extracted from refined vegetable oil. *J. Am. Oil Chem. Soc.*, *58*, 917-920

Yang, C.S., Strickhart, F.S. & Woo, G.K. (1974) Inhibition of the mono-oxygenase system by butylated hydroxyanisole and butylated hydroxytoluene. *Life Sci.*, *15*, 1497-1505

POTASSIUM BROMATE

1. Chemical and Physical Data

1.1 Synonyms and trade names

Chem. Abstr. Services Reg. No.: 7758-01-2
Chem. Abstr. Name: Bromic acid, potassium salt
IUPAC Systematic Name: Potassium bromate
Synonym: EEC No. E924

1.2 Structural and molecular formulae and molecular weight

$$K^+ \quad \underset{\underset{O}{\overset{\|}{}}}{\overset{\overset{O}{\overset{\|}{}}}{Br}} - O^-$$

KBrO₃   Mol. wt: 167.01

1.3 Chemical and physical properties of the pure substance

(*a*) *Description*: White crystals, crystalline powder or granules (Hawley, 1981; Windholz, 1983; Sax, 1984; American International Chemical, Inc., undated)

(*b*) *Melting-point*: Approximately 350°C (Windholz, 1983; Sax, 1984)

(*c*) *Density*: 3.27 (Sax, 1984; Weast, 1985)

(*d*) *Spectroscopy data*: Infrared spectral data (Sadtler Research Laboratories, 1967 [Y107K[a]]) have been reported.

---

[a]Spectrum number in Sadtler compilation

(e)   *Solubility*: Soluble in water (7.5 g/100 ml at 25°C; 49.8 g/100 ml at 100°C) (E.B. Knight, Inc., 1975; Weast, 1985); slightly soluble in ethanol; almost insoluble in acetone (Windholz, 1983; Weast, 1985)

(f)   *Stability*: Decomposes at temperatures above 370°C with the evolution of oxygen and toxic fumes containing potassium oxide and potassium bromide (Windholz, 1983; Sax, 1984)

(g)   *Reactivity*: Strong oxidizing agent; reacts vigorously with organic matter with reduction to bromide; also oxidizes some metals (Al, Cu) and some non-metals (As, P, Se, S) (Hawley, 1981; Sax, 1984)

1.4 Technical products and impurities

The Food Chemicals Codex (National Research Council, 1981) specifies that food-grade potassium bromate assay at not less than 99.0% and not more than 101.0% of potassium bromate after drying. Allowable limits of impurities present in the food-grade product are 3 mg/kg arsenic (see IARC, 1982) and 10 mg/kg heavy metals (as lead; see IARC, 1982).

Commercial potassium bromate from major producers may contain up to 0.02-0.05% bromides, 0.001-0.01% sulphates and 20 mg/kg iron. It is available in crystalline or powder form, and in mixtures with 5% magnesium carbonate or 50% calcium carbonate (AmeriBrom, Inc., undated; American International Chemical, Inc., undated; E.B. Knight, Inc., undated).

2. Production, Use, Occurrence and Analysis

2.1 Production and use

(a) Production

Potassium bromate can be produced by passing bromine through a solution of potassium hydroxide (Hawley, 1981). However, the compound is manufactured mainly by large-scale industrial electrolytic processes.

The largest primary producer of potassium bromate, with an annual capacity of 4.5 million kg, is located in Israel (Anon., 1983). Italy, the Netherlands and the UK each have one major producer of potassium bromate; the Federal Republic of Germany and Spain each have two potassium bromate manufacturers.

The US receives the majority of its potassium bromate from a domestic firm with the parent plant in Israel. Two other US firms are also reported to produce commercial quantities of potassium bromate.

In Japan, eight firms are reported to produce potassium bromate (The Chemical Daily Co., 1980).

(b)   Use

Potassium bromate is used primarily as a maturing agent for flour and as a dough conditioner in bread-making (AmeriBrom, Inc., undated). It has been used in the UK as a flour constituent for approximately 50 years (Fisher *et al.*, 1979). In 1974, the use of potassium bromate was reported to be widespread in Australia, Canada, the UK and the USA (Thewlis, 1974).

Potassium bromate is used in Japan in fish-paste products (Kurokawa *et al.*, 1983a). It is also a component of food for yeast (Kulp & Hepburn, 1978) and is used in the malting of beer (Sfat & Doncheck, 1981; WHO, 1983). It may be used in the manufacture of cheese (AmeriBrom, Inc., undated).

Potassium bromate also has several non-food uses. In analytical chemistry, it is used as an oxidizing agent (Hawley, 1981), a primary standard and a brominating agent (Stenger, 1978). It is also a component of home permanent-wave neutralizing compounds (Gosselin *et al.*, 1985).

(c)   Regulatory status and guidelines

The US Food and Drug Administration (1984) requires that brominated flour contain no more than 50 mg/kg potassium bromate. This standard is also adhered to in Japan and the UK (Ito, 1982), although a maximum of 15 mg/kg bromate has been suggested in the UK recently (British Industrial Biological Research Association, 1985).

The US Food and Drug Administration (1984) allows the use of potassium bromate in the malting of barley for the production of fermented beverages or distilled spirits. The amount of bromate in the malt may not exceed 75 mg/kg and the total of inorganic bromide residues in the fermented malt beverages from all sources, including the treated malt, is limited to 25 mg/kg of bromide. No bromide tolerance is established for distilled spirits, because of evidence that bromides do not pass over in the distillation process.

The Joint FAO/WHO Expert Committee on Food Additives (WHO, 1983) recommends temporarily a maximum level of potassium bromate used to treat flour of 75 mg/kg, provided that bakery products prepared from such treated flour contain negligible residues of potassium bromate.

The American Industrial Hygiene Association (1981) has recommended that workplace environmental exposures to potassium bromate dust in air not exceed 5 mg/m³ as an eight-hour time-weighted average.

2.2 Occurrence

(a)   Natural occurrence

Potassium bromate is not known to occur as a natural product.

(b)   Occupational exposure

In a production plant, eight-hour average concentrations of 0.9-34 mg/m³ potassium bromate have been measured. During packaging, area concentrations were in excess of 100 mg/m³, requiring the use of dust respirators (American Industrial Hygiene Association, 1981).

(c) Food and beverages

Potassium bromate is added to flour to enhance the maturing process, normally at a level of about 15 mg/kg, with a range of 5-45 mg/kg (Furia, 1980). Optimal levels for bulk fermentation of dough are up to 20 mg/kg. Bulk fermentation, however, has been replaced in many cases by mechanical processes which reduce total fermentation time by more than two-thirds; for these processes, the bromate level in dough is usually increased to about 45 mg/kg (Thewlis, 1974). Food for yeast, used in quantities ranging from 0.25 to 0.50% of the flour weight, typically contains about 0.3% potassium bromate (Kulp & Hepburn, 1978).

Bushuk and Hlynka (1960) demonstrated that potassium bromate present in flour at levels from 5 to 80 mg/kg could not be detected in bread throughout baking periods of 25 min; higher concentrations can result in the presence of unchanged bromate remaining in the finished bread (Thewlis, 1974). Concentrations of <50 mg/kg potassium bromate in flour are completely converted to potassium bromide during bread-making (Lee & Tkachuk, 1960; Thewlis, 1974).

Hidaka et al. (1983) measured residual levels of potassium bromate of <1 mg/kg in fish-paste products when <350 mg/kg of potassium bromate had been added to the ingredients prior to processing. Higher levels, however, have been reported in finished products. Watanabe et al. (1982) reported 10.1 mg/kg bromate in a sample of *chikuwa* fish paste; and Abe et al. (1981) analysed samples of several different kinds of fish-paste products and found concentrations ranging from about 10 mg/kg to more than 100 mg/kg.

(c) Other

Potassium bromate has been used as a neutralizer in home permanent-wave kits at concentrations of 10-25% (Gosselin et al., 1985). Due to a number of cases of accidental poisoning in children after ingestion of such solutions, Norris (1965) indicated that most manufacturers had replaced potassium bromate with less toxic substances. Potassium bromate is still used for this purpose, however, in some countries (Matsumoto et al., 1980; Gradus et al., 1984; Kuwahara et al., 1984).

2.3 Analysis

Several iodometric titration methods are suitable for the analysis of potassium bromate. Potassium bromate in bread and other food products has been determined by extraction and iodometric titration with thiosulphate or cysteine hydrochloride, titration to a starch/iodine endpoint (WHO, 1964; Barrett et al., 1971; Barakat et al., 1973) or back-titration of excess thiosulphate with iodate using calomel and a platinum electrode (Thewlis, 1974).

Watanabe et al. (1982) reported a method for determining bromate in bread and fish-paste products, with a detection limit of 1-2 mg/kg, involving aqueous extraction, separation of bromate from interfering ionic species by ion chromatography, and quantification by ion chromatography with electrochemical detection.

3. Biological Data Relevant to the Evaluation of Carcinogenic Risk to Humans

3.1 Carcinogenicity studies in animals

(a) Oral administration

Mouse: Groups of 60 male and 60 female Theiller's original strain mice [age unspecified] were fed diets composed of 79% bread crumbs made from flour that was either untreated, treated with 50 mg/kg (low dose) or 75 mg/kg (high dose) potassium bromate (containing 10% crystalline potassium bromate with unstated inorganic diluents; Fisher *et al.*, 1979) for 80 weeks, at which time the experiment was terminated. Mortality at the end of the study period was 62-65% in males and 48-57% in females; mortality was not reported to be treatment-related. Malignant tumours occurred in various tissues in 1/35 males and 4/53 females in the control group, in 1/46 males and 0/54 females in the low-dose group, and in 0/53 males and 4/52 females in the high-dose group (Ginocchio *et al.*, 1979). [The Working Group noted that, during the baking of bread, bromates are substantially degraded.]

Rat:Groups of 90 male and 90 female Wistar weanling rats were fed diets composed of 79% bread crumbs made from flour that was either untreated or treated with 50 mg/kg (low dose) or 75 mg/kg (high dose) potassium bromate (containing 10% crystalline potassium bromate with unstated inorganic diluents) for 104 weeks. Survival at the end of the study period was >60% in males and >50% in females; mortality was not treatment-related. Malignant tumours occurred in various tissues in 4/88 males and 6/89 females in the control group, in 6/90 males and 3/89 females in the low-dose group, and in 4/88 males and 3/88 females in the high-dose group (Fisher *et al.*, 1979). [The Working Group noted that, during the baking of bread, bromates are substantially degraded.]

Groups of 52-53 male and 52-53 female Fischer 344 rats, eight weeks of age, were administered 0, 250 or 500 mg/l potassium bromate (purity, >99.5%) in the drinking-water for 110 weeks (total doses: low-dose males, 9.6 g/kg bw; high-dose males, 21.3 g/kg bw; low-dose females, 9.6 g/kg bw; and high-dose females, 19.6 g/kg bw). A greater than 2% reduction in body-weight gain was observed in high-dose animals, especially in males. Survival rates were decreased in high-dose male rats but were similar in all other groups. The first tumours were a renal-cell tumour and an oligodendroglioma of the spinal cord in a male rat at week 14, and leukaemia in a female at week 58. Treatment-related increases in the incidence of tumours of the kidney were as follows: renal adenocarcinomas — males: controls, 3/53 (6%); low-dose, 24/53 (45%, $p < 0.001$); high-dose, 44/52 (85%, $p < 0.001$); and females: controls, 0/47; low-dose, 21/50 (40%, $p < 0.001$); high-dose, 36/49 (69%, $p < 0.001$); and renal adenomas — males: controls, 0/53; low-dose, 10/53 (19%, $p < 0.01$);

high-dose, 5/52 (10%, $p < 0.01$); and females: controls, 0/47; low-dose, 8/50 (15%, $p <$ 0.01); high-dose, 9/49 (17%, $p < 0.01$). These reported incidences were based on serial sections of the entire kidney. An increase in the incidence of mesotheliomas of the peritoneum was also observed in treated males: controls, 6/53 (11%); low-dose, 17/52 (33%, $p < 0.05$); and high-dose, 28/46 (59%, $p < 0.001$). No such tumour occurred in female rats. In female rats, the incidence of benign and malignant thyroid tumours was 3/52 controls, 10/52 low-dose, and 12/52 high-dose [trend test, $p < 0.01$]. In male rats, the incidence of benign and malignant tumours of the thyroid did not differ among groups (controls, 10/53; low-dose, 14/53; high-dose, 15/52) (Kurokawa et al., 1983a). [The same data were reported by Kurokawa et al. (1982) and Ohno et al. (1982).]

(b)   Skin application

Mouse: Groups of 19 and 20 female Sencar mice, six weeks of age, received either a single application to the skin of 20 nmol 7,12-dimethylbenz[a]anthracene in 0.2 ml acetone followed one week later by weekly applications of 0.2 ml of a 40 mg/ml solution of potassium bromate for 51 weeks, or weekly applications of 0.2 ml potassium bromate solution alone for 51 weeks. No skin tumour was found in either group (Kurokawa et al., 1984). [The Working Group noted that ionic compounds such as potassium bromate are poorly absorbed through the skin and that 12-O-tetradecanoylphorbol 13-acetate and benzoyl peroxide showed promoting activity when 7,12-dimethylbenz[a]anthracene was used as the initiator.]

(c)   Administration with known carcinogens

Rat: Groups of male Fischer 344 rats, seven weeks of age, were administered drinking-water as either distilled water alone for 26 weeks (group 1); 500 or 1000 mg/l N-nitrosoethyl-N-hydroxyethylamine (NEHEA) in distilled water for two weeks followed by distilled water for 24 weeks (groups 2 and 3); 500 or 1000 mg/l NEHEA in distilled water for two weeks followed by 500 mg/l potassium bromate (99.5% pure) in distilled water for 24 weeks (groups 4 and 5); or distilled water for two weeks followed by 500 mg/l potassium bromate in distilled water for 24 weeks (group 6). All animals were killed at the end of the 26 weeks. The incidences of renal-cell tumours were: group 1 (controls), 0/19; group 2, 4/23 (17%); group 3, 9/22 (41%); group 4, 10/20 (50%); group 5, 9/19 (47%); and group 6, 0/20. Incidences of dysplastic foci of the renal tubules were: group 1, 2/19 (11%); group 2, 15/23 (65%); group 3, 17/22 (77%); group 4, 19/20 (95%; $p < 0.05$ in comparison with group 2); group 5, 19/19 (100%); and group 6, 7/20 (35%) (Kurokawa et al., 1983b).

In a subsequent study, the enhancing effect of a broad range of doses (15-500 mg/l) of potassium bromate was studied when given after 500 mg/l NEHEA in the drinking-water for two weeks. With NEHEA alone, the incidence of renal-cell tumours was 3/15 (20%). When given with 500 mg/l potassium bromate, a non-statistically significant increase in the incidence of renal-cell tumours was observed (8/15, 53%). Enhancement of dysplastic foci was observed with doses of 30 mg/l and above (Kurokawa et al., 1985). [The authors concluded that potassium bromate had an enhancing effect on the induction by NEHEA of 'dysplastic' foci and kidney tumours. The Working Group noted, however, that studies on potassium bromate alone were of too short a duration to evaluate the carcinogenicity of this chemical, that the differences in the incidences of lesions in kidneys in appropriate groups of animals exposed to NEHEA with or without subsequent exposure to potassium bromate were not large, and the p values suggest borderline significance.]

3.2 Other relevant biological data

The literature on bromates and bromides is extensive. The Working Group confined its review to reports dealing primarily with potassium bromate. The biological effects of potassium bromate have been reviewed (WHO, 1964; International Programme on Chemical Safety, 1983).

[The Working Group noted that in experiments in which animals were fed bread made from flour treated with potassium bromate, the bromate at the levels tested would have been converted to bromide.]

(a) Experimental systems

Toxic effects

The acute hypotensive effects of potassium bromate in rabbits are due to both the potassium and the bromate ions. Rabbits did not survive single intravenous injections of 0.2 g potassium bromate solution for longer than 4 min, and did not survive six intravenous injections (total dose, 1 g) longer than 43 min. Stomach damage was ascribed to the bromate ion; kidney and stomach damage were seen in guinea-pigs and dogs in experiments carried out with sodium bromate (Santesson & Wickberg, 1913).

In guinea-pigs, subcutaneous injections of 100 mg/kg bw sodium bromate produced cochlear damage by 24 h. Animals killed at that time revealed hyaline droplet degeneration, cloudy swelling and necrosis of the epithelial cells in renal tubules, which were most severe in the proximal convoluted tubules. With 200 mg/kg bw, there was more rapid onset of similar effects (Matsumoto, 1973).

Mice (Theiller's original strain) fed for 80 weeks on diets containing 79% bread crumbs prepared from flour treated with 50 or 75 mg/kg potassium bromate showed no significant alteration of blood chemistry, renal function or histopathological parameters (Ginocchio *et al.*, 1979). No adverse effect was detected in Wistar rats fed similar diets for 104 weeks (Fisher *et al.*, 1979).

Dogs (greyhounds, red Irish setters and spaniels) of each sex fed diets containing flour treated with 200 mg/kg potassium bromate for 17 months showed no ill effect (Impey *et al.*, 1961).

Effects on reproduction and prenatal toxicity

No data were available to the Working Group.

Absorption, distribution, excretion and metabolism

When mice (Theiller's original strain) received diets containing 79% bread crumbs made from flour treated with 50 or 75 mg/kg potassium bromate, concentrations of 1 and 2 mg/kg bromine, respectively, were detected in adipose tissue (Ginocchio *et al.*, 1979).

Bromine did not accumulate in the adipose tissue of Wistar rats fed for 104 weeks on diets composed of 79% bread crumbs made from flour treated with 75 mg/kg potassium bromide (Fisher *et al.*, 1979).

Mutagenicity and other short-term tests

Potassium bromate was reported to give negative results in the *Bacillus subtilis rec$^{+/-}$* assay [figures not given] (Kawachi *et al.*, 1980). At concentrations of 3.0 mg/plate, potassium bromate was mutagenic to *Salmonella typhimurium* TA100 but not TA98 in the presence of an exogenous metabolic system (S9) from the liver of polychlorinated biphenyl-induced rats (Ishidate *et al.*, 1980, 1984).

Potassium bromate (0.085-0.25 mg/ml) induced chromosomal aberrations in cultured Chinese hamster CHL cells both in the presence and absence of polychlorinated biphenyl-induced rat-liver S9 (Ishidate & Yoshikawa, 1980; Ishidate *et al.*, 1981, 1984).

Chromatid breaks were induced in cultured Chinese hamster DON-6 cells by addition of 5×10^{14}M potassium bromate (Sasaki *et al.*, 1980).

An increase in the incidence of micronucleated polychromatic erythrocytes was observed in the bone marrow of mice treated intraperitoneally with 100 mg/kg bw potassium bromate (Hayashi *et al.*, 1982). It was reported that potassium bromate induced chromosomal aberrations in rats treated *in vivo* [details not given] (Kawachi *et al.*, 1980).

(b)   Humans

Toxic effects

A number of case reports of acute poisoning by potassium bromate solutions have been reviewed (Norris, 1965). In children 1.5 to three years of age, ingestion of 2-4 oz (57-113 g) of a 2% solution of potassium bromate caused nausea and vomiting, usually with abdominal pain; diarrhoea and haematemesis occurred in some cases (Parker & Barr, 1951; Gosselin *et al.*, 1976). In both children and adults, oliguria and death from renal failure have been observed (Dunsky, 1947; Ohashi *et al.*, 1971). Hearing loss and deafness have also been reported (Matsumoto, 1973; Quick *et al.*, 1975).

Effects on reproduction and prenatal toxicity

No data were available to the Working Group.

Absorption, distribution, excretion and metabolism

No data were available to the Working Group.

Mutagenicity and chromosomal effects

No data were available to the Working Group.

3.3 Case reports and epidemiological studies of carcinogenicity to humans

No data were available to the Working Group.

4. Summary of Data Reported and Evaluation

4.1 Exposure data

Potassium bromate is used in bread-making and in the production of fish paste and fermented beverages; however, manufacturing and baking practices are available that reportedly leave little or no residual bromate in the end product. Occupational exposure to potassium bromate occurs mainly in production plants. Consumers may be exposed through the use of home permanent-wave kits with potassium bromate neutralizer solutions.

4.2 Experimental data

Potassium bromate was tested for carcinogenicity in one experiment in rats by oral administration in the drinking-water, producing renal-cell adenomas and adenocarcinomas in animals of each sex, peritoneal mesotheliomas in males and thyroid tumours in females. Experiments in mice and rats fed diets containing bread baked from flour containing potassium bromate were considered to be inadequate to evaluate the carcinogenicity of potassium bromate itself.

The incidence of renal-cell tumours in rats induced by administration of N-nitrosoethyl-N-hydroxyethylamine was increased by subsequent administration of potassium bromate.

In rats, administration of potassium bromate in the drinking-water caused tubular lesions of the kidney which were classified as dysplastic foci.

No data were available to evaluate the reproductive effects or prenatal toxicity of potassium bromate to experimental animals.

Potassium bromate was mutagenic in *Salmonella typhimurium* in the presence of an exogenous metabolic system. The compound induced chromosomal aberrations in cultured Chinese hamster cells and micronuclei in mice treated *in vivo*.

4.3 Human data

No case report or epidemiological study of the carcinogenicity of potassium bromate was available to the Working Group.

Overall assessment of data from short-term tests: Potassium bromate[a]

	Genetic activity			Cell transformation
	DNA damage	Mutation	Chromosomal effects	
Prokaryotes		+		
Fungi/Green plants				
Insects				
Mammalian cells (*in vitro*)			+	
Mammals (*in vivo*)			+	
Humans (*in vivo*)				
Degree of evidence in short-term tests for genetic activity: **Sufficient**				Cell transformation: No data

[a]The groups into which the table is divided and the symbol used are defined on pp. 19-20 of the Preamble; the degrees of evidence are defined on pp. 20-21.

4.4 Evaluation[1,2]

There is *sufficient evidence*[3] for the carcinogenicity of potassium bromate in experimental animals.

No data were available on the carcinogenicity of potassium bromate to humans.

5. References

Abe, M., Ogawa, T. & Sakabe, Y. (1981) Contents of total bromide in fish paste products (Jpn.). *Nagoya-shi Eisei Kenkyusho HO, 28*, 48-50 [*Chem. Abstr., 99*, 52005u]

AmeriBrom, Inc. (undated) *Potassium Bromate Technical Bulletin*, New York

American Industrial Hygiene Association (1981) Workplace environmental exposure level guide. Potassium bromate. *Am. ind. Hyg. Assoc. J., 42*, A-53 - A-55

---

[1]For definition of the italicized term, see Preamble, p. 18.

[2]After the meeting, the Secretariat became aware of a study in which 9% of male hamsters administered potassium bromate in the drinking-water developed kidney tumours (Takamura *et al.*, 1986).

[3]In the absence of data on humans, it is reasonable, for practical purposes, to regard chemicals or exposures for which there is *sufficient evidence* of carcinogenicity in animals as if they presented a carcinogenic risk to humans.

American International Chemical, Inc. (undated) *Potassium Bromate Specification Sheet*, Natick, MA

Anon. (1983) Bromates. *Chem. Mark. Rep.*, *224*, 20

Barakat, M.Z., Abou-El Makarem, M. & Abdel-Aziz, S. (1973) Cysteinimetry. Determination of potassium bromate content of buffalo milk. *J. Sci. Food Agric.*, *24*, 1175-1180

Barrett, S., Croft, A.G. & Hartley, A. (1971) Determination of cysteine hydrochloride, ascorbic acid and potassium bromate in admixture in bread improver formulations. *J. Sci. Food Agric.*, *22*, 173-175

British Industrial Biological Research Association (1985) Code of practice for bromate in flour. *BIBRA Bull.*, *24*, 85

Bushuk, W. & Hlynka, I. (1960) Disappearance of bromate during baking of bread. *Cereal Chem.*, *37*, 573-575

The Chemical Daily Co. (1980) *JCW Chemicals Guide*, Tokyo, p. 291

Dunsky, I. (1947) Potassium bromate poisoning. *Am. J. Dis. Child.*, *74*, 730-734

Fisher, N., Hutchinson, J.B., Berry, R., Hardy, J., Ginocchio, A.V. & Waite, V. (1979) Long-term toxicity and carcinogenicity studies of the bread improver potassium bromate. 1. Studies in rats. *Food Cosmet. Toxicol.*, *17*, 33-39

Furia, T. (1980) *Food additives.* In: Mark, H.F., Othmer, D.F., Overberger, C.H. & Seaborg, G.T., eds, *Kirk-Othmer Encyclopedia of Chemical Technology*, 3rd ed., Vol. 11, New York, John Wiley & Sons, pp. 146-163

Ginocchio, A.V., Waite, V., Hardy, J., Fisher, N., Hutchinson, J.B. & Berry, R. (1979) Long-term toxicity and carcinogenicity studies of the bread improver potassium bromate. 2. Studies in mice. *Food Cosmet. Toxicol.*, *17*, 41-47

Gosselin, R.E., Hodge, H.C., Smith, R.P. & Gleason, M.N. (1976) *Clinical Toxicology of Commercial Products: Acute Poisoning*, 4th ed., Baltimore, MD, Williams & Wilkins, p. 66

Gosselin, R.E., Smith, R.P. & Hodge, H.C. (1985) *Clinical Toxicology of Commercial Products*, 5th ed., Baltimore, MD, Williams & Wilkins, p. VI-46

Gradus, D.B.-Z., Rhoads, M., Bergstrom, L.B. & Jordan, S.C. (1984) Acute bromate poisoning associated with renal failure and deafness presenting as hemolytic uremic syndrome. *Am. J. Nephrol.*, *4*, 188-191

Hawley, G.G., ed. (1981) *The Condensed Chemical Dictionary*, 10th ed., New York, Van Nostrand Reinhold, p. 846

Hayashi, M., Sofuni, T. & Ishidate, M., Jr (1982) High-sensitivity in micronucleus induction of a mouse strain (MS). *Mutat. Res.*, *105*, 253-256

Hidaka, T., Kirigaya, T., Kamijo, M., Suzuki, Y. & Kawamura, T. (1983) Studies on potassium bromate in foods. II. Behavior of potassium bromate added to bread and fish paste products during preparation (Jpn.). *Shokuhin Eiseigaku Zasshi*, *24*, 383-389 [*Chem. Abstr.*, *100*, 50167p]

IARC (1982) *IARC Monographs on the Evaluation of the Carcinogenic Risk of Chemicals to Humans*, Suppl. 4, *Chemicals, Industrial Processes and Industries Associated with Cancer in Humans, IARC Monographs, Volumes 1 to 29*, Lyon, pp. 50-51, 149-150

Impey, S.G., Moore, T. & Sharman, I.M. (1961) Effects of flour treatment on the suitability of bread as food for dogs. *J. Sci. Food Agric.*, *11*, 729-732

International Programme on Chemical Safety (1983) *Toxicological Evaluation of Certain Food Additives and Food Contaminants (WHO Food Add. Ser. No. 18)*, Geneva, pp. 110-117

Ishidate, M., Jr & Yoshikawa, K. (1980) Chromosome aberration tests with Chinese hamster cells in vitro with and without metabolic activation — a comparative study on mutagens and carcinogens. *Arch. Toxicol., Suppl. 4*, 41-44

Ishidate, M., Jr, Sofuni, T. & Yoshikawa, K. (1980) A primary screening for mutagenicity of food additives in Japan. *Mutagens Toxicol.*, *3*, 82-90

Ishidate, M., Jr, Sofuni, T. & Yoshikawa, K. (1981) Chromosomal aberration tests *in vitro* as a primary screening tool for environmental mutagens and/or carcinogens. *Gann Monogr.*, *27*, 95-108

Ishidate, M., Jr, Sofuni, T., Yoshikawa, K., Hayashi, M., Nohmi, T., Sawada, M. & Matsuoka, A. (1984) Primary mutagenicity screening of food additives currently used in Japan. *Food chem. Toxicol.*, *22*, 623-636

Ito, R. (1982) New considerations on hydrogen peroxide and related substances as food additives in view of carcinogenicity. *Paediatrician*, *II*, 222-224

Kawachi, T., Yahagi, T., Kada, T., Tazima, Y., Ishidate, M., Sasaki, M. & Sugimura, T. (1980) *Cooperative programme on short-term assays for carcinogenicity in Japan*. In: Montesano, R., Bartsch, H. & Tomatis, L., eds, *Molecular and Cellular Aspects of Carcinogen Screening Tests (IARC Scientific Publications No. 27)*, Lyon, International Agency for Research on Cancer, pp. 323-330

E.B. Knight, Inc. (1975) *Material Safety Data Sheet — Potassium Bromate (Form No. 101-39-75)*, Toms River, NJ

E.B. Knight, Inc. (undated) *Potassium Bromate Specification Sheet*, Toms River, NJ

Kulp, K. & Hepburn, F.N. (1978) *Bakery processes and leavening agents*. In: Mark, H.F., Othmer, D.F., Overberger, C.G. & Seaborg, G.T., eds, *Kirk-Othmer Encyclopedia of Chemical Technology*, 3rd ed., Vol. 3, New York, John Wiley & Sons, pp. 438-449

Kurokawa, Y., Hayashi, Y., Maekawa, A., Takahashi, M. & Kokubo, T. (1982) Induction of renal cell tumors in F-344 rats by oral administration of potassium bromate, a food additive. *Gann*, *73*, 335-338

Kurokawa, Y., Hayashi, Y., Maekawa, A., Takahashi, T., Kokuba, T. & Odashima, S. (1983a) Carcinogenicity of potassium bromate administered orally to F344 rats. *J. natl Cancer Inst.*, *71*, 965-972

Kurokawa, Y., Takahashi, M., Kokubo, T., Ohno, Y. & Hayashi, Y. (1983b) Enhancement by potassium bromate of renal tumorigenesis initiated by N-ethyl-N-hydroxyethyl-nitrosamine in F-344 rats. *Gann*, *74*, 607-610

Kurokawa, Y., Takamura, M., Matsushima, Y., Imazawa, T. & Hayashi, Y. (1984) Studies on the promoting and complete carcinogenic activities of some oxidizing chemicals in skin carcinogenesis. *Cancer Lett.*, *24*, 299-304

Kurokawa, Y., Aoki, S., Imazawa, T., Hayashi, Y., Matsushima, Y. & Takamura, N. (1985) Dose-related enhancing effect of potassium bromate on renal tumorigenesis in rats initiated with *N*-ethyl-*N*-hydroxyethylnitrosamine. *Jpn. J. Cancer Res. (Gann)*, *76*, 583-589

Kuwahara, T., Ikehara, Y., Kanatsu, K., Doi, T., Nagai, H., Nakayashiki, H., Tamura, T. & Kawai, C. (1984) 2 Cases of potassium bromate poisoning requiring long-term hemodialysis therapy for irreversible tubular damage. *Nephron*, *37*, 278-280

Lee, C.C. & Tkachuk, R. (1960) Addendum: disappearance of bromate during baking of bread. *Cereal Chem.*, *37*, 575-576

Matsumoto, I. (1973) Clinical and experimental studies on ototoxicity of bromate (Jpn.). *Otol. Fukuoka*, *19*, 220-236

Matsumoto, I., Morizono, T. & Paparella, M.M. (1980) Hearing loss following potassium bromate: two case reports. *Otolaryngol. Head Neck Surg.*, *88*, 625-629

National Research Council (1981) *Potassium bromate*. In: *Food Chemicals Codex*, 3rd ed., Washington DC, National Academy of Sciences, p. 240

Norris, J.A. (1965) Toxicity of home permanent waving and neutralizer solutions. *Food Cosmet. Toxicol.*, *3*, 93-97

Ohashi, N., Shiba, T., Kamiya, K. & Takamura, T. (1971) Acute renal failure following potassium bromate ('cold wave' neutralizer) poisoning (recovery from prolonged oliguria) (Jpn.). *Jpn. J. Urol.*, *62*, 639-646

Ohno, Y., Onodera, H., Takamura, N., Imazawa, T., Maekawa, A. & Kurokawa, Y. (1982) Carcinogenicity testing of potassium bromate in F-344 rats (Jpn.). *Eisei Shikenjo Hokoku*, *100*, 93-100

Parker, W.A. & Barr, J.R. (1951) Potassium bromate poisoning. *Br. med. J.*, *i*, 1363-1364

Quick, C.A., Chole, R.A. & Mauer, S.M. (1975) Deafness and renal failure due to potassium bromate poisoning. *Arch. Otolaryngol.*, *101*, 494-495

Sadtler Research Laboratories (1967) *Inorganics and Related Compounds — IR Grating Spectra*, Vol. 1, Philadelphia, PA

Santesson, C.G. & Wickberg, G. (1913) On the action of sodium bromate (Ger.). *Scand. Arch. Physiol.*, *30*, 337-374

Sasaki, M., Sugimura, K., Yoshida, M.A. & Abe, S. (1980) Cytogenetic effects of 60 chemicals on cultured human and Chinese hamster cells. *Kromosomo*, *II:20*, 574-584

Sax, N.I. (1984) *Dangerous Properties of Industrial Materials*, 6th ed., New York, Van Nostrand Reinhold Co., p. 518

Sfat, M.R. & Doncheck, J.A. (1981) *Malts and malting*. In: Mark, H.F., Othmer, D.F., Overberger, C.G. & Seaborg, G.T., eds, *Kirk-Othmer Encyclopoedia of Chemical Technology*, 3rd ed., Vol. 14, New York, John Wiley & Sons, pp. 810-823

Stenger, V.A. (1978) *Bromine compounds*. In: Mark, H.F., Othmer, D.F., Overberger, C.G. & Seaborg, G.T., eds, *Kirk-Othmer Encyclopedia of Chemical Technology*, 3rd ed., Vol. 4, New York, John Wiley & Sons, pp. 243-263

Takamura, N., Kurokawa, T., Matsushima, T., Imazawa, T., Onodera, H. & Hayashi, Y. (1986) Long-term oral administration of potassium bromate in male Syrian golden hamsters. *Sci. Rep. Res. Inst. Tokohu Univ. Ser. C, 32*, 43-46

Thewlis, B.H. (1974) The fate of potassium bromate when used as a breadmaking improver. *J. Sci. Food Agric., 25*, 1471-1475

US Food and Drug Administration (1984) Food and drugs. *US Code fed. Regul., Title 21*, Parts 137.155, 172.730

Watanabe, I., Tanaka, R. & Kashimoto, T. (1982) Determination of potassium bromate by ion chromatography (Jpn.). *Shokuhin Eiseigaku Zasshi, 23*, 135-141 [*Chem. Abstr., 97*, 180268c]

Weast, R.C., ed. (1985) *CRC Handbook of Chemistry and Physics*, 66th ed., Boca Raton, FL, CRC Press, p. B-126

WHO (1964) *7th Report of the Joint FAO/WHO Expert Committee on Food Additives. Specifications for the Identity and Purity of Food Additives and their Toxicological Evaluation: Emulsifiers, Stabilisers, Bleaching and Maturing Agents (WHO Tech. Rep. Ser. No. 281)*, Geneva, pp. 164-167

WHO (1983) *Evaluation of Certain Food Additives and Contaminants. Twenty-seventh Report of the Joint FAO/WHO Expert Committee on Food Additives (Tech. Rep. Series No. 696)*, Geneva, pp. 27-28

Windholz, M., ed. (1983) *The Merck Index*, 10th ed., Rahway, NJ, Merck & Co., p. 1099

AMINO ACID PYROLYSIS PRODUCTS IN FOOD

Glu-P-1 (2-AMINO-6-METHYLDIPYRIDO[1,2-*a*:3′,2′-*d*]IMIDAZOLE)

1. Chemical and Physical Data

1.1 Synonyms and trade names

Chem. Abstr. Services Reg. No.: 67730-11-4

Chem. Abstr. Name: 6-Methyldipyrido[1,2-*a*:3′,2′-*d*]imidazol-2-amine

IUPAC Systematic Name: 2-Amino-6-methyldipyrido[1,2-*a*:3′,2′-*d*]imidazole

1.2 Structural and molecular formulae and molecular weight

$C_{11}H_{10}N_4$ Mol. wt: 198.23

1.3 Chemical and physical properties of the pure substance

(*a*) *Description*: Yellow prisms (Takeda *et al.*, 1978)

(*b*) *Melting-point*: 226°C (Takeda *et al.*, 1978); 290-292°C (hydrobromide salt) (Takeda *et al.*, 1978; Sugimura *et al.*, 1981)

(*c*) *Spectroscopy data*: Ultraviolet, fluorescence (Peters *et al.*, 1981; Sugimura *et al.*, 1981), C-13 nuclear magnetic resonance (Aboul-Enein, 1983), proton nuclear magnetic resonance and mass spectral data (Sugimura *et al.*, 1981) have been reported.

(*d*) *Solubility*: Soluble in dimethyl sulphoxide and chloroform (Yamamoto *et al.*, 1978; Hayatsu *et al.*, 1983; Schunk *et al.*, 1984) (*e*) *Stability*: Stable under moderately acidic and alkaline conditions and in cold dilute aqueous solutions protected from light (Sugimura *et al.*, 1983)

(*f*) *Reactivity*: Rapidly converted to an azo dimer by dilute hypochlorite. Deactivated by weakly acidic nitrite solution with replacement of the 2-amino group by hydroxyl (Sugimura *et al.*, 1983)

2. Production, Use, Occurrence and Analysis

2.1 Production and use

(*a*) *Production*

Glu-P-1 was first isolated by Yamamoto *et al.* (1978) from the pyrolysis products of L-glutamic acid.

Takeda *et al.* (1978) reported the development of a reaction sequence for the synthesis of L-glutamic acid pyrolysis products, including Glu-P-1. In this process, 3-amino-8-methylimidazo[1,2-*a*]pyridine, 2-chloroacrylonitrile and aluminium chloride in nitrobenzene are heated at 100°C for 12 h. Glu-P-1 is isolated from the reaction products by multiple extractions, column chromatography on silica gel and crystallization from methanol-ethyl acetate.

Glu-P-1 is not produced in commercial or bulk quantities.

(*b*) *Use*

Glu-P-1 is not used commercially.

2.2 Occurrence

Glu-P-1 is not known to occur in nature.

Glu-P-1 has been identified among the pyrolysis products of L-glutamic acid at a level of 1 mg/kg (Yamamoto *et al.*, 1978). It has also been detected at low levels (estimate = 3-4 μg/100 mg) in casein pyrolysate (Yamaguchi *et al.*, 1979).

2.3 Analysis

Glu-P-1 was isolated from the pyrolysis products of L-glutamic acid by chloroform extraction, followed by column and thin-layer chromatography (Yamamoto *et al.*, 1978). The structure was determined by mass spectrometry, elemental analysis and X-ray crystallography.

Glu-P-1 can be adsorbed selectively from aqueous solutions onto cellulose or cotton to which C.I. Reactive Blue 21, a trisulpho-copper phthalocyanine dye, has been bound covalently. The adsorbed Glu-P-1 is eluted with ammoniacal methanol and quantified by adsorption spectrum (Hayatsu *et al.*, 1983).

Glu-P-1 has been separated from other amino acid pyrolysis products by gas chromatography using fused silica capillary columns and flame-ionization detection (Schunk *et al.*, 1984). High-performance liquid chromatography with ultraviolet and fluorescence detection has also been used to separate Glu-P-1 from Glu-P-2 and other protein and amino acid pyrolysates (Peters *et al.*, 1981).

3. Biological Data Relevant to the Evaluation of Carcinogenic Risk to Humans

3.1 Carcinogenicity studies in animals

Oral administration

Mouse: Groups of 40 male and 40 female CDF$_1$ [(BALB/cAnN × DBA/2N)F$_1$)] mice [age unspecified] were fed a pelleted diet containing 500 mg/kg Glu-P-1 hydrochloride (purity confirmed by high-performance liquid chromatography [percentage not indicated]) for 475 days, at which time the experiment was terminated. A group of 40 males and 40 females was fed basal diet alone and served as controls. [The Working Group noted that this group was used as the controls for several other experiments on similar chemicals.] The first blood-vessel tumour was observed on day 301 after the start of the experiment, at which time 34/40 treated males, 38/40 treated females, 39/40 control males and 40/40 control females were still alive. The mean survival of control females was 658 ± 55 days and that of control males 586 ± 109 days; mean survival for treated females was 398 ± 35 days and for males 331 ± 78 days. Blood-vessel tumours, which occurred at various sites and which were diagnosed as haemangioendotheliomas or haemangioendothelial sarcomas, were observed in 30/34 (88%) treated males and 31/38 (82%) treated females; no such tumour was found in control mice ($p < 0.001$). Most of the blood-vessel tumours were haemangioendothelial sarcomas (males, 27/30; females, 28/31). Liver tumours were also observed in 4/34 (12%) treated males and 37/38 (97%) treated females; no such tumour was found in control mice ($p < 0.001$ for females). Of the liver tumours observed in females, 13 were hepatocellular adenomas and 24 were hepatocellular carcinomas; only liver adenomas were observed in males (Ohgaki *et al.*, 1984).

Rat: Groups of 42 male and 42 female Fischer 344 rats, eight weeks of age, were fed a pelleted diet containing 500 mg/kg Glu-P-1 hydrochloride (purity confirmed by high-performance liquid chromatography [percentage not indicated]) for 104 weeks, at which time the experiment was terminated. A group of 50 males and 50 females were fed basal diet and served as controls. [The Working Group noted that this control group was also used in a test on Glu-P-2.] By weeks 50 to 60, approximately 50% of treated rats had died due to early development of tumours of the liver, intestine, Zymbal gland, brain and clitoral gland. The first liver tumour was observed in a female rat on day 277; liver tumours were observed in

35/42 (83%) treated males and 24/42 (57%) treated females. Most liver tumours were hepatocellular carcinomas. Three male rats had pulmonary metastases. The first tumour of the small intestine was observed in a male rat on day 300; by week 104, tumours of the small intestine (adenomas and adenocarcinomas) were observed in 26/42 (62%) treated males and 10/42 (24%) treated females. Tumours of the colon (adenomas and adenocarcinomas) were observed in 19/42 (45%) treated males and 7/42 (17%) treated females. Tumours of both the large and small intestines were found at multiple sites. Squamous-cell carcinomas of the Zymbal-gland, with local invasion, were observed in 18/42 (43%) treated males and 18/42 (43%) treated females. Clitoral-gland tumours were found in 5/42 (12%) treated females. [The increases in the incidences of tumours of the liver, intestines and Zymbal gland were statistically significant when compared to controls ($p < 0.001$), as was the increased incidence of clitoral-gland tumours ($p < 0.05$)]. Only two liver tumours were seen in male controls (Takayama *et al.*, 1984).

3.2 Other relevant biological data

(a) Experimental systems

Toxic effects

A group of male Fischer 344 rats received seven intraperitoneal injections of 20 mg/kg bw Glu-P-1 dissolved in dimethyl sulphoxide (DMSO) at one-week intervals; after one week of Glu-P-1 treatment they received a partial hepatectomy; during weeks 8 and 9 they were fed a diet containing 200 mg/kg 2-acetylaminofluorene; and, at the end of week 8, they were administered 1 ml/kg bw carbon tetrachloride by gavage. All animals were killed at the end of week 10. A control group received intraperitoneal injections of DMSO alone, followed by the same treatment. Statistically significant increases in the number and area of γ-glutamyl transpeptidase-positive liver-cell foci were observed in treated animals, compared to controls. When rats were fed diets containing 200 mg/kg 2-acetylaminofluorene for two weeks and administered 1 ml/kg bw carbon tetrachloride at the end of week 1, followed by seven intraperitoneal injections of 20 mg/kg bw Glu-P-1 in DMSO during weeks 4 to 9, with partial hepatectomy at the end of week 4, no increase in γ-glutamyl transpeptidase-positive liver-cell foci was found in treated animals compared to DMSO-treated controls (Tamano *et al.*, 1981).

Groups of male Fischer 344 rats received a partial hepatectomy, followed 18 h later by a single intraperitoneal injection of 2.5, 10 or 40 mg/kg bw Glu-P-1 dissolved in DMSO; animals were then fed a diet containing 200 mg/kg 2-acetylaminofluorene during weeks 3 and 4 and received 1 ml/kg bw carbon tetrachloride by gavage at the end of week 3. All animals were killed at the end of week 5. Dose-dependent increases in the number and area of γ-glutamyl transpeptidase-positive liver-cell foci were found in treated animals compared to controls that received an intraperitoneal injection of DMSO alone 18 h after partial hepatectomy, followed by treatment with 2-acetylaminofluorene (Tamano *et al.*, 1981).

Effects on reproduction and prenatal toxicity

No data were available to the Working Group.

Absorption, distribution, excretion and metabolism

The distribution of ^{14}C-Glu-P-1 was examined in male Fischer 344 rats after a single oral dose (21 mg/kg bw). At 24 and 48 h, the only organs with detectable radioactivity were liver and kidney. Radioactivity was found in urine (30%), faeces (50%) and bile (70%) at 24 h (Negishi *et al.*, 1984). In the bile, *N*-acetyl-Glu-P-1 was identified as one of the four putative metabolites of Glu-P-1. The fact that metabolic activation with bile from Glu-P-1-treated rats resulted in mutagenic effects in *Salmonella typhimurium* TA98 is evidence for bioactivation of this compound (Sato *et al.*, 1986). In male Fischer 344 rats that received 21 mg/kg bw ^{14}C-Glu-P-1 by gavage, 0.2% remained in the blood after 26 days. At 24 h, two-thirds of the radioactivity was bound to plasma albumin and the remainder to haemoglobin (Umemoto *et al.*, 1985).

The suggested overall metabolism of Glu-P-1 in mice and rats *in vivo*, leading to modification of DNA, is shown in Figure 1. Formation of the major oxidized metabolite, *N*-hydroxy-Glu-P-1, has been shown to be mediated by the hepatic microsomal cytochrome P450 system (Ishii *et al.*, 1981), although prostaglandin synthetase has been suggested as an alternative (Nemoto & Takayama, 1984). The cytochrome P450 isoenzymes induced by 3-methylcholanthrene or polychlorinated biphenyls were most active in this conversion (Nebert *et al.*, 1979; Ishii *et al.*, 1981; Watanabe *et al.*, 1982). The capacities of various species of cytochrome P450 purified from rat liver microsomes to convert Glu-P-1 to a direct mutagen were closely correlated with their *N*-hydroxylation activities (Kato *et al.*, 1983).

N-Hydroxy-Glu-P-1 is further activated chemically by acetylation, or *O*-acylation (possibly acetylation, aminoacylation, phosphorylation or sulphation) with cytosol enzymes, and the resulting *N*-*O*-acyl-Glu-P-1 reacts effectively with DNA (Hashimoto *et al.*, 1982a; Nagao *et al.*, 1983a). Thus, *N*-*O*-acyl-Glu-P-1 is an ultimate form of Glu-P-1 that reacts with DNA at the C8 position of guanine (Hashimoto *et al.*, 1982a).

Mutagenicity and other short-term tests

Glu-P-1 (tested in the range of 1-500 μg/plate) induced prophage λ in lysogenic *Escherichia coli* K12 in the presence of an exogenous metabolic system (S9) (Nagao *et al.*, 1983b). It was mutagenic in *Salmonella typhimurium* TA98 and TA100 in the presence of S9 from various mammalian species (Yamamoto *et al.*, 1978; Matsushima *et al.*, 1980; Takeda *et al.*, 1980; Ishii *et al.*, 1981; Peters *et al.*, 1981).

Glu-P-1 gave positive results in a wing spot test in *Drosophila melanogaster* (transheterozygous for the loci *mwh* and *flr*) raised in a medium containing 0.1-0.8 mg/g (Yoo *et al.*, 1985).

It was reported that Glu-P-1 (tested at up to 10[-3]M) did not induce unscheduled DNA synthesis in a short-term organ culture of rat tracheal epithelium [figures not given] (Ide *et al.*, 1981).

Fig. 1. Suggested metabolism of Glu-P-1 in mice and rats[a]

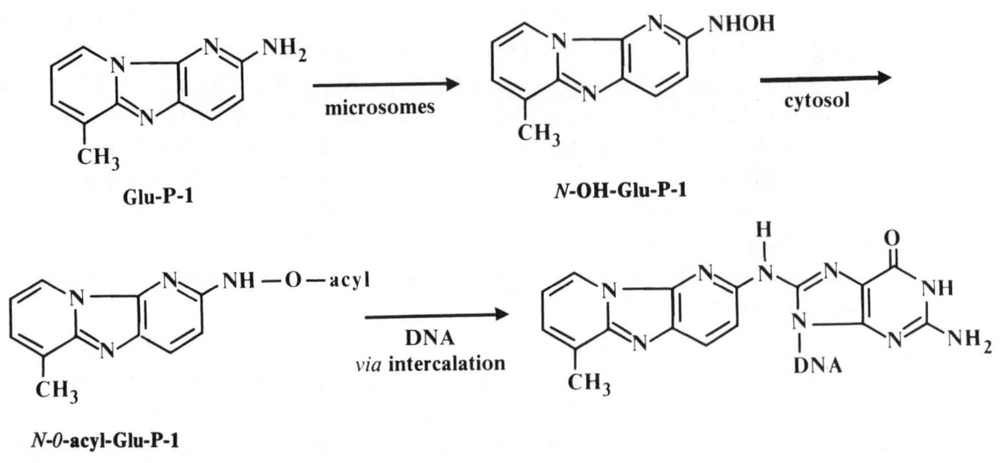

[a]From Hashimoto et al. (1982a)

Glu-P-1 (0.3-30 μg/ml) induced 8-azaguanine-resistant mutants in cultured embryonic human diploid cells (Kuroda, 1980), and, in the presence of polychlorinated biphenyl-induced rat liver S9, resulted in diphtheria toxin-resistant mutants in cultured Chinese hamster lung cells at 250-750 μg/ml (Nakayasu et al., 1983). However, it did not induce ouabain-resistant mutants in Chinese hamster V79 cells at a concentration of up to 100 μg/ml in the presence of a Syrian hamster embryo cell feeder layer (Takayama & Tanaka, 1983).

Glu-P-1 (0.25 and 0.5 mg/ml) induced chromosomal aberrations in cultured Chinese hamster lung cells without metabolic activation (Ishidate, 1983). At concentrations of $1 - 5 \times 10^{-5}$ M, Glu-P-1 induced a dose-dependent increase in the incidence of sister chromatid exchanges in human lymphoblastoid NL3 cells in the presence of polychlorinated biphenyl induced rat-liver S9 (Tohda et al., 1980).

Glu-P-1 (10 and 20 μg/ml) induced morphological transformation of Syrian hamster embryo cells in vitro in the presence of primary feeder cells (Takayama et al., 1979).

Following intraperitoneal administration of 25 mg/kg bw Glu-P-1 to male Wistar rats, modified DNA and RNA were isolated from liver (Hashimoto et al., 1982b).

Glu-P-1 (18 mg/kg bw administered intraperitoneally on days 8, 9 and 10 of pregnancy) gave positive results in the mouse spot test (Jensen, 1983).

(*b*)   *Humans*

No data were available to the Working Group.

3.3 Case reports and epidemiological studies of carcinogenicity in humans

No data were available to the Working Group.

4. Summary of Data Reported and Evaluation

4.1 Exposure data

Glu-P-1 (2-amino-6-methyldipyrido[1,2-*a*:3′,2′-*d*]imidazole) is found at low levels among the pyrolysis products of L-glutamic acid and casein, and human exposure may occur by ingestion of cooked foods containing these substances.

4.2 Experimental data

Glu-P-1 was tested for carcinogenicity in one experiment in mice and one experiment in rats by oral administration in the diet. It produced haemangioendotheliomas and haemangioendothelial sarcomas at various sites and hepatocellular adenomas in mice of each sex and liver carcinomas in female mice.In rats, it produced benign and malignant tumours of the liver, intestines and Zymbal gland in animals of each sex and tumours of the clitoral gland in females.

No data were available to evaluate the reproductive effects or prenatal toxicity of this compound to experimental animals.

Glu-P-1 induced prophage in bacteria. It was mutagenic in *Salmonella typhimurium* in the presence of an exogenous metabolic system, and gave positive results in the wing spot test in *Drosophila melanogaster*. Glu-P-1 induced mutations, chromosomal aberrations, sister chromatid exchanges and morphological transformation in cultured mammalian cells. It induced DNA damage in rats treated *in vivo* and positive results in the mouse spot test.

4.3 Human data

No case report or epidemiological study of the carcinogenicity of Glu-P-1 was available to the Working Group.

Overall assessment of data from short-term tests: Glu-P-1[a]

	Genetic activity			Cell transformation
	DNA damage	Mutation	Chromosomal effects	
Prokaryotes	+	+		
Fungi/Green plants				
Insects		+		
Mammalian cells (*in vitro*)		+	+	+
Mammals (*in vivo*)	+	+		
Humans (*in vivo*)				
Degree of evidence in short-term tests for genetic activity: **Sufficient**				Cell transformation: Positive

[a]The groups into which the table is divided and the symbol used are defined on pp. 19-20 of the Preamble; the degrees of evidence are defined on pp. 20-21.

4.4 Evaluation[1]

There is *sufficient evidence*[2] for the carcinogenicity of Glu-P-1 to experimental animals.

No data were available on the carcinogenicity of Glu-P-1 to humans.

5. References

Aboul-Enein, H.Y. (1983) Carbon-13 NMR of some mutagenic 2-aminodipyrido[1,2-a:3',2'-d]imidazoles. *Spectrosc. Lett.*, 16, 109-115

Hashimoto, Y., Shudo, K. & Okamoto, T. (1982a) Modification of DNA with potent mutacarcinogenic 2-amino-6-methyldipyrido[1,2-a:3',2'-d]imidazole isolated from a glutamic acid pyrolysate: structure of the modified nucleic acid base and initial chemical event caused by the mutagen. *J. Am. chem. Soc.*, 104, 7636-7640

[1]For definition of the italicized term, see Preamble, p. 18.

[2]In the absence of data on humans, it is reasonable, for practical purposes, to regard chemicals or exposures for which there is *sufficient evidence* of carcinogenicity in animals as if they presented a carcinogenic risk to humans.

Hashimoto, Y., Shudo, K. & Okamoto, T. (1982b) Modification of nucleic acids with muta-carcinogenic heteroaromatic amines in vivo: identification of modified bases in DNA extracted from rats injected with 3-amino-1-methyl-5H-pyrido[4,3-b]indole and 2-amino-6-methyldipyrido-[1,2-a:3',2'-d]imidazole. *Mutat. Res., 105*, 9-13

Hayatsu, H., Oka, T., Wakata, A., Ohara, Y., Hayatsu, T., Kobayashi, H. & Arimoto, S. (1983) Adsorption of mutagens to cotton bearing covalently bound trisulfo-copper-phthalocyanine. *Mutat. Res., 119*, 233-238

Ide, F., Ishikawa, T. & Takayama, S. (1981) Detection of chemical carcinogens by assay of unscheduled DNA synthesis in rat tracheal epithelium in short-term organ culture. *J. Cancer Res. clin. Oncol., 102*, 115-126

Ishidate, M., Jr (1983) *Chromosomal Aberration Test* in vitro, Tokyo, Realize Inc., p. 255

Ishii, K., Yamazoe, Y., Kamataki, T. & Kato, R. (1981) Metabolic activation of glutamic acid pyrolysis products, 2-amino-6-methyldipyrido[1,2-a:3'c1,2'-d]imidazole and 2-amino-dipyrido[1,2-a:3',2'-d]imidazole, by purified cytochrome P-450. *Chem.-biol. Interactions, 38*, 1-13

Jensen, N.J. (1983) Pyrolytic products from tryptophan and glutamic acid are positive in the mammalian spot test. *Cancer Lett., 20*, 241-244

Kato, R., Kamataki, T. & Yamazoe, Y. (1983) N-Hydroxylation of carcinogenic and mutagenic amines. *Environ. Health Perspect., 49*, 21-25

Kuroda, Y. (1980) Mutagenic activity of Trp-P-2 and Glu-P-1 on embryonic human diploid cells in culture. *Natl Inst. Genet. Jpn. annu. Rep., 31*, 45-46

Matsushima, T., Yahagi, T., Takamoto, Y., Nagao, M. & Sugimura, T. (1980) *Species differences in microsomal activation of mutagens and carcinogens, with special references to new potent mutagens from pyrolysates of amino acids and proteins.* In: Coon, M.J., Conney, A.H., Estabrook, R.W., Gelboin, H.V., Gillette, J.R. & O'Brien, P.J., eds, *Microsomes, Drug Oxidations and Chemical Carcinogenesis*, Vol. 2, New York, Academic Press, pp. 1093-1102

Nagao, M., Fujita, Y., Wakabayashi, K. & Sugimura, T. (1983a) Ultimate forms of mutagenic and carcinogenic heterocyclic amines produced by pyrolysis. *Biochem. biophys. Res. Commun., 114*, 626-631

Nagao, M., Sato, S. & Sugimura, T. (1983b) *Mutagens produced by heating foods.* In: Waller, G.R. & Feather, M.S., eds, *The Maillard Reaction in Foods and Nutrition (ACS Symposium Series 215)*, Washington DC, American Chemical Society, pp. 521-536

Nakayama, M., Nakasato, F., Sakamoto, H., Terada, M. & Sugimura, T. (1983) Mutagenic activity of heterocyclic amines in Chinese hamster lung cells with diphtheria toxin resistance as a marker. *Mutat. Res., 118*, 91-102

Nebert, D.W., Bigelow, S.W., Okey, A.B., Yahagi, T., Mori, Y., Nagao, M. & Sugimura, T. (1979) Pyrolysis products from amino acids and protein: highest mutagenicity requires cytochrome P_1-450. *Proc. natl Acad. Sci., 76*, 5929-5933

Negishi, C., Sato, S., Sugimura, T. & Rafter, J.J. (1984) *Distribution, excretion and metabolism of Glu-P-1, a carcinogenic glutamic acid pyrolysis product, in rat (Abstract No. 1).* In: *Proceedings of the Japanese Cancer Association, 43rd Annual Meeting,* Tokyo, Japanese Cancer Association, p. 29

Nemoto, N. & Takayama, S. (1984) Activation of 2-amino-6-methyldipyrido[1,2-*a*:3',2'-*d*]imidazole, a mutagenic pyrolysis product of glutamic acid, to bind to microsomal protein by NADPH-dependent and independent enzyme systems. *Carcinogenesis, 5,* 653-656

Ohgaki, H., Matsukura, N., Morino, K., Kawachi, T., Sugimura, T. & Takayama, S. (1984) Carcinogenicity in mice of mutagenic compounds from glutamic acid and soybean globulin pyrolysates. *Carcinogenesis, 5,* 815-819

Peters, J.H., Mortelmans, K.E., Reist, E.J., Sigman, C.C., Spanggord, R.J. & Thomas, D.W. (1981) Synthesis, chemical characterization, and mutagenic activities of pro-mutagens produced by pyrolysis of proteinaceous substances. *Environ. Mutagenesis, 3,* 639-649

Sato, S., Negishi, C., Umemoto, A. & Sugimura, T. (1986) Metabolic aspects of pyrolysis mutagens in food. *Environ. Health Perspect., 67* (in press)

Schunk, H., Hayashi, T. & Shibamoto, T. (1984) Analysis of mutagenic amino acid pyrolyzates with a fused silica capillary column. *J. high Resolut. Chromatogr. Chromatogr. Commun., 7,* 563-565

Sugimura, T., Nagao, M. & Wakabayashi, K. (1981) *Mutagenic heterocyclic amines in cooked food.* In: Egan, H., Fishbein, L., Castegnaro, M., O'Neill, I.K. & Bartsch, H., eds, *Environmental Carcinogens Selected Methods of Analysis,* Vol. 4, *Some Aromatic and Azo Dyes in the General and Industrial Environment (IARC Scientific Publications No. 40),* Lyon, International Agency for Research on Cancer, pp. 251-267

Sugimura, T., Sato, S. & Takayama, S. (1983) *New mutagenic heterocyclic amines found in amino acid and protein pyrolysates and in cooked food.* In: Wynder, E.L., Leveille, G.A., Weisburger, J.H. & Livingston, G.E., eds, *Environmental Aspects of Cancer: The Role of Macro and Micro Components of Foods,* Westport, CT, Food and Nutrition Press, pp. 167-186

Takayama, S. & Tanaka, M. (1983) Mutagenesis of amino acid pyrolysis products in Chinese hamster V79 cells. *Toxicol. Lett., 17,* 23-28

Takayama, S., Hirakawa, T., Tanaka, M., Kawachi, T. & Sugimura, T. (1979) In vitro transformation of hamster embryo cells with a glutamic acid pyrolysis product. *Toxicol. Lett., 4,* 281-284

Takayama, S., Masuda, M., Mogami, M., Ohgaki, H., Sato, S. & Sugimura, T. (1984) Induction of cancers in the intestine, liver and various other organs of rats by feeding mutagens from glutamic acid pyrolysate. *Gann, 75,* 207-213

Takeda, K., Shudo, K., Okamoto, T. & Kosuge, T. (1978) Synthesis of mutagenic principles isolated from L-glutamic acid pyrolysate. *Chem. pharm. Bull., 26,* 2924-2925

Takeda, K., Shudo, K., Okamoto, T., Nagao, M., Wakabayashi, K. & Sugimura, T. (1980) Effect of methyl substitution on mutagenicity of 2-aminodipyrido[1,2-*a*:3',2'-*d*]-imidazole, Glu-P-2. *Carcinogenesis*, *1*, 889-892

Tamano, S., Tsuda, H., Tatematsu, M., Hasegawa, R., Imaida, K. & Ito, N. (1981) Induction of γ-glutamyl transpeptidase positive foci in rat liver by pyrolysis products of amino acids. *Gann*, *72*, 747-753

Tohda, H., Oikawa, A., Kawachi, T. & Sugimura, T. (1980) Induction of sister-chromatid exchanges by mutagens from amino acid and protein pyrolysates. *Mutat. Res.*, *77*, 65-69

Umemoto, A., Negishi, C., Ishida, Y., Sato, S. & Sugimura, T. (1985) *Binding of Glu-P-1 metabolite to albumin and hemoglobin in rat* (Abstract No. 6). In: *Proceedings of the Japanese Cancer Association, 44th Annual Meeting*, Tokyo, Japanese Cancer Association, p. 2

Watanabe, J., Kawajiri, K., Yonekawa, H., Nagao, M. & Tagashira, Y. (1982) Immunological analysis of the roles of two major types of cytochrome P-450 in mutagenesis of compounds isolated from pyrolysates. *Biochem. biophys. Res. Commun.*, *104*, 193-199

Yamaguchi, K., Zenda, H., Shudo, K., Kosuge, T., Okamoto, T. & Sugimura, T. (1978) Isolation and structure determination of mutagenic substances of *L*-glutamic acid pyrolysate. *Proc. Jpn. Acad.*, *54B*, 248-250

Yamaguchi, K., Zenda, H., Shudo, K., Kosuge, T., Okamoto, T. & Sugimura, T. (1979) Presence of 2-aminodipyrido[1,2-*a*:3',2'-*d*]imidazole in casein pyrolysate. *Gann*, *70*, 849-850

Yamamoto, T., Tsuji, K., Kosuge, T., Okamoto, T., Shudo, K., Takeda, K., Iitaka, Y., Yamaguchi, K., Seino, Y., Yahagi, T., Nagao, M. & Sugimura, T. (1978) Isolation and structure determination of mutagenic substances of L-glutamic acid pyrolysate. *Proc. Jpn. Acad.*, *54B*, 2480250

Yoo, M.A., Ryo, H., Todo, T. & Kondo, S. (1985) Mutagenic potency of heterocyclic amines in the *Drosophila* wing spot test and its correlation to carcinogenic potency. *Jpn. J. Cancer Res. (Gann)*, *76*, 468-473

Glu-P-2 (2-AMINODIPYRIDO[1,2-*a*:3′,2′-*d*]IMIDAZOLE)

1. Chemical and Physical Data

1.1 Synonyms and trade names

Chem. Abstr. Services Reg. No.: 67730-10-3
Chem. Abstr. Name: Dipyrido[1,2-*a*:3′,2′-*d*]imidazol-2-amine
IUPAC Systematic Name: 2-Aminodipyrido[1,2-*a*:3′,2′-*d*]imidazole

1.2 Structural and molecular formulae and molecular weight

$C_{10}H_8N_4$ Mol. wt: 184.20

1.3 Chemical and physical properties of the pure substance

(*a*)   *Description*: Crystalline solid (Yamamoto *et al.*, 1978)

(*b*)   *Melting-point*: 286-287°C (hydrobromide salt) (Takeda *et al.*, 1978; Sugimura *et al.*, 1981)

(*c*)   *Spectroscopy data*: Ultraviolet (Yamaguchi *et al.*, 1980; Peters *et al.*, 1981; Sugimura *et al.*, 1981), fluorescence (Peters *et al.*, 1981; Sugimura *et al.*, 1981), C-13 nuclear magnetic resonance (Aboul-Enein, 1983) and proton nuclear magnetic resonance spectral data (Sugimura *et al.*, 1981) have been reported.

(*d*)   *Solubility*: Soluble in dimethyl sulphoxide and chloroform (Yamamoto *et al.*, 1978; Hayatsu *et al.*, 1983; Schunk *et al.*, 1984)

(*e*)   *Stability*: Stable under moderately acidic and alkaline conditions and in cold dilute aqueous solutions protected from light (Sugimura *et al.*, 1983)

(f)   *Reactivity*: Rapidly degraded by dilute hypochlorite; deactivated by weakly acidic nitrite solution with replacement of the 2-amino group by hydroxyl (Sugimura *et al.*, 1983)

2. Production, Use, Occurrence and Analysis

2.1 Production and use

(a)   Production

Glu-P-2 was first isolated by Yamamoto *et al.* (1978) from the pyrolysis products of L-glutamic acid.

Takeda *et al.* (1978) reported the development of a reaction sequence for the synthesis of L-glutamic acid pyrolysis products, including Glu-P-2. In this process, 3-aminoimidazo[1,2-*a*]pyridine, 2-chloroacrylonitrile and aluminium chloride in nitrobenzene are heated at 100°C for 12 h. Glu-P-2 is isolated from the reaction products by multiple extractions, column chromatography on silica gel and crystallization from methanol-ethyl acetate.

Glu-P-2 is not produced in commercial or bulk quantities.

(b)   Use

Glu-P-2 is not used commercially.

2.2 Occurrence

Glu-P-2 is not known to occur in nature.

Glu-P-2 has been detected in broiled (grilled) cuttlefish at a level of 350 μg/kg (Yamaguchi *et al.*, 1980) and among the pyrolysis products of L-glutamic acid at 1 mg/kg (Yamamoto *et al.*, 1978). It has been identified in the pyrolysate of casein (Yamaguchi *et al.*, 1979).

2.3 Analysis

Glu-P-2 was isolated from the pyrolysis products of L-glutamic acid by chloroform extraction, followed by column and thin-layer chromatography (Yamamoto *et al.*, 1978). The structure was determined by mass spectrometry, elemental analysis and X-ray crystallography.

Glu-P-2 can be adsorbed selectively from aqueous solutions onto cellulose or cotton to which C.I. Reactive Blue 21, a trisulpho-copper phthalocyanine dye, has been bound covalently. The adsorbed Glu-P-2 is eluted with ammoniacal methanol and quantified by adsorption spectrum (Hayatsu *et al.*, 1983).

Glu-P-2 has been separated from other amino acid pyrolysis products by gas chromatography using fused silica capillary columns and flame ionization detection

(Schunk *et al.*, 1984). High-performance liquid chromatography with ultraviolet and fluorescence detection has also been used to separate Glu-P-2 from Glu-P-1 and other protein and amino acid pyrolysates (Peters *et al.*, 1981).

3. Biological Data Relevant to the Evaluation of Carcinogenic Risk to Humans

3.1 Carcinogenicity studies in animals

Oral administration

Mouse: Groups of 40 male and 40 female CDF$_1$ [(BALB/cAnN × DBA/2N)F$_1$] mice [age unspecified] were fed a pelleted diet containing 500 mg/kg Glu-P-2 hydrochloride (purity confirmed by high-performance liquid chromatography [percentage not indicated]) for 588 days, at which time the experiment was terminated. A group of 40 males and 40 females was fed basal diet alone and served as controls. [The Working Group noted that this group was used as the controls for several experiments on similar chemicals.] On day 301 after the start of the experiment, 37/40 treated males, 36/40 treated females, 39/40 control males and 40/40 control females were still alive. The mean survival of control females was 658 ± 55 days and that of control males 586 ± 109 days; mean survival for treated females was 484 ± 46 days and for males 462 ± 72 days. Blood-vessel tumours were observed at various sites in 27/37 (73%) treated males and 20/36 (56%) treated females; no such tumour was found in control mice ($p < 0.001$). Most of the blood-vessel tumours were haemangioendothelial sarcomas (males, 25/27; females, 19/20). Liver tumours were also observed in 10/37 (27%) treated males and 36/36 (100%) treated females; no such tumour was found in control mice (males, $p < 0.002$; females, $p < 0.001$). Of the liver tumours observed in males, five were hepatocellular adenomas, four were hepatocellular carcinomas and one was a haemangioma; in females, six were hepatocellular adenomas and 30, hepatocellular carcinomas (Ohgaki *et al.*, 1984).

Rat: Groups of 42 male and 42 female Fischer 344 rats, eight weeks of age, were fed a pelleted diet containing 500 mg/kg Glu-P-2 hydrochloride (purity confirmed by high-performance liquid chromatography [percentage not indicated]) for 104 weeks, at which time the experiment was terminated. A group of 50 males and 50 females was fed basal diet alone and served as controls. [The Working Group noted that this control group was also used in a test on Glu-P-1.] By weeks 70 and 90, approximately 50% of treated rats had died, predominantly from tumours. The first liver tumour was observed in a female rat on day 519; liver tumours were observed in 11/42 (26%; [$p = 0.003$]) treated males and 2/42 (5%) treated females. Only two liver tumours were seen in male controls. Tumours of the small intestine (adenomas and adenocarcinomas) were induced in 14/42 (33%) [$p < 0.001$] treated males and 8/42 (19%) [$p = 0.001$] treated females. Tumours of the colon (adenomas and adenocarcinomas) were observed in 6/42 (14%) treated males [$p < 0.01$] and 8/42 (19%) treated females [$p = 0.001$]. Most intestinal tumours were solitary; no such tumour occurred in controls. Squamous-cell carcinomas of the Zymbal gland were observed in 1/42 (3%) treated males and 7/42 (17%) treated females [$p = 0.003$] compared with 0/50 controls. Clitoral-gland tumours were found in 11/42 (26%) [$p < 0.001$] treated females compared with 0/50 controls (Takayama et al., 1984).

3.2 Other relevant biological data

(a) Experimental systems

Toxic effects

A group of male Fischer 344 rats received seven intraperitoneal injections of 60 mg/kg bw Glu-P-2 dissolved in dimethyl sulphoxide (DMSO) at one-week intervals; after one week, they received partial hepatectomy; during weeks 8 and 9 they were fed a diet containing 200 mg/kg 2-acetylaminofluorene; and at the end of week 8, they were administered 1 ml/kg bw carbon tetrachloride by gavage. All animals were killed at the end of week 10. A control group received intraperitoneal injections of DMSO alone, followed by the same treatment. Statistically significant increases in the number and area of γ-glutamyl transpeptidase-positive liver-cell foci were observed in treated animals, compared to controls ($p < 0.001$). When rats were fed diets containing 200 mg/kg 2-acetylaminofluorene for two weeks and administered 1 ml/kg bw carbon tetrachloride at the end of week 1, followed by seven intraperitoneal injections of 60 mg/kg bw Glu-P-2 in DMSO during weeks 4 to 9, with partial hepatectomy at the end of week 4, statistically significant increases in the number and area of γ-glutamyl transpeptidase-positive liver-cell foci were also observed in treated animals compared to DMSO-treated controls (Tamano et al., 1981).

Groups of male Fischer 344 rats received a partial hepatectomy, followed 18 h later by a single intraperitoneal injection of 7.5, 30 or 120 mg/kg Glu-P-2 dissolved in DMSO; animals were then fed a diet containing 200 mg/kg 2-acetylaminofluorene during weeks 3 and 4 and administered 1 ml/kg bw carbon tetrachloride by gavage at the end of week 3. All animals were killed at the end of week 5. Dose-dependent increases in the number and area of γ-glutamyl transpeptidase-positive liver-cell foci were found in treated animals compared to controls that received an intraperitoneal injection of DMSO alone 18 h after partial hepatectomy, followed by treatment with 2-acetylaminofluorene (Tamano et al., 1981).

Effects on reproduction and prenatal toxicity
No data were available to the Working Group.

Absorption, distribution, excretion and metabolism

The metabolic activation of Glu-P-2 to mutagenic metabolites is mediated by the rat liver microsomal cytochrome P450 system (Ishii et al., 1981); the cytochrome P450 isoenzymes, induced by 3-methylcholanthrene or polychlorinated biphenyls, were most active in this respect (Nebert et al., 1979; Ishii et al., 1981; Watanabe et al., 1982). Three metabolites were obtained when Glu-P-2 was incubated with a reconstituted system containing a cytochrome P450 isoenzyme induced by polychlorinated biphenyls, but they were not characterized (Ishii *et al.*, 1981).

In a study to provide information on the metabolic steps involved in the formation of the active mutagenic form, it was observed that Glu-P-2 was not mutagenic to *Salmonella typhimurium* TA98/1,8-DNP$_6$ (defective in esterifying activity) in the presence of an exogenous metabolic system (S9 mix), while it was strongly mutagenic to the original TA98 with S9 mix, suggesting that the ultimate mutagenic form of Glu-P-2 is the sulphate ester of its *N*-hydroxy derivative (Nagao *et al.*, 1983a).

Mutagenicity and other short-term tests

Glu-P-2 (tested from 10-1000 μg/plate) induced prophage λ in lysogenic *Escherichia coli* K12 in the presence of an exogenous metabolic system (S9) (Nagao *et al.*, 1983b). It was mutagenic in *Salmonella typhimurium* TA1538, TA98 and TA100 in the presence of S9 from various species (Yamamoto *et al.*, 1978; Matsushima *et al.*, 1980; Takeda *et al.*, 1980; Ishii *et al.*, 1981; Peters *et al.*, 1981; N'Goy *et al.*, 1984).

Glu-P-2 gave positive results in a wing spot in *Drosophila melanogaster* (transhetero-zygous for the loci *mwh* and *flr*) raised in a medium containing 0.1-0.8 mg/g (Yoo *et al.*, 1985).

It was reported that Glu-P-2 (tested at up to 10^{-3}M) did not induce unscheduled DNA synthesis in a short-term organ culture of rat tracheal epithelium [figures not given] (Ide *et al.*, 1981).

Glu-P-2 (50-1500 μg/ml) induced diphtheria toxin-resistant mutants in cultured Chinese hamster lung cells in the presence of polychlorinated biphenyl-induced rat-liver S9 (Nakayasu *et al.*, 1983). It did not induce ouabain-resistant mutants in Chinese hamster V79 cells at concentrations of up to 100 μg/ml in the presence of a Syrian hamster embryo cell feeder layer (Takayama & Tanaka, 1983).

It was reported that Glu-P-2 induced chromosomal aberrations in Chinese hamster lung cells in the presence of an exogenous metabolic system (Ishidate, 1983). [The Working Group noted that a positive result was obtained at a single concentration of 2 mg/ml.] A borderline increase in the incidence of sister chromatid exchanges was observed when Glu-P-2 was tested in the presence of an exogenous metabolic system in cultured human lymphoblastoid NL3 cells (Tohda *et al.*, 1983) and in cultured human lymphocytes (N'Goy *et al.*, 1984).

(b) Humans

No data were available to the Working Group.

3.3 Case reports and epidemiological studies of carcinogenicity in humans

No data were available to the Working Group.

4. Summary of Data Reported and Evaluation

4.1 Exposure data

Glu-P-2 (2-aminodipyrido[1,2-*a*:3′,2′-*d*]imidazole) has been found in grilled fish and in L-glutamic acid and casein pyrolysates; therefore, consumption of grilled foods may result in human exposure.

4.2 Experimental data

Glu-P-2 was tested for carcinogenicity in one experiment in mice and one experiment in rats by oral administration in the diet. In mice, it produced haemangioendotheliomas and haemangioendothelial sarcomas at various sites and hepatocellular adenomas and carcinomas in animals of each sex. In rats, it produced benign and malignant tumours of the liver, intestines and Zymbal gland in animals of each sex and tumours of the clitoral gland in females.

No data were available to evaluate the reproductive effects or prenatal toxicity of this compound to experimental animals.

Glu-P-2 induced prophage in bacteria. It was mutagenic in *Salmonella typhimurium* in the presence of an exogenous metabolic system and in cultured mammalian cells, and gave positive results in the wing spot test in *Drosophila melanogaster*. Experiments for the induction of sister chromatid exchanges and chromosomal aberrations in cultured mammalian cells were inadequate.

4.3 Human data

No case report or epidemiological study of the carcinogenicity of Glu-P-2 was available to the Working Group.

4.4 Evaluation[1]

There is *sufficient evidence*[2] for the carcinogenicity of Glu-P-2 to experimental animals.

No data were available on the carcinogenicity of Glu-P-2 to humans.

---

[1]For definition of the italicized term, see Preamble, p. 18.

[2]In the absence of data on humans, it is reasonable, for practical purposes, to regard chemicals or exposures for which there is *sufficient evidence* of carcinogenicity in animals as if they presented a carcinogenic risk to humans.

Overall assessment of data from short-term tests: Glu-P-2[a]

	Genetic activity			Cell transformation
	DNA damage	Mutation	Chromosomal effects	
Prokaryotes	+	+		
Fungi/Green plants				
Insects		+		
Mammalian cells (*in vitro*)		+	?	
Mammals (*in vivo*)				
Humans (*in vivo*)				
Degree of evidence in short-term tests for genetic activity: **Sufficient**				Cell transformation: No data

[a]The groups into which the table is divided and the symbols used are defined on pp. 19-20 of the Preamble; the degrees of evidence are defined on pp. 20-21.

5. References

Aboul-Enein, H.Y. (1983) Carbon-13 NMR of some mutagenic 2-aminodipyrido[1,2-*a*:3′,2′-*d*]imidazoles. *Spectrosc. Lett.*, *16*, 109-115

Hayatsu, H., Oka, T., Wakata, A., Ohara, Y., Hayatsu, T., Kobayashi, H. & Arimoto, S. (1983) Adsorption of mutagens to cotton bearing covalently bound trisulfo-copper-phthalocyanine. *Mutat. Res.*, *119*, 233-238

Ide, F., Ishikawa, T. & Takayama, S. (1981) Detection of chemical carcinogens by assay of unscheduled DNA synthesis in rat tracheal epithelium in short-term organ culture. *J. Cancer Res. clin. Oncol.*, *102*, 115-126

Ishii, K., Yamazoe, Y., Kamataki, T. & Kato, R. (1981) Metabolic activation of glutamic acid pyrolysis products, 2-amino-6-methyldipyrido[1,2-*a*:3′,2′-*d*]imidazole and 2-amino-dipyrido[1,2-*a*:3′,2′-*d*]imidazole, by purified cytochrome P-450. *Chem.-biol. Interactions*, *38*, 1-13

Ishidate, M., ed. (1983) *Chromosomal Aberration Test* in vitro, Tokyo, Realize, Inc., p. 256

Matsushima, T., Yahagi, T., Takamoto, Y., Nagao, M. & Sugimura, T. (1980) *Species differences in microsomal activation of mutagens and carcinogens, with special reference to new potent mutagens from pyrolysates of amino acids and proteins.* In: Coon, M.J., Conney, A.H., Estabrook, R.W., Gelboin, H.V., Gillette, J.R. & O'Brien, P.J., eds, *Microsomes, Drug Oxidations and Chemical Carcinogenesis*, Vol. 2, New York, Academic Press, pp. 1093-1102

Nagao, M., Fujita, Y., Wakabayashi, K. & Sugimura, T. (1983a) Ultimate forms of mutagenic and carcinogenic heterocyclic amines produced by pyrolysis. *Biochem. biophys. Res. Commun.*, *114*, 626-631

Nagao, M., Sato, S. & Sugimura, T. (1983b) *Mutagens produced by heating foods.* In: Waller, G.R. & Feather, M.S., eds, *The Maillard Reaction in Foods and Nutrition* (*ACS Symposium Series 215*), Washington DC, American Chemical Society, pp. 521-536

Nakayasu, M., Nakasato, F., Sakamoto, H., Terada, M. & Sugimura, T. (1983) Mutagenic activity of heterocyclic amines in Chinese hamster lung cells with diphtheria toxin resistance as a marker. *Mutat. Res.*, *118*, 91-102

Nebert, D.W., Bigelow, S.W., Okey, A.B., Yahagi, T., Mori, Y., Nagao, M. & Sugimura, T. (1979) Pyrolysis products from amino acids and protein: highest mutagenicity requires cytochrome P_1-450. *Proc. natl Acad. Sci. USA*, *76*, 5929-5933

N'Goy, K., de Meester, C., Pairon, D., Fabry, L., Loukakou, B., N'Zouzi, C., Saint-Ruf, G., Mercier, M. & Poncelet, F. (1984) Mutagenicity of several derivatives of dipyrido[1,2-a:3',2',2'-d]imidazoles. *Mutat. Res.*, *136*, 23-31

Ohgaki, H., Matsukura, N., Morino, K., Kawachi, T., Sugimura, T. & Takayama, S. (1984) Carcinogenicity in mice of mutagenic compounds from glutamic acid and soybean globulin pyrolysates. *Carcinogenesis*, *5*, 815-819

Peters, J.H., Mortelmans, K.E., Reist, E.J., Sigman, C.C., Spanggord, R.J. & Thomas, D.W. (1981) Synthesis, chemical characterization, and mutagenic activities of pro-mutagens produced by pyrolysis of proteinaceous substances. *Environ. Mutagenesis*, *3*, 639-649

Schunk, H., Hayashi, T. & Shibamoto, T. (1984) Analysis of mutagenic amino acid pyrolyzates with a fused silica capillary column. *J. high Resolut. Chromatogr. Chromatogr. Commun.*, *7*, 563-565

Sugimura, T., Nagao, M. & Wakabayashi, K. (1981) *Mutagenic heterocyclic amines in cooked food.* In: Egan, H., Fishbein, L., Castegnaro, M., O'Neill, I.K. & Bartsch, H., eds, *Environmental Carcinogens. Selected Methods of Analysis*, Vol. 4, *Some Aromatic Amines and Azo Dyes in the General and Industrial Environment* (*IARC Scientific Publications No. 40*), Lyon, International Agency for Research on Cancer, pp. 251-267

Sugimura, T., Sato, S. & Takayama, S. (1983) *New mutagenic heterocyclic amines found in amino acid and protein pyrolysates and in cooked food.* In: Wynder, E.L., Leveille, G.A., Weisburger, J.H. & Livingston, G.E., eds., *Environmental Aspects of Cancer: The Role of Macro and Micro Components of Foods*, Westport, CT, Food and Nutrition Press, pp. 167-186

Takayama, S. & Tanaka, M. (1983) Mutagenesis of amino acid pyrolysis products in Chinese hamster V79 cells. *Toxicol. Lett.*, *17*, 23-28

Takayama, S., Masuda, M., Mogami, M., Ohgaki, H., Sato, S. & Sugimura, T. (1984) Induction of cancers in the intestine, liver and various other organs of rats by feeding mutagens from glutamic acid pyrolysate. *Gann*, *75*, 207-213

Takeda, K., Shudo, K., Okamoto, T. & Kosuge, T. (1978) Synthesis of mutagenic principles isolated from L-glutamic acid pyrolysate. *Chem. pharm. Bull.*, *26*, 2924-2925

Takeda, K., Shudo, K., Okamoto, T., Nagao, M., Wakabayashi, K. & Sugimura, T. (1980) Effect of methyl substitution on mutagenicity of 2-aminodipyrido[1,2-*a*:3′,2′-*d*]-imidazole, Glu-P-2. *Carcinogenesis*, *1*, 889-892

Tamano, S., Tsuda, H., Tatematsu, M., Hasegawa, R., Imaida, K. & Ito, N. (1981) Induction of γ-glutamyl transpeptidase positive foci in rat liver by pyrolysis products of amino acids. *Gann*, *72*, 747-753

Tohda, H., Tada, M., Sugawara, R. & Oikawa, A. (1983) Actions of amino-β-carbolines on induction of sister-chromatid exchanges. *Mutat. Res.*, *116*, 137-147

Watanabe, J., Kawajiri, K., Yonekawa, H., Nagao, M. & Tagashira, Y. (1982) Immuno-logical analysis of the roles of two major types of cytochrome P-450 in mutagenesis of compounds isolated from pyrolysates. *Biochem. biophys. Res. Commun.*, *104*, 193-199

Yamaguchi, K., Zenda, H., Shudo, K., Kosuge, T., Okamoto, T. & Sugimura, T. (1979) Presence of 2-aminodipyrido[1,2-*a*:3′,2′-*d*]imidazole in casein pyrolysate. *Gann*, *70*, 849-850

Yamaguchi, K., Shudo, K., Okamoto, T., Sugimura, T. & Kosuge, T. (1980) Presence of 2-aminodipyrido[1,2-*a*;3′,2′-*d*]imidazole in broiled cuttlefish. *Gann*, *71*, 743-744

Yamamoto, T., Tsuji, K., Kosuge, T., Okamoto, T., Shudo, K., Takeda, K., Iitaka, Y., Yamaguchi, K., Seino, Y., Yahagi, T., Nagao, M. & Sugimura, T. (1978) Isolation and structure determination of mutagenic substances of L-glutamic acid pyrolysate. *Proc. Jpn. Acad.*, *54B*, 248-250

Yoo, M.A., Ryo, H., Todo, T. & Kondo, S. (1985) Mutagenic potency of heterocyclic amines in the *Drosophila* wing spot test and its correlation to carcinogenic potency. *Jpn. J. Cancer Res. (Gann)*, *76*, 468-473

A-α-C (2-AMINO-9*H*-PYRIDO[2,3-*b*]INDOLE)

1. Chemical and Physical Data

1.1 Synonyms and trade names

Chem. Abstr. Services Reg. No.: 26148-68-5

Chem. Abstr. Name: 1*H*-Pyrido[2,3-*b*]indol-2-amine

IUPAC Systematic Name: 2-Amino-1*H*-pyrido[2,3-*b*]indole; 2-amino-9*H*-pyrido-[2,3-*b*]indole

Synonyms: AC; amino-α-carboline; 2-amino-α-carboline; Glob-P-2

1.2 Structural and molecular formulae and molecular weight

$C_{11}H_9N_3$ Mol. wt: 183.21

1.3 Chemical and physical properties of the pure substance

(*a*)   *Description*: Crystalline solid (Yoshida *et al.*, 1978)

(*b*)   *Melting-point*: 202°C (Yoshida *et al.*, 1980; Matsumoto *et al.*, 1981a; Sugimura *et al.*, 1981)

(*c*)   *Spectroscopy data*: Ultraviolet (Yoshida & Matsumoto, 1980; Peters *et al.*, 1981; Sugimura *et al.*, 1981; Tada *et al.*, 1983), infrared, C-13 nuclear magnetic resonance (Matsumoto *et al.*, 1979), proton nuclear magnetic resonance (Matsumoto *et al.*, 1979, 1981b; Sugimura *et al.*, 1981), fluorescence (Yoshida & Matsumoto, 1980; Peters *et al.*, 1981; Sugimura *et al.*, 1981) and mass spectral data (Matsumoto *et al.*, 1979; Yoshida & Matsumoto, 1980; Matsumoto *et al.*, 1981b; Sugimura *et al.*, 1981) have been reported.

(d)   *Solubility*: Soluble in methanol and dimethyl sulphoxide (Matsumoto *et al.*, 1981a; Hayatsu *et al.*, 1983)

(e)   *Stability*: Stable under moderately acidic and alkaline conditions and in cold dilute aqueous solutions protected from light (Sugimura *et al.*, 1983)

(f)   *Reactivity*: Rapidly degraded by dilute hypochlorite; deactivated by weakly acidic nitrite solution with replacement of the 2-amino group by hydroxyl (Sugimura *et al.*, 1983)

2. Production, Use, Occurrence and Analysis

2.1 Production and use

(a)   *Production*

A-α-C was first isolated by Yoshida *et al.* (1978) from the pyrolysis products of soya bean globulin.

The synthesis of A-α-C was reported by Matsumoto *et al.* (1979) using 6-bromo-2-picolinic acid as the initial precursor. This compound is reacted with *ortho*-phenylene-diamine to produce an intermediate, which upon treatment with nitrous acid is converted into a benzotriazolylpicolinic acid. In the presence of diphenyl phosphorazitate and triethylamine, the benzotriazolyl picolinic acid undergoes a Curtius rearrangement to yield 1-(2-amino-6-pyridyl)benzotriazole. Mixture of this compound with polyphosphoric acid at 175°C, and extraction of the reaction product with diethylether, produces crude A-α-C. Final purification is accomplished by Sephadex LH-20 chromatography.

A-α-C is not produced in commercial or bulk quantities.

(b)   *Use*

A-α-C is not used commercially.

2.2 Occurrence

A-α-C is not known to occur in nature.

A-α-C has been identified among the pyrolysis products of soya bean globulin at approximately 40 µg/g globulin (Yoshida *et al.*, 1978; Matsumoto *et al.*, 1981b).

Yields of A-α-C from the pyrolysis of albumin at temperatures of 300-700°C were approximately 5-80 µg/g (Yoshida *et al.*, 1980). A-α-C has been detected at 650 ng/g in grilled sliced beef, 180 ng/g in grilled chicken, 47 ng/g in grilled Chinese mushrooms and 1.5 ng/g in grilled onions (Matsumoto *et al.*, 1981a). The concentration of A-α-C in smoke condensate from various brands of cigarettes ranged from 25-258 ng/cigarette (Yoshida & Matsumoto, 1980; Matsumoto *et al.*, 1981a).

A-α-C was also detected after pyrolysis (550°C) of L-tryptophan (250-2500 μg/g), chicken meat (34 μg/g), horse mackerel (12 μg/g), casein (3.8 μg/g), globulin (1.5 μg/g), gluten (1.2 μg/g) and zein (0.05 μg/g) (Yoshida & Matsumoto, 1979; Yoshida et al., 1979; Tada et al., 1983).

2.3 Analysis

A-α-C was isolated from the basic fraction of soya bean globulin pyrolysate by successive chromatography on silica-gel, CM-Sephadex C-25 and Sephadex LH-20 columns, followed by separation of the amino-α-carbolines by thin-layer chromatography on silica gel plates. The structure of A-α-C was elucidated by high-resolution mass and nuclear magnetic resonance spectrometry (Matsumoto et al., 1981b) and X-ray crystallography (Yoshida et al., 1978).

A-α-C was determined in other protein pyrolysates and in tobacco smoke condensates by chloroform extraction, chromatography and quantitative fluorimetry (Yoshida et al., 1979; Yoshida & Matsumoto, 1980). High-performance liquid chromatography with Nucleosil C18 columns and spectrofluorimetry have also been used to separate and quantify A-α-C and MeA-α-C (2-amino-3-methyl-9H-pyrido[2,3-b]indole) (see p. 253) (Matsumoto et al., 1981a).

A-α-C can be adsorbed selectively from aqueous solutions onto cellulose or cotton to which C.I. Reactive Blue 21, a trisulpho-copper phthalocyanine dye, has been bound covalently. The adsorbed A-α-C is eluted with ammoniacal methanol and quantified by adsorption spectrum (Hayatsu et al., 1983).

3. Biological Data Relevant to the Evaluation
of Carcinogenic Risk to Humans

3.1 Carcinogenicity studies in animals

Oral administration[1]

Mouse: Groups of 40 male and 40 female CDF₁ [(BALB/cAnN × DBA/2N)F₁] mice [age unspecified] were fed a pelleted diet containing 800 mg/kg A-α-C acetate (purity confirmed by high-performance liquid chromatography [percentage not indicated]) for 685 days, at which time the experiment was terminated. A group of 40 males and 40 females fed basal diet alone and kept for 685 days served as controls. [The Working Group noted that this group was used as the controls for several experiments on similar chemicals.] On day 301 after the start of the experiment, 38/40 treated males, 34/40 treated females, 38/40 contral males and 40/40 control females were still alive. The mean survival was similar in

---

[1]The Working Group was aware of a study in progress in rats by oral administration (IARC, 1986).

treated and control mice. Blood-vessel tumours were observed at various sites in 20/38 (53%) treated males and 6/34 (18%) treated females; no such tumour was found in control mice (males, $p < 0.001$; females, $p < 0.02$). Most of these tumours were haemangio-endothelial sarcomas (males, 17/20; females, 6/6). Liver tumours were also observed in 15/38 (39%) treated males and 33/34 (97%) treated females; no such tumour was found in control mice ($p < 0.001$). Of the liver tumours observed in males, six were hepatocellular adenomas and nine were hepatocellular carcinomas; in females, three were hepatocellular adenomas and 30 were hepatocellular carcinomas (Ohgaki et al., 1984).

3.2 Other relevant biological data

(a)   Experimental systems

Toxic effects

A group of 16 male Fischer 344 rats received a partial hepatectomy, followed 18 h later by a single intraperitoneal injection of 50 mg/kg bw A-α-C in dimethyl sulphoxide (DMSO). Two weeks after the injection, the rats were fed basal diet containing 200 mg/kg 2-acetylaminofluorene for two weeks and received a single oral dose of 1 ml/kg bw carbon tetrachloride one week after the start of the 2-acetylaminofluorene treatment. A control group of 13 rats received partial hepatectomy and intraperitoneal injection of DMSO alone, followed by the same treatment as the experimental group. All animals were killed five weeks after the start of the experiment. A-α-C induced statistically significant increases in the number and area of γ-glutamyl transpeptidase-positive liver foci ($p < 0.001$) (Hasegawa et al., 1982).

Effects on reproduction and prenatal toxicity

No data were available to the Working Group.

Absorption, distribution, excretion and metabolism

The metabolic activation of A-α-C to mutagenic metabolites is mediated by the rat-liver microsomal cytochrome P450 system. Metabolism of A-α-C by hepatic microsomes from polychlorinated biphenyl-treated rats yielded five major metabolites, two of which were direct mutagens in Salmonella typhimurium TA98. The major mutagenic metabolite was determined to be the N-hydroxy derivative of A-α-C and the minor metabolite to be the nitroso derivative (Niwa et al., 1982). These and other data indicate that N-hydroxylation of A-α-C by the P448 type of cytochrome P450 is important for its mutagenic activation (Nebert et al., 1979; Niwa et al., 1982; Watanabe et al., 1982).

Mutagenicity and other short-term tests

A-α-C (tested in the range 20-1000 μg/plate) induced prophage λ in lysogenic Escherichia coli K12 (Nagao et al., 1983) and gave positive results in the Bacillus subtilis rec[+/−] assay in the presence of a metabolic system (S9) from livers of polychlorinated biphenyl (PCB)-induced rats (Matsumoto et al., 1981b). It was mutagenic to Salmonella *typhimurium* TA98 and TA100 in the presence of PCB-induced rat-liver S9 (Yoshida *et al.*, 1978; Matsumoto *et al.*, 1981b; Peters *et al.*, 1981; Niwa *et al.*, 1982).

A-α-C gave positive results in the wing spot test in *Drosophila melanogaster* (transheterozygous for the loci *mwh* and *flr*) raised in a medium containing 0.4 or 1 mg/g (Yoo *et al.*, 1985).

It was reported that A-α-C (tested at up to 10^{-3}M) did not induce unscheduled DNA synthesis in a short-term organ culture of rat tracheal epithelium [figures not given] (Ide *et al.*, 1981).

A-α-C (25 to 100 μg/ml) induced diphtheria toxin-resistant mutants in cultured Chinese hamster lung cells in the presence of PCB-induced rat-liver S9 (Nakayasu *et al.*, 1983).

A-α-C acetate induced polyploidy in cultured Chinese hamster lung cells in the absence of S9 at 0.0313 mg/ml and chromosomal aberrations at concentrations of 0.125 and 0.25 mg/ml when tested with PCB-induced rat-liver S9 (Ishidate, 1983). At concentrations of 10^{-6} to 10^{-4} M, A-α-C induced sister chromatid exchanges in human lymphoblastoid NL3 cells in the presence of PCB-induced rat-liver S9 (Tohda *et al.*, 1980).

(*b*)   *Humans*

No data were available to the Working Group.

3.3 Case reports and epidemiological studies of carcinogenicity in humans

No data were available to the Working Group.

4. Summary of Data Reported and Evaluation

4.1 Exposure data

A-α-C (2-amino-9H-pyrido[2,3-b]indole) has been found in a variety in grilled foods, in the pyrolysis products of proteins and in cigarette smoke. There is thus likely to be widespread human exposure to this compound.

4.2 Experimental data

A-α-C was tested for carcinogenicity in one experiment in mice by oral administration in the diet. It produced haemangioendothelial sarcomas and hepatocellular adenomas and carcinomas in animals of each sex (see also the 'General Remarks on the Substances Considered', p. 39).

No data were available to evaluate the reproductive effects or prenatal toxicity of this compound to experimental animals.

A-α-C induced prophage in bacteria. It induced DNA damage in *Bacillus subtilis* and mutations in *Salmonella typhimurium* in the presence of an exogenous metabolic system. It gave positive results in the wing spot test in *Drosophila melanogaster*. In cultured Chinese hamster lung cells, A-α-C induced mutations and chromosomal aberrations in the presence and polyploidy in the absence, of an exogenous metabolic system. It induced sister chromatid exchanges in human lymphoblastoid cells.

Overall assessment of data from short-term tests: A-α-C[a]

	Genetic activity			Cell transformation
	DNA damage	Mutation	Chromosomal effects	
Prokaryotes	+	+		
Fungi/Green plants				
Insects		+		
Mammalian cells (*in vitro*)		+	+	
Mammals (*in vivo*)				
Humans (*in vivo*)				
Degree of evidence in short-term tests for genetic activity: **Sufficient**				Cell transformation: No data

[a]The groups into which the table is divided and the symbol used are defined on pp. 19-20 of the Preamble; the degrees of evidence are defined on pp. 20-21.

4.3 Human data

No case report or epidemiological study of the carcinogenicity of A-α-C was available to the Working Group.

4.4 Evaluation[1]

There is *sufficient evidence*[2] for the carcinogenicity of A-α-C to experimental animals. No data were available on the carcinogenicity of A-α-C to humans.

[1]For definition of the italicized term, see Preamble, p. 18.
[2]In the absence of data on humans, it is reasonable, for practical purposes to regard chemicals or exposures for which there is *sufficient evidence* of carcinogenicity in animals as if they presented a carcinogenic risk to humans.

5. References

Hasegawa, R., Tsuda, H., Ogiso, T., Ohshima, M. & Ito, N. (1982) Initiating activities of pyrolysis products of L-lysine and soybean globulin assessed in terms of the induction of γ-glutamyl transpeptidase-positive foci in rat liver. *Gann*, *73*, 158-159

Hayatsu, H., Oka, T., Wakata, A., Ohara, Y., Hayatsu, T., Kobayashi, H. & Arimoto, S. (1983) Adsorption of mutagens to cotton bearing covalently bound trisulfo-copper-phthalocyanine. *Mutat. Res.*, *119*, 233-238

IARC (1986) *Information Bulletin on the Survey of Chemicals Being Tested for Carcinogenicity*, Vol. 12, Lyon, p. 85

Ide, F., Ishikawa, T. & Takayama, S. (1981) Detection of chemical carcinogens by assay of unscheduled DNA synthesis in rat tracheal epithelium in short term organ culture. *J. Cancer Res. clin. Oncol.*, *102*, 115-126

Ishidate, M., ed. (1983) *Chromosomal Aberration Test* in vitro, Tokyo, Realize Inc., p. 254

Matsumoto, T., Yoshida, D., Tomita, H. & Matsushita, H. (1979) Synthesis of 2-amino-9*H*-pyrido[2,3-*b*]indole isolated as a mutagenic principle from pyrolytic products of protein. *Agric. Biol. Chem.*, *43*, 675-677

Matsumoto, T., Yoshida, D. & Tomita, H. (1981a) Determination of mutagens amino-α-carbolines in grilled foods and cigarette smoke condensate. *Cancer Lett.*, *12*, 105-110

Matsumoto, T., Yoshida, D. & Tomita, H. (1981b) Synthesis and mutagenic activity of alkyl derivatives of 2-amino-9*H*-pyrido[2,3-*b*]indole. *Agric. Biol. Chem.*, *45*, 2031-2035

Nagao, M., Sato, S. & Sugimura, T. (1983) *Mutagens produced by heating foods*. In: Waller, G.R. & Feather, M.S., eds, *The Maillard Reaction in Foods and Nutrition* (*ACS Symposium Series 215*), Washington DC, American Chemical Society, pp. 521-536

Nakayasu, M., Nakasato, F., Sakamoto, H., Terada, M. & Sugimura, T. (1983) Mutagenic activity of heterocyclic amines in Chinese hamster lung cells with diphtheria toxin resistance as a marker. *Mutat. Res.*, *118*, 91-102

Nebert, D.W., Bigelow, S.W., Okey, A.B., Yahagi, T., Mori, Y., Nagao, M. & Sugimura, T. (1979) Pyrolysis products from amino acids and protein: highest mutagenicity requires cytochrome P_1-450. *Proc. natl Acad. Sci. USA*, *76*, 5929-5933

Niwa, T., Yamazoe, Y. & Kato, R. (1982) Metabolic activation of 2-amino-9*H*-pyrido[2,3-*b*]indole by rat-liver microsomes. *Mutat. Res.*, *95*, 159-170

Ohgaki, H., Matsukura, N., Morino, K., Kawachi, T., Sugimura, T. & Takayama, S. (1984) Carcinogenicity in mice of mutagenic compounds from glutamic acid and soy bean globulin pyrolysates. *Carcinogenesis*, *5*, 815-819

Peters, J.H., Mortelmans, K.E., Reist, E.J., Sigman, C.C., Spanggord, R.J. & Thomas, D.W. (1981) Synthesis, chemical characterization, and mutagenic activities of pro-mutagens produced by pyrolysis of proteinaceous substances. *Environ. Mutagenesis*, *3*, 636-649

Sugimura, T., Nagao, M. & Wakabayashi, K. (1981) *Mutagenic heterocyclic amines in cooked food.* In: Egan, H., Fishbein, L., Castegnaro, M., O'Neill, I.K. & Bartsch, H., eds, *Environmental Carcinogens. Selected Methods of Analysis,* Vol. 4, *Some Aromatic and Azo Dyes in the General and Industrial Environment (IARC Scientific Publications No. 40),* Lyon, International Agency for Research on Cancer, pp. 251-267

Sugimura, T., Sato, S. & Takayama, S. (1983) *New mutagenic heterocyclic amines found in amino acid and protein pyrolysates and in cooked food.* In: Wynder, E.L., Leveille, G.A., Weisburger, J.H. & Livingston, G.E., eds, *Environmental Aspects of Cancer: The Role of Macro and Micro Components of Foods,* Westport, CT, Food and Nutrition Press, pp. 167-186

Tada, M., Saeki, H. & Oikawa, A. (1983) The identification of 3-amino-9H-pyrido[3,4-b]indole derivatives in L-tryptophan pyrolysates. *Bull. chem. Soc. Jpn.,* 56, 1450-1454

Tohda, H., Oikawa, A., Kawachi, T. & Sugimura, T. (1980) Induction of sister-chromatid exchanges by mutagens from amino acid and protein pyrolysates. *Mutat. Res.,* 77, 65-69

Watanabe, J., Kawajiri, K., Yonekawa, H., Nagao, M. & Tagashira, Y. (1982) Immuno-logical analysis of the roles of two major types of cytochrome P-450 in mutagenesis of compounds isolated from pyrolysates. *Biochem. biophys. Res. Commun.,* 104, 193-199

Yoo, M.A., Ryo, H., Todo, T. & Kondo, S. (1985) Mutagenic potency of heterocyclic amines in the *Drosophila* wing spot test and its correlation to carcinogenic potency. *Jpn. J. Cancer Res. (Gann),* 76, 468-473

Yoshida, D. & Matsumoto, T. (1979) Isolation of 2-amino-9H-pyrido[2,3-b]indole and 2-amino-3-methyl-9H-pyrido[2,3-b]indole as mutagens from pyrolysis product of tryptophan. *Agric. Biol. Chem.,* 43, 1155-1156

Yoshida, D. & Matsumoto, T. (1980) Amino-α-carbolines as mutagenic agents in cigarette smoke condensate. *Cancer Lett.,* 10, 141-149

Yoshida, D., Matsumoto, T., Yoshimura, R. & Matsuzaki, T. (1978) Mutagenicity of amino-α-carbolines in pyrolysis products of soybean globulin. *Biochem. biophys. Res. Commun.,* 83, 915-920

Yoshida, D., Nishigata, H. & Matsumoto, T. (1979) Pyrolytic yields of 2-amino-9H-pyrido[2,3-b]indole and 3-amino-1-methyl-5H-pyrido[4,3-b]indole as mutagens from proteins. *Agric. Biol. Chem.,* 43, 1769-1770

Yoshida, D., Matsumoto, T. & Nishigata, H. (1980) Effect of heating methods on mutagenic activity and yield of mutagenic compounds in pyrolysis products of protein. *Agric. Biol. Chem.,* 44, 253-25

MeA-α-C (2-AMINO-3-METHYL-9H-PYRIDO[2,3-b]INDOLE)

1. Chemical and Physical Data

1.1 Synonyms and trade names

Chem. Abstr. Services Reg. No.: 68006-83-7

Chem. Abstr. Name: 3-Methyl-1H-pyrido[2,3-b]indol-2-amine

IUPAC Systematic Names: 2-Amino-3-methyl-1H-pyrido[2,3-b]indole; 2-amino-3-methyl-9H-pyrido[2,3-b]indole

Synonyms: Glob-P-1; Me-amino-α-carboline; MeAC; methyl-amino-α-carboline

1.2 Structural and molecular formulae and molecular weight

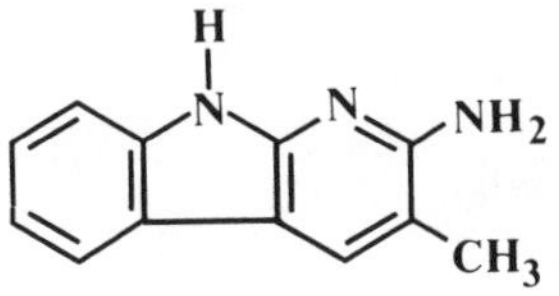

$C_{12}H_{11}N_3$

Mol. wt: 197.24

1.3 Chemical and physical properties of the pure substance

(a) *Description*: Colourless needles (Matsumoto *et al.*, 1981a)

(b) *Melting-point*: 215-218°C (Matsumoto *et al.*, 1981a); 211-214°C (Sugimura *et al.*, 1981)

(c) *Spectroscopy data*: Ultraviolet (Yoshida & Matsumoto, 1980; Peters *et al.*, 1981), proton nuclear magnetic resonance (Matsumoto *et al.*, 1981a), fluorescence (Yoshida & Matsumoto, 1980; Peters *et al.*, 1981; Sugimura *et al.*, 1981) and mass spectral data (Yoshida & Matsumoto, 1980; Matsumoto *et al.*, 1981a; Sugimura *et al.*, 1981) have been reported.

(d) *Solubility*: Soluble in methanol and dimethyl sulphoxide (Matsumoto *et al.*, 1981b; Hayatsu *et al.*, 1983; Schunk *et al.*, 1984)

(e) *Stability*: Stable under moderately acidic and alkaline conditions and in cold dilute aqueous solutions protected from light (Sugimura *et al.*, 1983) (f)*Reactivity*: Rapidly degraded by dilute hypochlorite; deactivated by weakly acidic nitrite solution with replacement of the 2-amino group by hydroxyl (Sugimura *et al.*, 1983)

2. Production, Use, Occurrence and Analysis

2.1 Production and use

(a)   Production

MeA-α-C was first isolated by Yoshida *et al.* (1978) from the pyrolysis products of soya bean globulin.

Synthesis of the alkyl derivatives of A-α-C (2-amino-9*H*-pyrido[2,3-*b*]indole), including MeA-α-C, was reported by Matsumoto *et al.* (1981a). Methylpropanedinitrile is reduced with lithium aluminium hydride to its corresponding enaminonitrile, which is condensed with 2-aminoindole to produce MeA-α-C. Final purification is achieved by ethyl acetate extraction and Sephadex LH-20 chromatography, followed by high-performance liquid chromatography.

MeA-α-C is not produced in commercial or bulk quantities.

(b)   Use

MeA-α-C is not used commercially.

2.2 Occurrence

MeA-α-C is not known to occur in nature.

MeA-α-C has been identified among the pyrolysis products of soya bean globulin at 80 μg/g globulin (Yoshida *et al.*, 1978; Matsumoto *et al.*, 1981a). It has also been detected in L-tryptophan pyrolysates (550°C) at 20 μg/g (Yoshida & Matsumoto, 1979). In grilled foods, it was detected at levels of 63.5 ng/g in beef slices, 15.1 ng/g in chicken and 5.4 ng/g in Chinese mushrooms (Matsumoto *et al.*, 1981b). The concentration of MeA-α-C in smoke condensate from various brands of cigarettes ranged from 6.2-37 ng/cigarette (Yoshida & Matsumoto, 1980; Matsumoto *et al.*, 1981b).

2.3 Analysis

MeA-α-C was isolated from the basic fraction of soya bean globulin pyrolysate by successive chromatography on silica gel, CM-Sephadex C-25 and Sephadex LH-20 columns, followed by separation of the amino-α-carbolines by thin-layer chromatography on silica-gel plates. The structure of MeA-α-C was elucidated by high-resolution mass and nuclear magnetic resonance spectroscopy (Matsumoto *et al.*, 1981a) and X-ray crystallography (Yoshida *et al.*, 1978).

MeA-α-C was determined in tobacco smoke condensates by chloroform extraction, chromatography and quantitative fluorimetry (Yoshida & Matsumoto, 1980). High-performance liquid chromatography with Nucleosil C18 columns and spectrofluorimetry have also been used to separate and quantify MeA-α-C and A-α-C (see p. 245) (Matsumoto et al., 1981b).

MeA-α-C can be adsorbed selectively from aqueous solutions onto cellulose or cotton to which C.I. Reactive Blue 21, a trisulpho-copper phthalocyanine dye, has been bound covalently. The adsorbed MeA-α-C is eluted with ammoniacal methanol and quantified by adsorption spectrum (Hayatsu et al., 1983).

3. Biological Data Relevant to the Evaluation of Carcinogenic Risk to Humans

3.1 Carcinogenicity studies in animals

Oral administration

Mouse: Groups of 40 male and 40 female CDF$_1$ [(BALB/cAnN × DBA/2N)F$_1$] mice [age unspecified] were fed a pelleted diet containing 800 mg/kg MeA-α-C acetate (purity confirmed by high-performance liquid chromatography [percentage not indicated]) for 588 days, at which time the experiment was terminated. A group of 40 males and 40 females fed basal diet alone and kept for 685 days served as controls. [The Working Group noted that this group was used as the controls for several experiments on similar chemicals]. On day 301, 37/40 treated males, 33/40 treated females, 39/40 control males and 40/40 control females were still alive. The mean survival of control females was 658 ± 55 days and that of control males 586 ± 109 days; mean survival for treated females was 492 ± 77 days and for males 445 ± 44 days. Haemangioendothelial sarcomas were observed at multiple sites in 35/37 (95%) treated males and 28/33 (85%) treated females; no such tumour was found in control mice ($p < 0.001$). Liver tumours were also observed in 21/37 (57%) treated males and 28/33 (85%) treated females, and no such tumour was found in control mice ($p < 0.001$). Of the liver tumours observed in males, 12 were hepatocellular adenomas and nine were hepatocellular carcinomas; in females, 13 were hepatocellular adenomas and 15 hepatocellular carcinomas (Ohgaki et al., 1984).

3.2 Other relevant biological data

(a) Experimental systems

Toxic effects

A group of 19 male Fischer 344 rats received a partial hepatectomy followed 18 h later by a single intraperitoneal injection of 80 mg/kg bw MeA-α-C in dimethyl sulphoxide (DMSO). Two weeks after the injection, the rats were fed basal diet containing 200 mg/kg 2-acetylaminofluorene for two weeks and received a single oral dose of 1 ml/kg bw carbon tetrachloride one week after the start of the 2-acetylaminofluorene treatment. A control group of 13 rats received partial hepatectomy and intraperitoneal injection of DMSO alone, followed by the same treatment as the experimental group. All animals were killed five weeks after the start of the experiment. MeA-α-C induced statistically significant increases in the number and area of γ-glutamyl transpeptidase-positive liver foci (Hasegawa et al., 1982).

Effects on reproduction and prenatal toxicity

No data were available to the Working Group.

Absorption, distribution, excretion and metabolism

The metabolic activation of MeA-α-C to mutagenic metabolites is mediated by the rat-liver microsomal cytochrome P450 system. Mutagenic activation of this compound by an S9 fraction prepared from the livers of rats treated with polychlorinated biphenyls was inhibited by more than 70% by antibody against the major type of cytochrome P450 of rat liver microsomes induced by 3-methylcholanthrene (MC), while it was not inhibited appreciably by antibody to the major type of cytochrome P450 induced by phenobarbital. Thus, MeA-α-C appears to be activated selectively by MC-P448 to form a mutagenic intermediate in rat liver microsomes (Watanabe et al., 1982). A species of mouse-liver microsomal cytochrome P450, P_1450, induced by benzo[a]pyrene and controlled by the regulatory gene of the Ah locus, was far more efficient than other forms of cytochrome P450 in metabolizing MeA-α-C to its active mutagenic form (Nebert et al., 1979). The metabolites of MeA-α-C formed by rat or mouse liver microsomal enzymes have not been characterized.

In a study to provide information on the metabolic steps involved in the formation of the active mutagenic form, it was observed that MeA-α-C was weakly mutagenic to Salmonella typhimurium TA98/1,8-DNP$_6$ (defective in esterifying activity) in the presence of S9 mix, while it was strongly mutagenic to the original TA98 with S9 mix, suggesting that the ultimate mutagenic form of MeA-α-C is the sulphate ester of its N-hydroxy derivative (Nagao et al., 1983a).

Mutagenicity and other short-term tests

MeA-α-C (tested at concentrations of 20-1000 μg/plate) induced prophage λ in lysogenic Escherichia coli K12 (Nagao et al., 1983b) and gave positive results in the Bacillus subtilis rec$^{+/-}$ assay (Matsumoto et al., 1981a) in the presence of a metabolic system (S9) from the livers of polychlorinated biphenyl (PCB)-induced rats. It was mutagenic to Salmonella typhimurium TA98 and TA100 in the presence of PCB-induced rat-liver S9 (Yoshida et al., 1978; Matsumoto et al., 1981a; Peters et al., 1981).

MeA-α-C gave positive results in the wing spot test in Drosophila melanogaster (transheterozygous for the loci mwh and flr) raised in a medium containing 0.4 or 1 mg/g (Yoo et al., 1985).

It induced polyploidy in cultured Chinese hamster lung cells at concentrations of 0.0625 and 0.125 mg/ml in the absence of S9, and induced chromosomal aberrations at concentrations of 0.5 and 1.25 mg/ml in the presence of PCB-induced rat liver S9 (Ishidate, 1983).

(b) *Humans*

No data were available to the Working Group.

3.3 Case reports and epidemiological studies of carcinogenicity in humans

No data were available to the Working Group.

4. Summary of Data Reported and Evaluation

4.1 Exposure data

MeA-α-C (2-amino-3-methyl-9H-pyrido[2,3-b]indole has been found in grilled foods, in the pyrolysis products of proteins and in cigarette smoke. There is thus likely to be widespread human exposure to this compound.

4.2 Experimental data

MeA-α-C was tested for carcinogenicity in one experiment in mice by oral administration in the diet. It produced haemangioendothelial sarcomas at various sites and hepatocellular adenomas and carcinomas in animals of each sex (see also 'General Remarks on the Substances Considered', p. 39).

No data were available to evaluate the reproductive effects or prenatal toxicity of this compound to experimental animals.

MeA-α-C induced prophage in bacteria. It induced DNA damage in *Bacillus subtilis* and was mutagenic in *Salmonella typhimurium* in the presence of an exogenous metabolic system. It gave positive results in the wing spot test in *Drosophila melanogaster*. In cultured Chinese hamster lung cells, MeA-α-C induced polyploidy in the absence, and chromosomal aberrations in the presence, of an exogenous metabolic system.

4.3 Human data

No case report or epidemiological study of the carcinogenicity of MeA-α-C was available to the Working Group.

4.4 Evaluation[1]

There is *sufficient evidence*[2] for the carcinogenicity of MeA-α-C to experimental animals.

No data were available on the carcinogenicity of MeA-α-C to humans.

---

[1]For definition of the italicized term, see Preamble, p. 18.

[2]In the absence of data on humans, it is reasonable, for practical purposes, to regard chemicals or exposures for which there is *sufficient evidence* of carcinogenicity in animals as if they presented a carcinogenic risk to humans.

Overall assessment of data from short-term tests: MeA-α-C[a]

	Genetic activity			Cell transformation
	DNA damage	Mutation	Chromosomal effects	
Prokaryotes	+	+		
Fungi/Green plants				
Insects		+		
Mammalian cells (*in vitro*)			+	
Mammals (*in vivo*)				
Humans (*in vivo*)				
Degree of evidence in short-term tests for genetic activity: **Sufficient**				Cell transformation: No data

[a]The groups into which the table is divided and the symbol used are defined on pp. 19-20 of the Preamble; the degrees of evidence are defined on pp. 20-21.

5. References

Hasegawa, R., Tsuda, H., Ogiso, T., Ohshima, M. & Ito, N. (1982) Initiating activities of pyrolysis products of L-lysine and soybean globulin assessed in terms of the induction of γ-glutamyl transpeptidase-positive foci in rat liver. *Gann, 73*, 158-159

Hayatsu, H., Oka, T., Wakata, A., Ohara, Y., Hayatsu, T., Kobayashi, H. & Arimoto, S. (1983) Adsorption of mutagens to cotton bearing covalently bound trisulfo-copper-phthalocyanine. *Mutat. Res., 119*, 233-238

Ishidate, M., ed. (1983) *Chromosomal Aberration Test* in vitro, Tokyo, Realize Inc., p. 253

Matsumoto, T., Yoshida, D. & Tomita, H. (1981a) Synthesis and mutagenic activity of alkyl derivatives of 2-amino-9*H*-pyrido[2,3-*b*]indole. *Agric. Biol. Chem., 45*, 2031-2035

Matsumoto, T., Yoshida, D. & Tomita, H. (1981b) Determination of mutagens, amino-α-carbolines in grilled foods and cigarette smoke condensate. *Cancer Lett., 12*, 105-110

Nagao, M., Fujita, Y., Wakabayashi, K. & Sugimura, T. (1983a) Ultimate forms of mutagenic and carcinogenic heterocyclic amines produced by pyrolysis. *Biochem. biophys. Res. Commun., 114*, 626-631

Nagao, M., Sato, A. & Sugimura, T. (1983b) *Mutagens produced by heating foods.* In: Waller, G.R., & Feather, M.S., eds, *The Maillard Reaction in Foods and Nutrition (ACS Symposium Series 215)*, Washington DC, American Chemical Society, pp. 521-536

Nebert, D.W., Bigelow, S.W., Okey, A.B., Yahagi, T., Mori, Y., Nagao, M. & Sugimura, T. (1979) Pyrolysis products from amino acids and protein: highest mutagenicity requires cytochrome P_1-450. *Proc. natl Acad. Sci. USA, 76,* 5929-5933

Ohgaki, H., Matsukura, N., Morino, K., Kawachi, T., Sugimura, T. & Takayama, S. (1984) Carcinogenicity in mice of mutagenic compounds from glutamic acid and soybean globulin pyrolysates. *Carcinogenesis, 5,* 815-819

Peters, J.H., Mortelmans, K.E., Reist, E.J., Sigman, C.C., Spanggord, R.J. & Thomas, D.W. (1981) Synthesis, chemical characterization, and mutagenic activities of promutagens produced by pyrolysis of proteinaceous substances. *Environ. Mutagenesis, 3,* 639-649

Schunk, H., Hayashi, T. & Shibamoto, T. (1984) Analysis of mutagenic amino acid pyrolyzates with a fused silica capillary column. *J. high Resolut. Chromatogr. Chromatogr. Commun., 7,* 563-565

Sugimura, T., Nagao, M. & Wakabayashi, K. (1981) *Mutagenic heterocyclic amines in cooked food.* In: Egan, H., Fishbein, L., Castegnaro, M., O'Neill, I.K. & Bartsch, H., eds, *Environmental Carcinogens. Selected Methods of Analysis,* Vol. 4, *Some Aromatic and Azo Dyes in the General and Industrial Environment (IARC Scientific Publications No. 40)*, Lyon, International Agency for Research on Cancer, pp. 251-267

Sugimura, T., Sato, S. & Takayama, S. (1983) *New mutagenic heterocyclic amines found in amino acid and protein pyrolysates and in cooked food.* In: Wynder, E.L., Leveille, G.A., Weisburger, Y.H. & Livingston, G.E., eds, *Environmental Aspects of Cancer: The Role of Macro and Micro Components of Foods*, Westport, CT, Food and Nutrition Press, pp. 167-186

Watanabe, J., Kawajiri, K., Yonekawa, H., Nagao, M. & Tagashira, Y. (1982) Immunological analysis of the roles of two major types of cytochrome P-450 in mutagenesis of compounds isolated from pyrolysates. *Biochem. biophys. Res. Commun., 104,* 193-199

Yoo, M.A., Ryo, H., Todo, T. & Kondo, S. (1985) Mutagenic potency of heterocyclic amines in the *Drosophila* wing spot test and its correlation to carcinogenic potency. *Jpn. J. Cancer Res. (Gann), 76,* 468-473

Yoshida, D. & Matsumoto, T. (1979) Isolation of 2-amino-9*H*-pyrido[2,3-*b*]indole and 2-amino-3-methyl-9*H*-pyrido[2,3-*b*]indole as mutagens from pyrolysis product of tryptophan. *Agric. Biol. Chem., 43,* 1155-1156

Yoshida, D. & Matsumoto, T. (1980) Amino-α-carbolines as mutagenic agents in cigarette smoke condensate. *Cancer Lett., 10,* 141-149

Yoshida, D., Matsumoto, T., Yoshimura, R. & Matsuzaki, T. (1978) Mutagenicity of amino-α-carbolines in pyrolysis products of soybean globulin. *Biochem. biophys. Res. Commun., 83,* 915-920

IQ (2-AMINO-3-METHYLIMIDAZO[4,5-*f*]QUINOLINE)

1. Chemical and Physical Data

1.1 Synonyms and trade names

Chem. Abstr. Services Reg. No.: 76180-96-6
Chem. Abstr. Name: 3-Methyl-3*H*-imidazo[4,5-*f*]quinolin-2-amine
IUPAC Systematic Name: 2-Amino-3-methyl-3*H*-imidazo[4,5-*f*]quinoline

1.2 Structural and molecular formulae and molecular weight

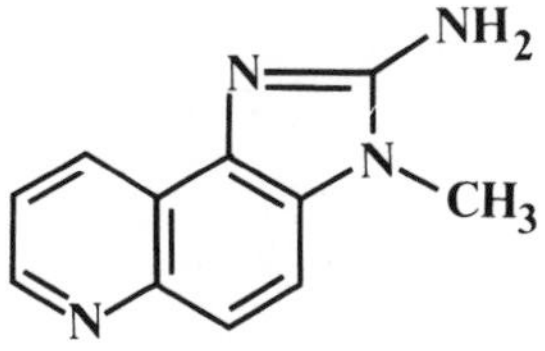

$C_{11}H_{10}N_4$

Mol. wt: 198.23

1.3 Chemical and physical properties of the pure substance

(*a*)   *Description*: Crystalline solid (Kasai *et al.*, 1981)

(*b*)   *Melting-point*: > 300°C (Kasai *et al.*, 1981; Sugimura *et al.*, 1981; Lee *et al.*, 1982)

(*c*)   *Spectroscopy data*: Ultraviolet (Sugimura *et al.*, 1981), Fourier-transform infrared (Kasai *et al.*, 1981), proton nuclear magnetic resonance (Sugimura *et al.*, 1981) and mass spectral data (Spingarn *et al.*, 1980) have been reported.

(d)   *Solubility*: Soluble in methanol, ethanol and dimethyl sulphoxide (Kasai *et al.*, 1980a, 1981; Lee *et al.*, 1982; Schunk *et al.*, 1984)

(*e*)   *Stability*: Stable under moderately acidic and alkaline conditions and in cold dilute aqueous solutions protected from light (Sugimura *et al.*, 1983)

(*f*)   *Reactivity*: Rapidly degraded by dilute hypochlorite; not deactivated by weakly acidic nitrite solutions (Sugimura *et al.*, 1983)

2. Production, Use, Occurrence and Analysis

2.1 Production and use

(a) Production

The isolation and identification of IQ was first reported by Kasai et al. (1980b). Its structure was confirmed by chemical synthesis, in which 5,6-diaminoquinoline was reacted with cyanogen bromide and the resulting cyclic intermediate was converted to IQ by heating the tetramethylammonium salt of this compound under reduced pressure. Final purification was accomplished by sublimation, silica-gel column chromatography and crystallization from aqueous methanol (Kasai et al., 1980a, 1981).

Although this synthesis yields primarily the 3-N-methyl derivative, other methyl derivatives are also produced in the last step. Synthetic routes to IQ that avoid formation of the other isomers (by making the last step cyclization rather than methylation) were devised by Lee et al. (1982) and by Adolfsson and Olsson (1983).

IQ is not produced in commercial or bulk quantities.

(b) Use

IQ is not used commercially.

2.2 Occurrence

IQ is not known to occur in nature.

It was originally isolated from broiled fish and has also been detected in fried ground beef and beef extracts; ranges are given in Table 1. IQ has also been found in a mixture of creatine and proline heated to 180°C (Yoshida et al., 1984) and in fried bacon (Miller, 1984).

2.3 Analysis

IQ has been isolated from broiled sun-dried sardines, ground and extracted with methanol. The neutral fraction obtained from the extract was subjected to Diaion HP-20 column chromatography, chloroform-methanol-water partitioning, and Sephadex LH-20 column chromatography. The resulting mutagenic fraction was separated into IQ and MeIQ (2-amino-3,4-dimethylimidazo[4,5-f]quinoline) (see p. 275) by silica-gel column chromatography and further purified by reverse-phase high-performance liquid chromatography (HPLC). The structure was mainly deduced from proton nuclear magnetic resonance and high-resolution mass spectral data (Kasai et al., 1980b, 1981).

IQ has been isolated from beef extract by dichloromethane extraction, column chromatography on Adsorbosil-5 and Sephadex LH20 and HPLC, with analysis by mass spectrometry, ultraviolet spectrophotometry and/or mutagenesis assay (Hargraves et al., 1982; Hargraves & Pariza, 1983; Turesky et al., 1983). The authors reported that this

Table 1. Concentrations of IQ in foods

Sample	Concentration (ng/g)	Reference
Beef extract		
for bacteriological media	41-142	Turesky *et al.* (1983)
	20-40	Hayatsu *et al.* (1983)
bacteriological and food-grade	42	Takahashi *et al.* (1985)
food-grade	~ 4	Hargraves & Pariza (1983)
Ground beef (fried)		
fat content unspecified	~ 0.02	Hargraves & Pariza (1983)
	~ 0.6	Nagao *et al.* (1983a)
10-28% fat (240°C)	0.5-20	Barnes *et al.* (1983)
15% fat (250°C)	0.02	Felton *et al.* (1984)
Sardines (sun-dried, broiled)	~ 20	Kasai *et al.* (1980b)
	158	Nagao *et al.* (1983a)

technique did not detect IQ in extracts of fried ground beef [although analysis of the data suggests that as much as 0.02 ng/g may have been present] (Hargraves *et al.*, 1982; Hargraves & Pariza, 1983). Using another procedure, however, IQ was detected in fried ground beef at levels in the range of 0.02 ng/g following dichloromethane extraction, chromatography on XAD-2 resin, preparative reverse-phase HPLC, and analysis by high-resolution gas chromatography/mass spectroscopy (Felton *et al.*, 1984). Using the method of standard additions, preparative thin-layer chromatography followed by reverse-phase HPLC was reported to detect levels as low as 0.1 ng/g IQ in fried ground beef (Barnes *et al.*, 1983).

IQ can be adsorbed selectively from aqueous solutions onto cellulose or cotton to which C.I. Reactive Blue 21, a trisulpho-copper phthalocyanine dye, has been bound covalently. The adsorbed IQ is eluted with ammoniacal methanol and quantified by assay for mutagenic activity (Hayatsu *et al.*, 1983). More recently, this 'blue-cotton' adsorption technique has been used as the first step in a simplified procedure for the detection of IQ in beef extracts, with a sensitivity of approximately 0.1 ng. Analysis involves extraction of acidified adsorbates with dichloromethane, silica-gel chromatography, and assay by HPLC with electrochemical detection (Takahashi *et al.*, 1985).

IQ has also been separated from other heterocyclic amines formed upon pyrolysis of amino acids by gas chromatography with fused silica capillary columns (Schunk *et al.*, 1984).

3. Biological Data Relevant to the Evaluation
of Carcinogenic Risk to Humans

3.1 Carcinogenicity studies in animals

(a) Oral administration

Mouse: Groups of 40 male and 40 female CDF_1 mice [(BALB/cAnN × DBA/2N)F_1], seven weeks of age, were fed a pelleted diet containing 300 mg/kg IQ (purity, >99.6%, checked by high-performance liquid chromatography, with <0.4% impurities) for 675 days, at which time the experiment was terminated. A group of 40 males and 40 females fed basal diet alone served as controls. The numbers of survivors on day 394, when leukaemia was found in a female control, were similar in the four groups: 39/40 treated males, 36/40 treated females, 33/40 control males and 38/40 control females. The incidences of liver tumours (hepatocellular adenomas and hepatocellular carcinomas) in treated mice were 16/39 (41%; $p < 0.005$) in males and 27/36 (75%; $p < 0.001$) in females; of these, eight in males and 22 in females were hepatocellular carcinomas. The incidences of adenomas and adenocarcinomas of the lung were 27/39 (69%) in males and 15/36 (42%) in females; those of squamous-cell papillomas and carcinomas of the forestomach were 16/39 (41%) in males and 11/36 (31%) in females. The incidences of liver, lung and forestomach tumours in controls were: males, 2/33, 7/33 and 1/33; females, 0/38, 7/38 and 0/38, respectively. One male and three female controls had liver haemangioendotheliomas; these tumours were not seen in treated animals (Ohgaki *et al.*, 1984).

Rat: In a study cited in a preliminary report, groups of 40 male and 40 female Fischer 344 rats, eight weeks of age, were fed a pelleted diet containing 300 mg/kg IQ (purity confirmed by high-performance liquid chromatography [percentage not indicated]) for 300 days. A control group of 50 males and 50 females was fed basal diet alone. The times of appearance of the first tumours in males were day 255 for those of the colon, day 239 for those of the small intestine and day 288 for those of the liver. Twenty males and four females from the treated group [but no control] were killed at 300 days, because of ill health due to occurrence of tumours. The incidences of tumours in treated animals at day 300 were as follows: squamous-cell carcinomas of the Zymbal gland: 18/20 (90%) males and 4/4 (100%) females; tumours of the colon: 9/20 (45%) males (two adenomas, seven adenocarcinomas); adenocarcinomas of the small intestine, 5/20 (25%) males; hepatocellular carcinomas, 8/20 (40%) males; carcinomas of the skin, 4/20 (20%) males; and squamous-cell carcinomas of the oral cavity, 2/20 (10%) males. Squamous-cell carcinomas of the clitoral gland were found in 2/4 (50%) treated females (Takayama *et al.*, 1984). [The Working Group noted that no control animal was examined.]

A group of 32 female Sprague-Dawley rats, six weeks of age, received 0.35 mmol [70 mg]/kg bw IQ hydrochloride in 5% Emulphor by gavage thrice weekly during weeks 1-4, twice weekly during weeks 5-8 and weekly during weeks 9-31 and were maintained without further treatment until sacrifice at week 52. A group of 27 rats received 0.25 ml 5% Emulphor according to the same schedule, and a further group of nine animals served as untreated controls. Adenocarcinomas of the mammary gland were observed in 0/9 untreated controls, 0/27 vehicle controls and 14/32 (44%; $p < 0.05$) treated animals. Liver tumours were observed in 0/9 untreated controls, 0/27 vehicle controls and 6/32 (three neoplastic nodules, two hepatocellular carcinomas and two haemangioendotheliomas) treated animals. Squamous-cell carcinomas of the Zymbal gland were found in 11/32 (34%) treated animals, but no such tumour occurred in controls [$p = 0.002$; Fisher exact test] (Tanaka *et al.*, 1985; Weisburger *et al.*, 1986).

(b) Skin application

A group of 30 female Sencar mice, 49-51 days of age, received topical applications of 6 μmol [1.2 mg] IQ (no impurity were detected by high-performance liquid chromatography) in 0.1 ml dimethyl sulphoxide on the dorsal skin thrice weekly for two weeks, followed ten days later by applications of 2.1 mg 12-*O*-tetradecanoyphorbol 13-acetate (TPA) in 0.1 ml acetone twice a week for 20 weeks. A control group of 20 animals was treated with applications of dimethyl sulphoxide alone, followed by TPA treatment. Skin tumours were observed in 2/30 treated mice and 1/30 controls (Barnes *et al.*, 1985; Weisburger *et al.*, 1986). [The Working Group noted the short duration of the study.]

3.2 Other relevant biological data

(a) Experimental systems

Toxic effects

Female Sprague-Dawley rats (six weeks of age) administered a total dose of 15 mmol/kg bw [3000 mg/kg bw] IQ by gavage over 30 weeks exhibited a weight gain over one year which was 94% that of the controls. In addition, after one year, the treated group had altered liver-cell foci, atypical hyperplastic acinar-cell lesions in the pancreas and altered proliferative foci in the adrenal cortex, none of which was present in the control group (Tanaka *et al.*, 1985).

The activation of oncogenes in hepatocellular carcinomas induced by IQ in Fischer 344 rats was studied by transfecting DNA from the tumours into NIH 3T3 cells. In one hepatocellular carcinoma out of five tested, activated *H-ras*-1 oncogene was identified, as well as another oncogene not belonging to the *ras*-gene family (Ishikawa *et al.*, 1985).

Effects on reproduction and prenatal toxicity

No data were available to the Working Group.

Absorption, distribution, excretion and metabolism

The absorption and excretion of [2-^{14}C]-IQ (specific activity, 2.03 Ci/mol) was studied in Sprague-Dawley rats of each sex. After a single oral dose (10^7 dpm; 4 mg/kg bw), excretion was rapid, 46-68% being excreted in the faeces and 37-49% in the urine within 72 h. About 70% of the radioactivity was found in the bile after 24 h in a separate study. While no mutagenic activity was detected in urine or faeces, after metabolic activation, the bile had mutagenic activity (Sjödin & Jägerstad, 1984).

Male NMRI mice were injected intravenously with 25 μCi [2-^{14}C]-IQ (specific activity, 18.8 Ci/mol). After short survival times, whole-body autoradiograms showed widespread distribution, the liver and kidney being identified as sites of retention of non-extractable residues. The uptake of IQ by retina and other pigmented tissues of female C3H mice injected intravenously with IQ exceeded that of any other tissue, at all survival times studied, demonstrating an affinity of IQ for melanine (Bergman, 1985).

When female NMRI mice were injected intravenously with 25 μCi [2-^{14}C]-IQ (8.8 mg/kg bw; specific activity, 18.8 Ci/mol) on day 16 of gestation, IQ crossed the placenta and reached the fetus. After 20 min, uptake in the fetal liver was observed; at 4 h, amniotic fluid, fetal urinary bladder and intestinal contents were heavily labelled. By 24 h, radioactivity was found in fetal intestines and amniotic fluid (Bergman, 1985).

When IQ was incubated with rat-liver microsomes, the formation of *N*-hydroxy-IQ, a directly-acting mutagen, was shown to be mediated by a cytochrome P450-dependent system (Yamazoe *et al.*, 1983). The cytochrome P450 isoenzymes most active in this transformation were those induced by polychlorinated biphenyls (PCB) and 3-methyl-cholanthrene (Watanabe *et al.*, 1982; Yamazoe *et al.*, 1983). When microsomal ability to activate IQ to a mutagen was compared using hepatic microsomes obtained from mice, rats and rabbits not exposed to inducing agents, more than a nine-fold difference was observed (Yamazoe *et al.*, 1983). The metabolite, *N*-hydroxy-IQ, was found to bind rapidly and covalently to calf thymus DNA (Okamoto *et al.*, 1981).

In a study to provide information on the metabolic steps involved in the formation of the active mutagenic form, it was observed that IQ was not mutagenic to *Salmonella typhimurium* TA98/1,8-DNP$_6$ (defective in esterifying activity) in the presence of an exogenous metabolic system (S9 mix), while it was strongly mutagenic to the original TA98 with S9 mix. The mutagenicity of IQ to TA98 was inhibited by pentachlorophenol, an aryl sulphotransferase inhibitor. These data suggest that the ultimate form of IQ is probably the sulphate ester of *N*-hydroxy-IQ (Nagao *et al.*, 1983b). The addition of L-buthionine sulphoximine, an inhibitor of glutathione synthesis, enhanced binding of IQ to primary hepatocyte monolayer cultures, suggesting that conjugation with glutathione may be involved in the deactivation of IQ *in vivo* (Loretz & Pariza, 1984).

Mutagenicity and other short-term tests

IQ (tested at concentrations of 1-100 μg/plate) induced prophage λ in lysogenic *Escherichia coli* K12 in the presence of an exogenous metabolic system (S9) from the livers of polychlorinated biphenyl (PCB)-induced rats (Nagao *et al.*, 1983a). It was mutagenic to *Salmonella typhimurium* TA1537, TA1538, TA1978, TA98 and TA100 in the presence of S9 from various species (Kasai *et al.*, 1981; Nagao *et al.*, 1981; Gayda & Pariza, 1983; Nagao *et al.*, 1983a,b; Thompson *et al.*, 1983; Grivas & Jägerstad, 1984; Barnes *et al.*, 1985; Wild *et al.*, 1985). However, IQ was not mutagenic to strain TA1535. In an intrasanguineous host-mediated assay in mice, IQ induced a dose-dependent increase in mutations (strain TA98) when administered intraperitoneally or orally (Wild *et al.*, 1985). Urine from rats treated intravenously with IQ was mutagenic in strains TA98 and TA100 but not in TA1535 or TA1537 in the presence of S9 (Barnes & Weisburger, 1985).

IQ gave positive results in the wing spot test in *Drosophila melanogaster* (transhetero-zygous for the loci *mwh* and *flr*) raised in a medium containing 0.1-1.0 mg/g (Yoo *et al.*, 1985). It also induced sex-linked recessive lethal mutations in *Drosophila melanogaster* (Wild *et al.*, 1985).

IQ induced single-strand DNA breaks in mouse leukaemia cells in the presence of PCB-induced rat-liver S9 at concentrations of $10^{-5}M$ and $10^{-4}M$, and in rat hepatocytes isolated from 3,3',4,4'-tetrachloroazobenzene-induced rat liver at concentrations of 5×10^{-6} and 5×10^{-5} M (Caderni *et al.*, 1983). In rat hepatocytes, IQ induced unscheduled DNA synthesis at concentrations of 1.25×10^{-6} and 1.25×10^{-5} M (Barnes *et al.*, 1985). It also induced unscheduled DNA synthesis in primary cultures of rat and hamster hepatocytes, but not guinea-pig hepatocytes, at doses of 3, 10 and 30 μM (Loury & Byard, 1985).

IQ (5-40 μg/ml) induced diphtheria toxin-resistant mutants in Chinese hamster lung cells in the presence of PCB-induced rat-liver S9 (Nakayasu *et al.*, 1983). It induced mutations in repair-deficient, but not wild-type, cultured Chinese hamster ovary cells at doses of up to 300 μg/ml in the presence of PCB-induced hamster-liver S9 (Thompson *et al.*, 1983). However, at concentrations up to 50 μg/ml, it did not induce ouabain-resistant mutants in Chinese hamster V79 cells in the presence or absence of a Syrian hamster embryo feeder layer (Takayama & Tanaka, 1983).

IQ induced sister chromatid exchanges in repair-deficient cultured Chinese hamster ovary cells and in wild-type cells in the presence of PCB-induced hamster-liver S9, but did not induce chromosomal aberrations in either cell type at concentrations of up to 300 μg/ml (Thompson *et al.*, 1983).

IQ was reported to cause morphological transformation in the BALBc/3T3 mouse cell line (Cortesi & Dolara, 1983). [The Working Group noted that only one experiment was carried out and that a small number of transformed foci was induced.]

When given by intraperitoneal injection to male C57BL/6 mice at concentrations of 20-160 mg/kg bw, IQ did not increase the incidence of chromosomal aberrations but caused a 1.44-fold increase in sister chromatid exchanges (Minkler & Carrano, 1984). [The Working Group noted that this was a borderline increase.]

IQ did not induce unscheduled DNA synthesis in male rats when given by gavage at concentrations of 77-230 mg/kg bw (Furihata & Matsushima, 1982). [The Working Group noted that the experiment was designed to investigate one organ only.]

No micronuclei were induced in the bone marrow of NMRI mice after intraperitoneal administration of 198 or 594 mg/kg bw or after administration by gavage of 198 mg/kg bw (Wild *et al.*, 1985).

Gene mutation was not observed in the spot test in mice exposed to 20 mg/kg bw IQ *in utero* nor in the melanocyte test following treatment *in utero* with up to 400 mg/kg bw (Wild *et al.*, 1985).

(*b*) *Humans*

No data were available to the Working Group.

3.3 Case reports and epidemiological studies of carcinogenicity in humans

No data were available to the Working Group.

4. Summary of Data Reported and Evaluation

4.1 Exposure data

IQ (2-amino-3-methylimidazo[4,5-*f*]quinoline) has been found in grilled fish, fried beef and some beef extracts. Consumption of these foods may result in human exposure.

4.2 Experimental data

IQ was tested for carcinogenicity in one experiment in mice by oral administration in the diet and in one experiment in female rats by oral intubation. Hepatocellular adenomas and carcinomas, adenomas and adenocarcinomas of the lung, and squamous-cell papillomas and carcinomas of the forestomach were reported in mice. Rats developed adeno-carcinomas of the mammary gland and squamous-cell carcinomas of the Zymbal gland.

In an experiment in progress described in a preliminary report, male and female rats administered IQ in the diet developed tumours at various sites, but no data on controls were available.

IQ crosses the placenta of mice.

IQ induced prophage in bacteria and was mutagenic to *Salmonella typhimurium* in the presence of an exogenous metabolic system. It gave positive results in the wing spot test in *Drosophila melanogaster* and induced sex-linked recessive lethal mutations. IQ induced DNA damage, mutations and sister chromatid exchanges in mammalian cells *in vitro*. It did not induce mutations or chromosomal effects *in vivo*.

4.3 Human

No case report or epidemiological study of the carcinogenicity of IQ was available to the Working Group.

4.4 Evaluation[1]

There is *sufficient evidence*[2] for the carcinogenicity of IQ to experimental animals.

No data were available on the carcinogenicity of IQ to humans.

---

[1]For definition of the italicized term, see Preamble, p. 18.

[2]In the absence of adequate data on humans, it is reasonable, for practical purposes, to regard chemicals or exposures for which there is *sufficient evidence* of carcinogenicity in animals as if they represented a carcinogenic risk to humans.

Overall assessment of data from short-term tests: IQ[a]

	Genetic activity			Cell transformation
	DNA damage	Mutation	Chromosomal effects	
Prokaryotes	+	+		
Fungi/Green plants				
Insects		+		
Mammalian cells (*in vitro*)	+	+	+	
Mammals (*in vivo*)		–	–	
Humans (*in vivo*)				
Degree of evidence in short-term tests for genetic activity: **Sufficient**				Cell transformation: Inadequate

[a]The groups into which the table is divided and the symbols used are defined on pp. 19-20 of the Preamble; the degrees of evidence are defined on pp. 20-21.

5. References

Adolfsson, L. & Olsson, K. (1983) A convenient synthesis of mutagenic 3*H*-imidazo-[4,5-*f*]quinolin-2-amines and their 2-^{14}C-labelled analogues. *Acta chem. scand.*, *37B*, 157-159

Barnes, W.S. & Weisburger, J.H. (1985) Fate of the food mutagen 2-amino-3-methyl-imidazo[4,5-*f*]quinoline (IQ) in Sprague-Dawley rats. I. Mutagens in the urine. *Mutat. Res.*, *156*, 83-91

Barnes, W.S., Maher, J.C. & Weisburger, J.H. (1983) High-pressure liquid chromatography method for analysis of 2-amino-3-methylimidazo[4,5-*f*]-quinoline, a mutagen formed during the cooking of food. *J. agric. Food Chem.*, *31*, 883-886

Barnes, W.S., Lovelette, C.A., Tong, C., Williams, G.M. & Weisburger, J.H. (1985) Genotoxicity of the food mutagen 2-amino-3-methylimidazo[4,5-*f*]quinoline (IQ) and analogs. *Carcinogenesis*, *6*, 441-444

Bergman, K. (1985) Autoradiographic distribution of ^{14}C-labeled 3*H*-imidazo[4,5-*f*]quinoline-2-amines in mice. *Cancer Res.*, *45*, 1351-1356

Caderni, G., Kreamer, B.L. & Dolara, P. (1983) DNA damage of mammalian cells by the beef extract mutagen 2-amino-3-methylimidazo[4,5-*f*]quinoline. *Food Chem. Toxicol.*, *21*, 641-643

Cortesi, E. & Dolara, P. (1983) Neoplastic transformation of BALB 3T3 mouse embryo fibroblasts by the beef extract mutagen 2-amino-3-methylimidazo[4,5-*f*]quinoline. *Cancer Lett.*, *20*, 43-47

Felton, J.S., Knize, M.G., Wood, C., Wuebbles, B.J., Healy, S.K., Stuermer, D.H., Bjeldanes, L.F., Kimble, B.J. & Hatch, F.T. (1984) Isolation and characterization of new mutagens from fried ground beef. *Carcinogenesis*, *5*, 95-102

Furihata, C. & Matsushima, T. (1982) *Unscheduled DNA synthesis in rat stomach —short-term assay of potential stomach carcinogens*. In: Bridges, B.A., Butterworth, B.E. & Weinstein, B.I., eds, *Indicators of Genotoxic Exposure (Banbury Report No. 13)*, Cold Spring Harbor, NY, Cold Spring Harbor Laboratory, pp. 123-135

Gayda, D.P. & Pariza, M.W. (1983) Activation of 2-amino-3-methylimidazo[4,5-*f*]-quinoline and 2-aminofluorene for bacterial mutagenesis by primary monolayer cultures of adult rat hepatocytes. *Mutat. Res.*, *118*, 7-14

Grivas, S. & Jägerstad, M. (1984) Mutagenicity of some synthetic quinolines and quinoxalines related to IQ, MeIQ or MeIQx in Ames test. *Mutat. Res.*, *137*, 29-32

Hargraves, W.A., Dietrich, R. & Pariza, M.W. (1982) *A new chromatographic method for separating mutagens from commercial beef extract and fried ground beef*. In: Stich, H.F., ed., *Carcinogens and Mutagens in the Environment*, Vol. 1, Boca Raton, FL, CRC Press, pp. 223-229

Hargraves, W.A. & Pariza, M.W. (1983) Purification and mass spectral characterization of bacterial mutagens from commercial beef extract. *Cancer Res.*, *43*, 1467-1472

Hayatsu, H., Matsui. Y., Ohara, Y., Oka, T. & Hayatsu, T. (1983) Characterization of mutagenic fractions in beef extract and in cooked ground beef. Use of blue-cotton for efficient extraction. *Gann*, *74*, 472-482

Ishikawa, F., Takaku, F., Nagao, M., Ochiai, M., Hayashi, K., Takayama, S. & Sugimura, T. (1985) Activated oncogenes in a rat hepatocellular carcinoma induced by 2-amino-3-methylimidazo-[4,5-*f*]quinoline. *Jpn. J. Cancer Res. (Gann)*, *76*, 425-428

Kasai, H., Nishimura, S., Wakabayashi, K., Nagao, M. & Sugimura, T. (1980a) Chemical synthesis of 2-amino-3-methylimidazo[4,5-*f*]quinoline (IQ), a potent mutagen isolated from broiled fish. *Proc. Jpn. Acad.*, *56B*, 382-384

Kasai, H., Yamaizumi, Z., Wakabayashi, K., Nagao, M., Sugimura, T., Yokoyama, S., Miyazawa, T., Spingarn, N.E., Weisburger, J.H. & Nishimura, S. (1980b) Potent novel mutants produced by broiling fish under normal conditions. *Proc. Jpn. Acad.*, *56B*, 278-283

Kasai, H., Yamaizumi, Z., Nishimura, S., Wakabayashi, K., Nagao, M., Sugimura, T., Spingarn, N.E., Weisburger, J.H., Yokoyama, S. & Miyazawa, T. (1981) A potent mutagen in broiled fish. Part 1. 2-Amino-3-methyl-3*H*-imidazo[4,5-*f*]quinoline. *J. chem. Soc. Perkin Trans. 1*, 2290-2293

Lee, C.-S., Hasimoto, Y., Shudo, K. & Okamoto, T. (1982) Synthesis of mutagenic heteroaromatics: 2-aminoimidazo[4,5-*f*]quinolines. *Chem. pharm. Bull.*, *30*, 1857-1859

Loretz, L.J. & Pariza, M.W. (1984) Effect of glutathione levels, sulfate levels, and metabolic inhibitors on covalent binding of 2-amino-3-methylimidazo[4,5-*f*]quinoline and 2-acetylaminofluorene to cell macromolecules in primary monolayer cultures of adult rat hepatocytes. *Carcinogenesis*, *5*, 895-899

Loury, D.J. & Byard, J.L. (1985) Genotoxicity of the cooked-food mutagens IQ and MeIQ in primary cultures of rat, hamster, and guinea pig hepatocytes. *Environ. Mutagenesis*, *7*, 245-254

Miller, A.J. (1984) Detection, characterization, and presumptive identification of a bacterial mutagen from thermally processed bacon. *Diss. Abstr.*, *45*, 1418B

Minkler, J.L. & Carrano, A.V. (1984) In vivo cytogenetic effects of the cooked-food-related mutagens Trp-P-2 and IQ in mouse bone marrow. *Mutat. Res.*, *140*, 49-53

Nagao, M., Sato, S. & Sugimura, T. (1983a) *Mutagens produced by heating foods*. In: Waller, G.R. & Feather, M.S., eds, *The Maillard Reaction in Foods and Nutrition (ACS Symposium Series 125)*, Washington DC, American Chemical Society, pp. 521-536

Nagao, M., Fujita, Y., Wakabayashi, K. & Sugimura, T. (1983b) Ultimate forms of mutagenic and carcinogenic heterocyclic amines produced by pyrolysis. *Biochem. biophys. Res. Commun.*, *114*, 626-631

Nagao, M., Wakabayashi, K., Kasai, H., Nishimura, S. & Sugimura, T. (1981) Effect of methyl substitution on mutagenicity of 2-amino-3-methylimidazo[4,5-*f*]quinoline, isolated from broiled sardine. *Carcinogenesis*, *2*, 1147-1149

Nakayasu, M., Nakasato, F., Sakamoto, H., Terada, M. & Sugimura, T. (1983) Mutagenic activity of heterocyclic amines in Chinese hamster lung cells with diphtheria toxin resistance as a marker. *Mutat. Res.*, *118*, 91-102

Ohgaki, H., Kusama, K., Matsukura, N., Morino, K., Hasegawa, H., Sato, S., Takayama, S. & Sugimura, T. (1984) Carcinogenicity in mice of a mutagenic compound, 2-amino-3-methylimidazo[4,5-*f*]quinoline, from broiled sardine, cooked beef and beef extract. *Carcinogenesis*, *5*, 921-924

Okamoto, T., Shudo, K., Hashimoto, Y., Kosuge, T., Sugimura, T. & Nishimura, S. (1981) Identification of a reactive metabolite of the mutagen, 2-amino-3-methylimidazolo-[4,5-*f*]-quinoline. *Chem. pharm. Bull.*, *29*, 590-593

Schunk, H., Hayashi, Y. & Shibamoto, T. (1984) Analysis of mutagenic amino acid pyrolyzates with a fused silica capillary column. *J. high Resolut. Chromatogr. Chromatogr. Commun.*, *7*, 563-565

Sjödin, P. & Jägerstad, M. (1984) A balance study of ^{14}C-labelled 3*H*-imidazo[4,5-*f*]-quinolin-2-amines (IQ and MeIQ) in rats. *Food chem. Toxicol.*, *22*, 207-210

Spingarn, N.E., Kasai, H., Vuolo, L.L., Nishimura, S., Yamaizumi, Z., Sugimura, T., Matsushima, T. & Weisburger, J.H. (1980) Formation of mutagens in cooked food. III. Isolation of a potent mutagen from beef. *Cancer Lett.*, *9*, 177-183

Sugimura, T., Nagao, M. & Wakabayashi, K. (1981) *Mutagenic heterocyclic amines in cooked food.* In: Egan, H., Fishbein, L., Castegnaro, M., O'Neill, I.K. & Bartsch, H., eds, *Environmental Carcinogens. Selected Methods of Analysis*, Vol. 4, *Some Aromatic and Azo Dyes in the General and Industrial Environment* (*IARC Scientific Publications No. 40*), Lyon, International Agency for Research on Cancer, pp. 251-267

Sugimura, T., Sato, S. & Takayama, S. (1983) *New mutagenic heterocyclic amines found in amino acid and protein pyrolysates and in cooked food.* In: Wynder, E.L., Leveille, G.A., Weisburger, J.H. & Livingston, G.E., eds, *Environmental Aspects of Cancer: The Role of Macro and Micro Components of Foods*, Westport, CT, Food and Nutrition Press, pp. 167-186

Takahashi, M., Wakabayashi, K., Nagao, M., Yamamoto, M., Masui, T., Goto, T., Kinae, N., Tomita, I. & Sugimura, T. (1985) Quantification of 2-amino-3-methylimidazo-[4,5-*f*]quinoline (IQ) and 2-amino-3,8-dimethylimidazo[4,5-f]quinoxaline (MeIQx) in beef extracts by liquid chromatography with electrochemical detection (LCEC). *Carcinogenesis, 6*, 1195-1199

Takayama, S. & Tanaka, M. (1983) Mutagenesis of amino acid pyrolysis products in Chinese hamster V79 cells. *Toxicol. Lett., 17*, 23-28

Takayama, S., Nakatsuru, Y., Masuda, M., Ohgaki, H., Sato, S. & Sugimura, T. (1984) Demonstration of carcinogenicity in F344 rats of 2-amino-3-methylimidazo[4,5-*f*]-quinoline from broiled sardine, fried beef and beef extract. *Gann, 75*, 467-470

Tanaka, T., Barnes, W.S., Williams, G.M. & Weisburger, J.H. (1985) Multipotential carcinogenicity of the fried food mutagen 2-amino-3-methylimidazo[4,5-*f*]quinoline in rats. *Jpn. J. Cancer Res. (Gann), 76*, 570-576

Thompson, L.H., Carrano, A.V., Salazar, E., Felton, J.S. & Hatch, F.T. (1983) Comparative genotoxic effects of the cooked-food-related mutagens Trp-P-2 and IQ in bacteria and cultured mammalian cells. *Mutat. Res., 117*, 243-257

Turesky, R.J., Wishnok, J.S., Tannenbaum, S.R., Pfund, R.A. & Buchi, G.H. (1983) Qualitative and quantitative characterization of mutagens in commercial beef extract. *Carcinogenesis, 4*, 863-866

Watanabe, J., Kawajiri, K., Yonekawa, H., Nagao, M. & Tagashira, Y. (1982) Immuno-logical analysis of the roles of two major types of cytochrome P-450 in mutagenesis of compounds isolated from pyrolysates. *Biochem. biophys. Res. Commun., 104*, 193-199

Weisburger, J.M., Barnes, W.S., Lovellette, C.A., Tong, C., Tanaka, T. & Williams, G.M. (1986) Genotoxicity, carcinogenicity and mode of action of the fried food mutagen 2-amino-3-methylimidazo[4,5-*f*]quinoline (IQ) *Environ. Health Perspect., 67*, 121-127

Wild, D., Gocke, E., Harnasch, D., Kaiser, G. & King, M.-T. (1985) Differential mutagenic activity of IQ (2-amino-3-methylimidazo[4,5-*f*]quinoline) in *Salmonella typhimurium* strains in vitro and in vivo, in *Drosophila*, and in mice. *Mutat. Res., 156*, 93-102

Yamazoe, Y., Shimada, M., Kamataki, T. & Kato, R. (1983) Microsomal activation of 2-amino-3-methylimidazo[4,5-*f*]-quinoline, a pyrolysate of sardine and beef extracts, to a mutagenic intermediate. *Cancer Res., 43*, 5768-5774

Yoo, M.A., Ryo, H., Todo, T. & Kondo, S. (1985) Mutagenic potency of heterocyclic amines in the *Drosophila* wing spot test and its correlation to carcinogenic potency. *Jpn. J. Cancer Res. (Gann)*, *76*, 468-473

Yoshida, D., Saito, Y. & Mizusaki, S. (1984) Isolation of 2-amino-3-methylimidazo[4,5-*f*]-quinoline as a mutagen from the heated product of a mixture of creatinine and proline. *Agric. Biol. Chem.*, *48*, 241-243

MeIQ (2-AMINO-3,4-DIMETHYLIMIDAZO[4,5-*f*]QUINOLINE

1. Chemical and Physical Data

1.1 Synonyms and trade names

Chem. Abstr. Services Reg. No.: 77094-11-2
Chem. Abstr. Name: 3,4-Dimethyl-3*H*-imidazo[4,5-*f*]quinolin-2-amine
IUPAC Systematic Name: 2-Amino-3,4-dimethyl-3*H*-imidazo[4,5-*f*]quinoline

1.2 Structural and molecular formulae and molecular weight

$C_{12}H_{12}N_4$ Mol. wt: 212.25

1.3 Chemical and physical properties of the pure substance

(a) *Description*: Brown crystalline solid (Lee *et al.*, 1982; Adolfsson & Olsson, 1983)

(b) *Melting-point*: 294-296°C (Lee *et al.*, 1982); 296-298°C (Adolfsson & Olsson, 1983)

(c) *Spectroscopy data*: Ultraviolet (Kasai *et al.*, 1980a), proton nuclear magnetic resonance (Sugimura *et al.*, 1981) and mass spectral data (Hargraves & Pariza, 1983) have been reported.

(d) *Solubility*: Soluble in methanol, ethanol and dimethyl sulphoxide (Lee *et al.*, 1982; Adolfsson & Olsson, 1983; Schunk *et al.*, 1984)

(e) *Stability*: Stable under moderately acidic and alkaline conditions and in cold dilute aqueous solutions protected from light (Sugimura *et al.*, 1983)

(f) *Reactivity*: Rapidly degraded by dilute hypochlorite; not deactivated by weakly acidic nitrite solutions (Sugimura *et al.*, 1983)

2. Production, Use, Occurrence and Analysis

2.1 Production and use

(a) Production

The isolation and identification of MeIQ was first reported by Kasai *et al.* (1980b). Its structure was confirmed by chemical synthesis, in which 6-acetamido-7-methylquinoline was nitrated and the resulting *N*-nitroacetamido derivative was hydrolysed, with rearrangement to 6-amino-5-nitro-7-methylquinoline. Reduction of the nitro group, reaction with cyanogen bromide and methylation yielded a mixture of the *N*-3-methyl (MeIQ) and *N*-1-methyl derivatives of 2-amino-4-methylimidazo[4,5-*f*]quinoline. High-performance liquid chromatography was used to separate these compounds and isolate MeIQ (Kasai *et al.*, 1980a).

Alternative syntheses of MeIQ, which avoid formation of other methyl isomers (by making the last step cyclization rather than methylation), were devised by Lee *et al.* (1982) and by Adolfsson and Olsson (1983).

MeIQ is not produced in commercial or bulk quantities.

(b) Use

MeIQ is not used commercially.

2.2 Occurrence

MeIQ is not known to occur in nature.

MeIQ has been detected in grilled sun-dried sardines at 20 to 72 ng/g (Kasai *et al.*, 1980b; Nagao *et al.*, 1983a). It has been tentatively identified in beef extract used in bacteriological media (Hargraves & Pariza, 1983).

2.3 Analysis

MeIQ has been isolated from broiled sun-dried sardines, ground and extracted with methanol. The neutral fraction obtained from the extract was subjected to Diaion HP-20 column chromatography, chloroform-methanol-water partitioning and Sephadex LH-20 column chromatography. The resulting mutagenic fraction was separated into IQ (p. 261) and MeIQ by silica-gel column chromatography and further purified by reverse-phase high-performance liquid chromatography. The structure was deduced mainly from proton nuclear magnetic resonance and high-resolution mass spectral data (Kasai *et al.*, 1980b).

MeIQ has also been separated from heterocyclic amines formed upon the pyrolysis of other amino acids by gas chromatography with fused silica capillary columns (Schunk *et al.*, 1984).

3. Biological Data Relevant to the Evaluation of Carcinogenic Risk to Humans

3.1 Carcinogenicity studies in animals

Oral administration

Mouse: In a study described in a preliminary report, groups of 40 male and 40 female CDF_1 [(BALB/cAnN × DBA/2N)F_1] mice, six weeks of age, were given 0 or 0.04% MeIQ in a pelleted diet. The mean body weights of treated mice were consistently 30% lower than those of controls. The first forestomach tumour was observed in a male mouse given MeIQ for 46 weeks and the first liver tumour in a male mouse at 71 weeks. At week 83 of the experiment, 16/40 males and 22/40 females in the treated group were autopsied; squamous-cell carcinomas of the forestomach were found in 10/16 males and 11/22 females (six and four of the tumours, respectively, metastasizing to the liver). Liver tumours were found in 1/16 males (one cholangiocarcinoma) and 9/22 females (three adenomas and six carcinomas). No liver or forestomach tumour was seen in controls (Ohgaki *et al.*, 1985a).

In an abstract describing the same study, it was reported that mice fed 0.01% MeIQ in the diet developed forestomach tumours later and at a lower incidence than mice fed 0.04% (Ohgaki *et al.*, 1985b).

3.2 Other relevant biological data

(*a*)   *Experimental systems*

Toxic effects
No data were available to the Working Group.

Effects on reproduction and prenatal toxicity
No data were available to the Working Group.

Absorption, distribution, excretion and metabolism
The absorption and excretion of [2-^{14}C]-labelled MeIQ (specific activity, 2.03 Ci/mol) was studied in Sprague-Dawley rats of each sex. After a single oral dose (10×10^6 dpm; 4 mg/kg bw), excretion was rapid, 56-66% being excreted in the faeces and 42-49% in the urine within 72 h. In a separate study, about 80% of the radioactivity was found in the bile after 24 h. While no mutagenic activity was detected in urine or faeces, mutagenicity requiring metabolic activation was seen in bile (Sjödin & Jägerstad, 1984).

Male NMRI mice were injected intravenously with 25 μCi [2-^{14}C]-MeIQ (specific activity, 24 Ci/mol). After short survival times, whole-body autoradiograms showed widespread distribution, the liver and kidney being identified as sites of retention of non-extractable residues. The uptake of MeIQ in retina and other pigmented tissues of female C3H mice injected intravenously with MeIQ exceeded that of any other tissue, at all survival times studied, demonstrating an affinity of MeIQ for melanin (Bergman, 1985).

When female NMRI mice were injected intravenously with 25 μCi [2-^{14}C]-MeIQ (6.6 mg/kg bw; specific activity, 24.0 Ci/mol) on day 16 of gestation, MeIQ crossed the placenta and reached the fetus. Uptake by fetal liver was observed after 20 min; at 4 h, amniotic fluid, fetal urinary bladder and intestinal contents were heavily labelled. By 24 h, some radioactivity still remained in fetal intestines and amniotic fluid (Bergman, 1985).

The metabolic activation of MeIQ to directly mutagenic compounds was shown to be mediated by a rat-liver microsomal cytochrome P450 system. The cytochrome P450 isoenzyme induced by 3-methylcholanthrene appeared to be most active in this transformation (Watanabe *et al.*, 1982).

In a study designed to provide information on the metabolic steps involved in the formation of the active mutagenic form, it was observed that MeIQ was not mutagenic to *Salmonella typhimurium* TA98/1,8-DNP$_6$ (defective in esterifying activity) in the presence of an exogenous metabolic system (S9 mix), while it was strongly mutagenic to the original TA98 with S9 mix, suggesting that the ultimate mutagenic form of MeIQ is the sulphate ester of its *N*-hydroxy derivative (Nagao *et al.*, 1983b).

Mutagenicity and other short-term tests

MeIQ (tested at concentrations of 0.1-1 μg/plate) induced prophage λ in lysogenic *Escherichia coli* K12 in the presence of an exogenous metabolic system (S9) (Nagao *et al.*, 1983a). It was mutagenic to *Salmonella typhimurium* TA98 and TA100 in the presence of polychlorinated biphenyl (PCB)-induced rat-liver S9 (Kasai *et al.*, 1980b; Nagao *et al.*, 1981; Grivas & Jägerstad, 1984).

MeIQ gave positive results in the wing spot test in *Drosophila melanogaster* (transheterozygous for the loci *mwh* and *flr*) raised in medium containing 0.1 or 0.4 mg/g (Yoo *et al.*, 1985).

It induced unscheduled DNA synthesis at doses of 3, 10 and 30 μM in primary cultures of rat, hamster and guinea-pig hepatocytes (Loury & Byard, 1985).

MeIQ (6-50 μg/ml) induced diphtheria toxin-resistant mutants in Chinese hamster lung cells in the presence of PCB-induced rat-liver S9 (Nakayasu *et al.*, 1983). At concentrations of up to 50 μg/ml, it was reported not to induce ouabain-resistant mutants in Chinese hamster V79 cells in the presence or absence of a Syrian hamster embryo feeder layer (Takayama & Tanaka, 1983).

(b)   Humans

No data were available to the Working Group.

3.3 Case reports and epidemiological studies of carcinogenicity in humans

No data were available to the Working Group.

4. Summary of Data Reported and Evaluation

4.1 Exposure data

MeIQ (2-amino-3,4-dimethylimidazo[4,5-*f*]quinoline) has been found in grilled fish, and consumption of this food may result in human exposure.

4.2 Experimental data

In a preliminary report of an ungoing study, MeIQ was tested for carcinogenicity in mice by oral administration in the diet. Although squamous-cell carcinomas of the forestomach were reported in animals of each sex and liver-cell carcinomas in females, the data were inadequate for evaluation.

MeIQ crosses the placenta of mice.

MeIQ induced prophage in bacteria and was mutagenic to *Salmonella typhimurium* in the presence of an exogenous metabolic system. It gave positive results in the wing spot test in *Drosophila melanogaster*. It induced DNA damage and, in the presence of an exogenous system, mutations in cultured mammalian cells.

Overall assessment of data from short-term tests: MeIQ[a]

	Genetic activity			Cell transformation
	DNA damage	Mutation	Chromosomal effects	
Prokaryotes	+	+		
Fungi/Green plants				
Insects		+		
Mammalian cells (*in vitro*)	+	+		
Mammals (*in vivo*)				
Humans (*in vivo*)				
Degree of evidence in short-term tests for genetic activity: **Sufficient**				Cell transformation: No data

[a]The groups into which the table is divided and the symbol used are defined on pp. 19-20 of the Preamble; the degrees of evidence are defined on pp. 20-21.

4.3 Human data

No case report or epidemiological study of the carcinogenicity of MeIQ was available to the Working Group.

4.4 Evaluation[1]

There is *inadequate evidence* for the carcinogenicity of MeIQ in experimental animals. No evaluation could be made of the carcinogenicity of MeIQ to humans.

5. References

Adolfsson, L. & Olsson, K. (1983) A convenient synthesis of mutagenic 3*H*-imidazo[4,5-*f*]-quinoline-2-amines and their 2-^{14}C-labelled analogues. *Acta chem. scand.*, *37*B, 157-159

Bergman, K. (1985) Autoradiographic distribution of ^{14}C-labeled 3*H*-imidazo[4,5-*f*]-quinoline-2-amines in mice. *Cancer Res.*, *45*, 1351-1356

Grivas, S. & Jägerstad, M. (1984) Mutagenicity of some synthetic quinolines and quinoxalines related to IQ, MeIQ or MeIQx in Ames test. *Mutat. Res.*, *137*, 29-32

Hargraves, W.A. & Pariza, M.W. (1983) Purification and mass spectral characterization of bacterial mutagens from commercial beef extract. *Cancer Res.*, *43*, 1467-1472

Kasai, H., Yamaizumi, Z., Wakabayashi, K., Nagao, M., Sugimura, T., Yokoyama, S., Miyazawa, T. & Nishimura, S. (1980a) Structure and chemical synthesis of MeIQ, a potent mutagen isolated from broiled fish. *Chem. Lett.*, 1391-1394

Kasai, H., Yamaizumi, Z., Wakabayashi, K., Nagao, M., Sugimura, T., Yokoyama, S., Miyazawa, T., Spingarn, N.E., Weisburger, J.H. & Nishimura, S. (1980b) Potent novel mutagens produced by broiling fish under normal conditions. *Proc. Jpn. Acad.*, *56*B, 278-283

Lee, C.-S., Hashimoto, Y., Shudo, K. & Okamoto, T. (1982) Synthesis of mutagenic heteroaromatics: 2-aminoimidazo[4,5-*f*]quinolines. *Chem. pharm. Bull.*, *30*, 1857-1859

Loury, D.J. & Byard, J.L. (1985) Genotoxicity of the cooked-food mutagens IQ and MeIQ in primary cultures of rat, hamster, and guinea pig hepatocytes. *Environ. Mutagenesis*, *7*, 245-254

Nagao, M., Sato, S. & Sugimura, T. (1983a) *Mutagens produced by heating foods*. In: Waller, G.R. & Feather, M.S., eds, *The Maillard Reaction in Foods and Nutrition (ACS Symposium Series 215)*, Washington DC, American Chemical Society, pp. 521-536

---

[1]For definition of the italicized term, see Preamble, p. 18.

Nagao, M., Fujita, Y., Wakabayashi, K. & Sugimura, T. (1983b) Ultimate forms of mutagenic and carcinogenic heterocyclic amines produced by pyrolysis. *Biochem. biophys. Res. Commun.*, *114*, 626-631

Nagao, M., Wakabayashi, K., Kasai, H., Nishimura, S. & Sugimura, T. (1981) Effect of methyl substitution on mutagenicity of 2-amino-3-methylimidazo[4,5-*f*]quinoline, isolated from broiled sardine. *Carcinogenesis*, *2*, 1147-1149

Nakayasu, M., Nakasato, F., Sakamoto, H., Terada, M. & Sugimura, T. (1983) Mutagenic activity of heterocyclic amines in Chinese hamster lung cells with diphtheria toxin resistance as a marker. *Mutat. Res.*, *118*, 91-102

Ohgaki, H., Hasegawa, H., Kato, T., Suenaga, M., Ubukata, M., Sato, S., Takayama, S. & Sugimura, T. (1985a) Induction of tumors in the forestomach and liver of mice by feeding 2-amino-3,4-dimethyl-imidazo[4,5-*f*]quinoline (MeIQ). *Proc. Jpn. Acad.*, *61B*, 137-139

Ohgaki, H., Hasegawa, H., Kato, T., Suenaga, M., Sato, S., Takayama, S. & Sugimura, T. (1985b) *Carcinogenicity in mice and rats of IQ, MeIQ and MeIQx* (Abstract). In: Hayashi, J., Nagao, M., Sugimura, T., Takayama, S., Tomatis, L., Wattenburg, L.W. & Wogan, G., eds, *Diet, Nutrition and Cancer*, Tokyo, Gakkai Shuppan, pp. 29-30

Schunk, H., Hayashi, T. & Shibamoto, T. (1984) Analysis of mutagenic amino acid pyrolyzates with a fused silica capillary column. *J. high Resolut. Chromatogr. Chromatogr. Commun.*, *7*, 563-565

Sjödin, P. & Jägerstad, M. (1984) A balance study of ^{14}C-labelled 3*H*-imidazo[4,5-*f*]-quinolin-2-amines (IQ and MeIQ) in rats. *Food Chem. Toxicol.*, *22*, 207-210

Sugimura, T., Nagao, M. & Wakabayashi, K. (1981) *Mutagenic heterocyclic amines in cooked food*. In: Egan, H., Fishbein, L., Castegnaro, M., O'Neill, I.K. & Bartsch, H., eds, *Environmental Carcinogens. Selected Methods of Analysis*, Vol. 4, *Some Aromatic and Azo Dyes in the General and Industrial Environment (IARC Scientific Publications No. 40)*, Lyon, International Agency for Research on Cancer, pp. 251-267

Sugimura, T., Sato, S. & Takayama, S. (1983) *New mutagenic heterocyclic amines found in amino acid and protein pyrolysates and in cooked food*. In: Wynder, E.L., Leveille, G.A., Weisburger, J.H. & Livingston, G.E., eds, *Environmental Aspects of Cancer: The Role of Macro and Micro Components of Foods*, Westport, CT, Food and Nutrition Press, pp. 167-186

Takayama, S. & Tanaka, M. (1983) Mutagenesis of amino acid pyrolysis products in Chinese hamster V79 cells. *Toxicol. Lett.*, *17*, 23-28

Watanabe, J., Kawajiri, K., Yonekawa, H., Nagao, M. & Tagashira, Y. (1982) Immunological analysis of the roles of two major types of cytochrome P-450 in mutagenesis of compounds isolated from pyrolysates. *Biochem. biophys. Res. Commun.*, *104*, 193-199

Yoo, M.A., Ryo, H., Todo, T. & Kondo, S. (1985) Mutagenic potency of heterocyclic amines in the *Drosophila* wing spot test and its correlation to carcinogenic potency. *Jpn. J. Cancer Res. (Gann)*, *76*, 468-473

MeIQx (2-AMINO-3,8-DIMETHYLIMIDAZO[4,5-f]QUINOXALINE)

1. Chemical and Physical Data

1.1 Synonyms and trade names

Chem. Abstr. Services Reg. No.: 77500-04-0
Chem. Abstr. Name: 3,8-Dimethyl-3*H*-imidazo[4,5-*f*]quinoxalin-2-amine
IUPAC Systematic Name: 2-Amino-3,8-dimethyl-3*H*-imidazo[4,5-*f*]quinoxaline

1.2 Structural and molecular formulae and molecular weight

$C_{11}H_{11}N_5$ Mol wt: 213.24

1.3 Chemical and physical properties of the pure substance

(a) *Spectroscopy data*: Ultraviolet (Kasai *et al.*, 1981a), proton nuclear magnetic resonance and mass spectral data (Kasai *et al.*, 1981b) have been reported.

(b) *Solubility*: Soluble in methanol (Kasai *et al.*, 1981a)

(c) *Stability*: Stable under moderately acidic and alkaline conditions and in cold dilute aqueous solutions protected from light (Sugimura *et al.*, 1983)

(d) *Reactivity*: Rapidly degraded by dilute hypochlorite; not deactivated by weakly acidic nitrite solutions (Sugimura *et al.*, 1983)

2. Production, Use, Occurrence and Analysis

2.1 Production and use

(a) Production

The isolation and identification of MeIQx were first reported by Kasai *et al.* (1981b). Its structure was confirmed by chemical synthesis, in which 6-amino-3-methyl-5-nitroquinoxaline was methylated, reduced to the diamine and cyclized with cyanogen bromide to form MeIQx (Kasai *et al.*, 1981a; Sugimura *et al.*, 1983).

MeIQx is not produced in commercial or bulk quantities.

(b) Use

MeIQx is not used commercially.

2.2 Occurrence

MeIQx is not known to occur in nature.

MeIQx has been detected in fried ground beef in the range of 0.45-2.4 ng/ g (Hargraves & Pariza, 1983; Hayatsu *et al.*, 1983; Nagao *et al.*, 1983a; Felton *et al.*, 1984), in food-grade beef extract at a level of 3-28 ng/ g (Hargraves & Pariza, 1983; Takahashi *et al.*, 1985) and in bacteriological-grade beef extract in the range of 59-527 ng/ g (Hayatsu *et al.*, 1983; Turesky *et al.*, 1983; Takahashi *et al.*, 1985). It has also been found in mixtures of creatinine, glucose and glycine heated at 128°C in diethylene glycol (Jägerstad *et al.*, 1984).

2.3 Analysis

MeIQx was initially isolated and purified by acid-base partitioning and Sephadex LH-20 column chromatography. Reverse-phase high-performance liquid chromatography (HPLC) on octadecyl silylated columns was subsequently used to separate MeIQx from IQ (2-amino-3-methylimidazo[4,5-*f*]quinoline) (see p. 261). The structure was mainly deduced from proton nuclear magnetic resonance and high-resolution mass spectral data and by comparison with synthetic MeIQx (Kasai *et al.*, 1981b).

MeIQx has been isolated from beef extract and fried ground beef by dichloromethane extraction, column chromatography on Adsorbosil-5 and Sephadex LH20 and HPLC, with analysis by mass spectrometry, ultraviolet spectrophotometry and/ or mutagenesis assay (Hargraves *et al.*, 1982; Hargraves & Pariza, 1983; Turesky *et al.*, 1983).

Felton *et al.* (1984) detected MeIQx at 1 ng/ g in fried ground beef by dichloromethane extraction, chromatography on XAD-2 resin, preparative reverse-phase HPLC and analysis by high-resolution gas chromatography/ mass spectroscopy.

MeIQx can be adsorbed selectively from aqueous solutions onto cellulose or cotton to which C.I. Reactive Blue 21, a trisulpho-copper phthalocyanine dye, has been bound covalently. The adsorbed MeIQx is eluted with ammoniacal methanol and quantified by assay for mutagenic activity (Hayatsu *et al.*, 1983). More recently, this 'blue cotton' adsorption technique has been used as the first step in a simplified procedure for the detection of MeIQx in beef extracts, with a sensitivity of approximately 0.1 ng. Analysis involves extraction of acidified adsorbates with dichloromethane, silica-gel chromatography, and assay by HPLC with electrochemical detection (Takahashi *et al.*, 1985).

3. Biological Data Relevant to the Evaluation of Carcinogenic Risk to Humans

3.1 Carcinogenicity studies in animals

Oral administration

Mouse: It was reported in an abstract that groups [numbers unspecified] of CDF_1 mice were fed diets containing MeIQx [dose unspecified]. At experimental week 70, 4/16 treated males and 7/18 treated females were found to have liver tumours. The incidence of liver tumours in the control group was not stated (Ohgaki *et al.*, 1985). [The Working Group noted the incomplete reporting of the results.]

3.2 Other relevant biological data

(a)   Experimental systems

Toxic effects
No data were available to the Working Group.

Effects on reproduction and prenatal toxicity
No data were available to the Working Group.

Absorption, distribution, excretion and metabolism
In a study designed to provide information on the metabolic steps involved in the formation of the active mutagenic form, it was observed that MeIQx was not mutagenic to *Salmonella typhimurium* $TA98/1,8-DNP_6$ (defective in esterifying activity) in the presence of an exogenous metabolic system (S9) mix, while it was strongly mutagenic to strain TA98 with S9 mix, suggesting that the ultimate mutagenic form of MeIQx is the sulphate ester of its *N*-hydroxy derivative (Nagao *et al.*, 1983b).

Mutagenicity and other short-term tests
MeIQx was mutagenic in *Salmonella typhimurium* TA98 and TA100 in the presence of an exogenous metabolic system (S9) from the livers of polychlorinated biphenyl-induced rats (Kasai *et al.*, 1981a; Grivas & Jägerstad, 1984).

It gave positive results in the wing spot test in *Drosophila melanogaster* (transhetero-zygous for the loci *mwh* and *flr*) raised in a medium containing 0.1 or 0.2 mg/g (Yoo *et al.*, 1985).

MeIQx (25-100 µg/ml) induced diphtheria toxin-resistant mutants in cultured Chinese hamster lung cells in the presence of polychlorinated biphenyl-induced rat liver S9 (Nakayasu *et al.*, 1983).

(b) Humans

No data were available to the Working Group.

3.3 Case reports and epidemiological studies of carcinogenicity in humans

No data were available to the Working Group.

4. Summary of Data Reported and Evaluation

4.1 Exposure data

MeIQx (2-amino-3,8-dimethylimidazo[4,5-*f*]quinoxaline) has been found in fried beef and some beef extracts, and consumption of these foods may result in human exposure.

4.2 Experimental data

In a preliminary report of one study, MeIQx was tested for carcinogenicity in mice by oral administration. The data were inadequate for evaluation.

No data were available to evaluate the reproductive effects or prenatal toxicity of this compound to experimental animals.

MeIQx was mutagenic to *Salmonella typhimurium* and gave positive results in the wing spot test in *Drosophila melanogaster*. It was mutagenic in cultured Chinese hamster lung cells in the presence of an exogenous metabolic system.

4.3 Human data

No case report or epidemiological study of the carcinogenicity of MeIQx was available to the Working Group.

4.4 Evaluation[1]

There is *inadequate evidence* for the carcinogenicity of MeIQx in experimental animals.

No evaluation could be made of the carcinogenicity of MeIQx to humans.

---

[1]For definition of the italicized term, see Preamble, p. 18.

Overall assessment of data from short-term tests: MeIQx[a]

	Genetic activity			Cell transformation
	DNA damage	Mutation	Chromosomal effects	
Prokaryotes		+		
Fungi/Green plants				
Insects		+		
Mammalian cells (in vitro)		+		
Mammals (in vivo)				
Humans (in vivo)				
Degree of evidence in short-term tests for genetic activity: **Limited**				Cell transformation: No data

[a]The groups into which the table is divided and the symbol used are defined on pp. 19-20 of the Preamble; the degrees of evidence are defined on pp. 20-21.

5. References

Felton, J.S., Knize, M.F., Wood, C., Wuebbles, B.J., Healy, S.K., Stuermer, D.H., Bjeldanes, L.F., Kimble, B.J. & Hatch, F.T. (1984) Isolation and characterization of new mutagens from fried ground beef. *Carcinogenesis*, *5*, 95-102

Grivas, S. & Jägerstad, M. (1984) Mutagenicity of some synthetic quinolines and quinoxalines related to IQ, MeIQ or MeIQx in Ames test. *Mutat. Res.*, *137*, 29-32

Hargraves, W.A. & Pariza, M.W. (1983) Purification and mass spectral characterization of bacterial mutagens from commercial beef extract. *Cancer Res.*, *43*, 1467-1472

Hargraves, W.A., Dietrich, R. & Pariza, M.W. (1982) *A new chromatographic method for separating mutagens from commercial beef extract and fried ground beef.* In: Stich, H.F., ed., *Carcinogens and Mutagens in the Environment*, Vol. 1, Boca Raton, FL, CRC Press, pp. 223-229

Hayatsu, H., Matsui, Y., Ohara, Y., Oka, T. & Hayatsu, T. (1983) Characterization of mutagenic fractions in beef extract and in cooked ground beef. Use of blue-cotton for efficient extraction. *Gann*, *74*, 472-482

Jägerstad, M., Olsson, K., Grivas, S., Negishi, C., Wakabayashi, K., Tsuda, M., Sato, S. & Sugimura, T. (1984) Formation of 2-amino-3,8-dimethyl-imidazo[4,5-*f*]quinoxaline in a model system by heating creatinine, glycine and glucose. *Mutat. Res.*, *126*, 239-244

Kasai, H., Shiomi, T., Sugimura, T. & Nishimura, S. (1981a) Synthesis of 2-amino-3,8-dimethylimidazo[4,5-*f*]quinoxaline (Me-IQx), a potent mutagen isolated from fried beef. *Chem. Lett.*, 675-678

Kasai, H., Yamaizumi, Z., Shiomi, T., Yokoyama, S., Miyazawa, T., Wakabayashi, K., Nagao, M., Sugimura, T. & Nishimura, S. (1981b) Structure of a potent mutagen isolated from fried beef. *Chem. Lett.*, 485-488

Nagao, M., Sato, S. & Sugimura, T. (1983a) *Mutagens produced by heating foods.* In: Waller, G.R. & Feather, M.S., eds, *The Maillard Reaction in Foods and Nutrition (ACS Symposium Series 215)*, Washington DC, American Chemical Society, pp. 521-536

Nagao, M., Fujita, Y., Wakabayashi, K. & Sugimura, T. (1983b) Ultimate forms of mutagenic and carcinogenic heterocyclic amines produced by pyrolysis. *Biochem. biophys. Res. Commun.*, *114*, 626-631

Nakayasu, M., Nakasato, F., Sakamoto, H., Terada, M. & Sugimura, T. (1983) Mutagenic activity of heterocyclic amines in Chinese hamster lung cells with diphtheria toxin resistance as a marker. *Mutat. Res.*, *118*, 91-102

Ohgaki, H., Hasegawa, H., Kato, T., Suenaga, M., Sato, S., Takayama, S. & Sugimura, T. (1985) *Carcinogenicity in mice and rats of IQ, MeIQ and MeIQx* (Abstract). In: Hayashi, J., Nagao, M., Sugimura, T., Takayama, S., Tomatis, L., Wattenberg, L.W. & Wogan, G., eds, *Diet, Nutrition and Cancer*, Tokyo, Gakkai Shuppan, pp. 29-30

Sugimura, T., Sato, S. & Takayama, S. (1983) *New mutagenic heterocyclic amines found in amino acid and protein pyrolysates and in cooked food.* In: Wynder, E.L., Leveille, G.A., Weisburger, J.H. & Livingston, G.E., eds, *Environmental Aspects of Cancer: The Role of Macro and Micro Components of Foods*, Westport, CT, Food and Nutrition Press, pp. 167-186

Takahashi, M., Wakabayashi, K., Nagao, M., Yamamoto, M., Masui, T., Goto, T., Kinae, N., Tomita, I. & Sugimura, T. (1985) Quantification of 2-amino-3-methylimidazo-[4,5-*f*]quinoline (IQ) and 2-amino-3,8-dimethylimidazo[4,5-*f*]quinoxaline (MeIQx) in beef extracts by liquid chromatography with electrochemical detection (LCEC). *Carcinogenesis*, *6*, 1195-1199

Turesky, R.J., Wishnok, J.S., Tannenbaum, S.R., Pfund, R.A. & Buchi, G.H. (1983) Qualitative and quantitative characterization of mutagens in commercial beef extract. *Carcinogenesis*, *4*, 863-866

Yoo, M.A., Ryo, H., Todo, T. & Kondo, S. (1985) Mutagenic potency of heterocyclic amines in the *Drosophila* wing spot test and its correlation to carcinogenic potency. *Jpn. J. Cancer Res. (Gann)*, *76*, 468-473

FUROCOUMARINS

ANGELICIN AND SOME SYNTHETIC DERIVATIVES

1. Chemical and Physical Data

Angelicin

1.1 Synonyms and trade names

Chem. Abstr. Services Reg. No.: 523-50-2

Chem. Abstr. Name: 2*H*-Furo[2,3-*h*][1]benzopyran-2-one

IUPAC Systematic Names: 2*H*-Furo[2,3-*h*][1]benzopyran-2-one; 4-hydroxy-5-benzo-furanacrylic acid, δ-lactone

Synonyms: Angecin; furo[2,3-*h*]coumarin; furo[5′,4′:7,8]coumarin; 3-(4-hydroxy-5-benzofuranyl)-2-propenoic acid, δ-lactone; isopsoralen

1.2 Structural and molecular formulae and molecular weight

$C_{11}H_6O_3$ Mol. wt: 186.17

1.3 Chemical and physical properties of the pure substance

(*a*)   *Description*: White crystalline solid with a slight hay-like odour

(*b*)   *Melting-point*: 140°C (Royer *et al.*, 1978)

(c) *Spectroscopy data*: Ultraviolet (Perel'son & Sheinker, 1967; Mantulin & Song, 1973; Royer *et al.*, 1978; Guiotto *et al.*, 1981; Song *et al.*, 1981; Dall'Acqua *et al.*, 1984), infrared, proton nuclear magnetic resonance (Royer *et al.*, 1978), ^{13}C nuclear magnetic resonance (Bose *et al.*, 1979; Rodighiero *et al.*, 1984a), fluorescence (Mantulin & Song, 1973; Song *et al.*, 1981; Dall'Acqua *et al.*, 1984) and mass spectral data (ICIS Chemical Information System, 1984 [MSSS]) have been reported.

(d) *Solubility*: Very slightly soluble in water (20 mg/l); soluble in methanol (Baccichetti *et al.*, 1984) and ethanol (Mullen *et al.*, 1984)

1.4 Technical products and impurities

No data were available to the Working Group.

Angelicin derivatives

Synonyms, Chemical Abstracts and IUPAC Systematic Names, structural and molecular formulae and molecular weights of the synthetic alkyl angelicins considered in this monograph are given in Table 1. Table 2 illustrates the numbering systems used for these derivatives.

2. Production, Use, Occurrence and Analysis

2.1 Production and use

(a) *Production*

Several synthetic routes for the preparation of angelicin have been described. Royer *et al.* (1978) reported the synthesis of angelicin beginning with resorcinol and proceeding through 4-hydroxybenzofuran and 5-formyl-4-hydroxybenzofuran as intermediates. An alternative pathway exists in which the direct condensation of umbelliferone (7-hydroxy-coumarin) and 4-chloro-1,3-dioxolan-2-one at 150-165°C produces 20% angelicin and 15% psoralen (Reisch & Mester, 1979).

Recent interest has been directed toward the synthesis of methylated angelicin derivatives. An early paper described the production of methyl analogues of angelicin from *ortho*-allyl-7-hydroxycoumarins. Initially, 7-allyloxy-4-methylcoumarin undergoes a Claisen rearrangement to produce 8-allyl-7-hydroxy-4-methylcoumarin. This product is subsequently acetylated, brominated and cyclized to form 4,5'-dimethylangelicin (Kaufman, 1961). 4,5'-Dimethylpsoralen has been identified as an impurity in some preparations of 4,5'-dimethylangelicin (Rodighiero *et al.*, 1981a).

Table 1. Alkyl angelicins

Chemical name [Chem. Abstr. Services Reg. No.]	Chem. Abstr. Name [Synonym] IUPAC Systematic Names	Structural and molecular formulae and molecular weight
5-Methylangelicin [73459-03-7]	5-Methyl-2H-furo[2,3-h][1]-benzopyran-2-one [5-Methylisopsoralen, 5-MA] 4-Hydroxy-6-methyl-5-benzo-furanacrylic acid, δ-lactone; 5-methyl-2H-furo[2,3-h][1]-benzopyran-2-one	$C_{12}H_8O_3$ Mol. wt: 200.19
4,4'-Dimethylangelicin [22975-76-4]	4,9-Dimethyl-2H-furo[2,3-h]-[1]benzopyran-2-one [4,4'-DMA] 4-Hydroxy-β,3-dimethyl-5-benzo-furanacrylic acid, δ-lactone; 4,9-dimethyl-2H-furo[2,3-h][1]-benzopyran-2-one	$C_{13}H_{10}O_3$ Mol. wt: 214.22
4,5'-Dimethylangelicin [4063-41-6]	4,8-Dimethyl-2H-furo[2,3-h]-[1]benzopyran-2-one [4,5'-DMA] 4-Hydroxy-β,2-dimethyl-5-benzo-furanacrylic acid, δ-lactone; 4,8-dimethyl-2H-furo[2,3-h]-[1]benzopyran-2-one	$C_{13}H_{10}O_3$ Mol. wt: 214.22
4,4',6-Trimethylangelicin [90370-29-9]	4,6,9-Trimethyl-2H-furo-[2,3-h][1]benzopyran-2-one [4,4',6-TMA] 4-Hydroxy-β,3,7-trimethyl-5-benzo-furanacrylic acid, δ-lactone; 4,6,9-trimethyl-2H-furo-[2,3-h][1]benzo-pyran-2-one	$C_{14}H_{12}O_3$ Mol. wt: 228.25

Table 1 (contd)

Chemical name [Chem. Abstr. Services Reg. No.]	Chem. Abstr. Name [Synonym] IUPAC Systematic Names	Structural and molecular formulae and molecular weight
4'-Methylangelicin [78982-40-8]	9-Methyl-2*H*-furo[2,3-*h*][1]-benzopyran-2-one [4'-MA] 4-Hydroxy-3-methyl-5-benzo-furanacrylic acid, δ-lactone; 9-methyl-2*H*-furo[2,3-*h*][1]-benzopyran-2-one	$C_{12}H_8O_3$ Mol. wt: 200.19

Table 2. Numbering systems for angelicin derivatives

Numbering system for Chemical Abstracts and IUPAC Systematic Names

Numbering system for common name

Numbering system for alternative IUPAC Systematic Name (as δ-lactone)

More recent synthetic schemes have been developed to minimize the occurrence of bifunctional methylpsoralens that are present as contaminants. The critical step in this procedure is separation of the 6-allyl isomers from 8-allylumbelliferones by high-performance liquid chromatography (Rodighiero *et al.*, 1981a). This purification step can be eliminated in the synthesis of 6-methylangelicins by using *O*-allylumbelliferones methylated in the 6-position as the starting material (Guiotto *et al.*, 1984).

In a method for the synthesis of angelicins without methyl groups on the furan ring, such as 5-methylangelicin, 8-allylumbelliferones are ozonized to the corresponding 8-coumarinyl acetaldehydes and then cyclized (Guiotto *et al.*, 1981). The search for new methyl derivatives of angelicin has recently led to the synthesis of 4'-methylangelicin (Dall'Acqua *et al.*, 1983) and 4,4',6-trimethylangelicin (Guiotto *et al.*, 1984).

Angelicin is not currently produced in commercial quantities but is available from a pharmaceutical firm in India (Dall'Acqua *et al.*, 1984).

(b) Use

Angelicin and its methylated derivatives are not currently in widespread use as therapeutic agents, but are being investigated for potential use in the photochemotherapy of psoriasis (Dall'Acqua *et al.*, 1983; Baccichetti *et al.*, 1984; Guiotto *et al.*, 1984).

2.2 Occurrence

Angelicin and its methoxy derivatives have been isolated and detected in various Umbelliferae, including angelica (*Angelica atropurpurea*), parsnip (*Pastinaca sativa*) and several hogweed (*Heracleum*) species. The distribution is presented in Table 3.

Levels have been quantified: angelicin and pimpinellin have been detected in the fresh fruiting heads of *Heracleum mantegazzianum* at 292 and 79 mg/100 g, respectively (Beyrich, 1968); angelicin, sphondin and isobergapten have been detected at 0.5 mg/g and pimpinellin at 1.6 mg/g in the root of *H. sphondylium* (van der Sluis *et al.*, 1981). Levels in roots of *H. laciniatum* were approximately 0.05, 0.09, 0.08 and 0.06 mg/g of root for angelicin, sphondin, isobergapten and pimpinellin, respectively (Kavli *et al.*, 1983a).

Methylangelicins are not known to occur as natural products.

2.3 Analysis

Angelicin has been separated from methoxyangelicins and other furocoumarins by thin-layer chromatography (TLC) and high-performance liquid chromatography (HPLC). TLC detection methods have included fluorescence scanning *in situ* (Kavli *et al.*, 1983a), ultraviolet light (van der Sluis *et al.*, 1981), and the susceptibility of microorganisms to photo-induced toxicity (Ashwood-Smith *et al.*, 1983). Sensitivity has been reported in the nanogram range, i.e., generally between 0.01-20 ng, depending on the detection system and the angelicin derivative under consideration.

Table 3. Occurrence of angelicin and other furocoumarins in some plant species[a]

Species	Angelicin	Isobergapten[b]	Pimpinellin[c]	Sphondin[d]	Reference
Angelica atropurpurea[e]	P	−	T	T	Berenbaum (1981)
Heracleum dissectum[f]	P	−	P	P	Beyrich (1968)
H. laciniatum[g]	P	P	P	P	Kavli et al. (1983a, 1984)
H. lanatum[e]	T	T	P	P	Berenbaum (1981)
H. mantegazzianum[e]	T	T	P	−	Berenbaum (1981)
H. mantegazzianum[h]	P	−	−	−	Beyrich (1968)
H. sibiricum[f]	P	P	P	P	Beyrich (1968)
H. sosnowskyi[f]	P	P	P	P	Beyrich (1968)
H. sphondylium[i]	P	P	P	P	van der Sluis et al. (1981)
Pastinaca sativa[j]	P	−	−	P	Berenbaum (1981)

[a]P, present; T, trace; −, not found

[b]5-Methoxyangelicin

[c]5,6-Dimethoxyangelicin

[d]6-Methoxyangelicin

[e]In seeds and leaves; present: detected by high-performance liquid chromatography (HPLC) and confirmed by thin-layer chromatography (TLC); trace: detected by HPLC, not detectable by TLC; −: not detected by HPLC or TLC

[f]Plant part unspecified

[g]In root extract; determined by TLC or HPLC

[h]In the fresh fruiting head; determined by isolation and comparison with authentic compounds

[i]In fresh roots; determined by gas chromatography and HPLC

[j]Only in seeds; see footnote e

Reverse-phase HPLC has been used to separate all of the methoxy angelicins from psoralens and other furocoumarins (Vande Casteele et al., 1983; Kavli et al., 1984; Thompson & Brown, 1984).

3. Biological Data Relevant to the Evaluation of Carcinogenic Risk to Humans

3.1 Carcinogenicity studies in animals

Skin application

[The Working Group noted that the various compounds tested were not pure. The degree of purity of angelicin was unspecified; it was established that the purity of the methylangelicin derivatives tested was >99%. The impurities in the methyl derivatives are their linear isomers; the most probable impurity in angelicin is its linear isomer, psoralen. Angular and linear isomers are quantitatively and qualitatively different with respect to their binding to DNA in the presence of ultraviolet A radiation (see section 3.2(a), *Mutagenicity and other short-term tests*). Their presence in the tested compounds can markedly affect the photobiological activity and may thus have influenced the results. In all of these studies, although control groups are described for each test, they are the same animals.]

Angelicin

Mouse: A group of 40 male Skh:hairless-1 albino mice, six weeks old, were given thrice-weekly applications of 0.05 ml of a 0.1% solution of angelicin [purity unspecified] in ethanol on the skin of the back for 12-15 months [time unspecified]. The animals were immobilized for 45 min and irradiated with long-wave ultraviolet irradiation (UVA) (six FR 40T12/PUVA Sylvania Lifeline bulbs emitting radiation of 320-400 nm, with a maximum wavelength of 355 nm; wavelengths <320 nm were eliminated with a Mylar filter [irradiance unspecified]). The radiation dose per treatment was $2.5\text{-}5.0 \times 10^4$ J/m^2 (total dose, >250 × 10^4 J/m^2). Four groups of 20 animals each received treatment with angelicin solution alone or UVA irradiation alone (total doses, 148, 250 and 751.5×10^4 J/m^2). No skin tumour was observed with angelicin alone or with UVA alone. In a fifth control group of 40 animals treated with a 0.1% solution of methoxsalen (because of the photocarcinogenic potential of this chemical [see IARC, 1980]) in ethanol followed by 1.0×10^4 J/m^2 UVA irradiation (total dose, 220×10^4 J/m^2), there was a 70% tumour incidence [mortality rate unspecified], and the time required to produce a tumour incidence of 50% being 60 weeks. Skin tumour yield in animals treated with angelicin and UVA was 20% [mortality rate unspecified] at 60 weeks; the time required to produce a tumour incidence of 50% in surviving animals was therefore >60 weeks. Histological analysis of tumours revealed well-differentiated invasive squamous-cell carcinomas (Mullen *et al.*, 1984).

5-Methylangelicin

Mouse: In the same study, groups of 40 male Skh:hairless-1 albino mice, six weeks old, were given thrice-weekly applications of 0.05 ml of a 0.01% or 0.1% solution of 5-methylangelicin [purity unspecified] in ethanol on the skin of the back for 12-15 months [time unspecified]. The animals were immobilized and irradiated, as described above, to give a radiation dose per treatment of 1×10^4 J/m^2 [total doses, 136.5×10^4 J/m^2 (0.01% solution) and 107×10^4 J/m^2 (0.1% solution)]. Four groups of 20 animals each received treatment with 0.1% 5-methylangelicin solution alone or UVA irradiation alone (148, 250 and 751.5×10^4 J/m^2); no skin tumour was observed in any of these groups. In a fifth control group of 40 animals treated with a 0.1% ethanol solution of methoxsalen followed by 1.0×10^4 J/m^2 UVA irradiation (total dose, 220×10^4 J/m^2), there was a 70% tumour yield [mortality rate unspecified] with time required to produce a tumour incidence of 50% of 60 weeks. Skin tumour (invasive squamous-cell carcinomas) yields and times required to produce a

50% tumour incidence in animals in the groups treated with 0.01% 5-methylangelicin plus 136×10^4 J/m² UVA radiation, and 0.1% 5-methylangelicin plus 107×10^4 J/m² UVA radiation were 78 and 97%, and 53 and 33 weeks, respectively (Mullen *et al.*, 1984).

4,4'-Dimethylangelicin

No data were available to the Working Group.

4,5'-Dimethylangelicin

Mouse: In the same study, further groups of 40 male Skh:hairless-1 albino mice, six weeks old, were given thrice-weekly applications of 0.05 ml of a 0.1% solution of 4,5'-dimethylangelicin [purity unspecified] in ethanol on the skin of the back for 12-15 months, immobilized and irradiated, as described above, to give radiation doses per treatment of 2.5 and 7.5×10^4 J/m² (total doses, 289 and 758×10^4 J/m²), respectively. Four groups of 20 animals each received treatment with 0.1% 4,5'-dimethylangelicin solution alone or UVA irradiation alone (148, 250 and 751.5×10^4 J/m², respectively); no skin tumour was observed in any of the these groups. In a fifth control group of 40 animals treated with a 0.1% ethanol solution of methoxsalen followed by 1.0×10^4 J/m² UVA irradiation (total dose, 220×10^4 J/m²), there was a 70% tumour yield [mortality rate unspecified] with time required to produce a tumour incidence of 50% of 60 weeks. Skin tumour (invasive squamous-cell carcinomas) yields and times required to produce a 50% tumour incidence in animals in the groups treated with 0.1% 4,5-dimethylangelicin plus 289×10^4 J/m² or 758×10^4 J/m² were 97.3 and 100%, and 40 and 42 weeks, respectively (Mullen *et al.*, 1984).

4,4',6-Trimethylangelicin

No data were available to the Working Group.

3.2 Other relevant biological data

(*a*)   *Experimental systems*

The photobiology and photochemistry of psoralens, with emphasis on angelicins, have been reviewed (Averbeck, 1984; Ben-Hur & Song, 1984; Pathak, 1984; Rodighiero *et al.*, 1984b).

Toxic effects

The oral and intraperitoneal LD_{50} values for *angelicin* in rats were 322 mg/kg bw and 165 mg/kg bw, respectively, and the intraperitoneal LD_{50} in mice was 254 mg/kg bw (Chandhoke & Ghatak, 1975). The oral LD_{50} values for *5-methylangelicin* and *4,5'-dimethylangelicin* in mice were reported to be 2000 and 2500 mg/kg bw, respectively (Baccichetti *et al.*, 1982) and that of *4,4',6-trimethylangelicin* in methylcellulose was >2000 mg/kg bw (Dall'Acqua *et al.*, 1985).

Administration of *4,5'-dimethylangelicin* and subsequent irradiation with UVA did not produce changes in the skin of guinea-pigs (Bordin *et al.*, 1979). *Angelicin* and *4,5'-*dimethylangelicin plus UVA irradiation (306-428 nm; maximum, 345 nm) killed cultured human lymphocytes. Blast transformation stimulated by phytohaemagglutinin did not alter this effect (Barth *et al.*, 1983).

In the presence of UVA, topical or oral application of *4,4'-dimethylangelicin* inhibited epidermal DNA synthesis in mice *in vivo* (Dall'Acqua *et al.*, 1983). Treatment with *4,5'-*dimethylangelicin plus UVA inhibited DNA synthesis in Ehrlich ascites tumour cells (Bordin *et al.*, 1978; Dall'Acqua *et al.*, 1981) and epidermal DNA synthesis in NCL mice after topical or oral application (Bordin *et al.*, 1981). Interaction of *4,4',6-trimethylangelicin* with UVA resulted in effective inhibition of DNA synthesis in Ehrlich ascites cells (Baccichetti *et al.*, 1984) and in epidermal cells of NCL mice after oral or topical treatment (Carlassare *et al.*, 1984). Treatment with *5-methylangelicin* and UVA irradiation inhibited DNA synthesis in Ehrlich ascites tumour cells. Topical or oral administration of *5-methylangelicin* and UVA irradiation inhibited epidermal DNA synthesis in mice *in vivo* (Bordin *et al.*, 1981).

Oral administration of *angelicin* to male CD-1 mice caused a significant increase in hepatic microsomal protein. There was no effect on the activities of aryl hydrocarbon hydroxylase, ethylmorphine *N*-demethylase or cytochrome P450 (Bickers & Pathak, 1984).

Effects on reproduction and prenatal toxicity
No data were available to the Working Group.

Absorption, distribution, excretion and metabolism
No data were available to the Working Group.

Mutagenicity and other short-term tests
The angular and linear derivatives of angelicin are quantitatively and qualitatively different with respect to their binding to DNA in the presence of UVA, as indicated in Table 4. The table also includes data on psoralen derivatives, for comparison.

Angelicin
Angelicin formed a molecular complex with DNA *in vitro* in the dark (Dall'Acqua *et al.*, 1978).

Angelicin photobound covalently to DNA *in vitro* forming monoadducts but not DNA interstrand cross-links; binding was UVA dose-dependent (Rodighiero *et al.*, 1969, 1970; Dall'Acqua *et al.*, 1971a,b; Rodighiero *et al.*, 1971; Musajo *et al.*, 1974; Bordin *et al.*, 1975; Dall'Acqua *et al.*, 1981). Photobinding of angelicin to DNA, which in some studies was shown to be dependent on UVA dose, was observed in *Saccharomyces cerevisiae* (Chandra *et al.*, 1973; Averbeck *et al.*, 1975, 1976), in *Escherichia coli* (Chandra *et al.*, 1973; Bordin *et al.*, 1976) and in Ehrlich ascites tumour cells (Bordin *et al.*, 1975, 1978). Photobinding but not DNA interstrand cross-linking was observed in DNA of phage λ during ω reactivation (Belogurov & Zavilgelsky, 1981), in mouse embryo fibroblasts (Szafarz *et al.*, 1983) and in VA-13 human fibroblasts (Kaye *et al.*, 1980; Hanawalt *et al.*, 1981).

Table 4. Binding of angelicin and its derivatives and isomers to DNA

Compound	Rate constant for DNA binding with UVA		Rate constant for DNA cross-link formation with UVA	
	(min^{-1})	Reference	(min^{-1})	Reference
Angelicin	1.1×10^{-2}	Dall'Acqua et al. (1981)	0	Dall'Acqua et al. (1981)
Psoralen	4.0×10^{-2}	Dall'Acqua et al. (1974a)	3.79×10^{-3}	Dall'Acqua et al. (1974b)
5-Methylangelicin	3.4×10^{-2}	Dall'Acqua et al. (1981)	0	Dall'Acqua et al. (1981)
5-Methylpsoralen	7.8×10^{-2}	Dall'Acqua et al. (1974a)	8.53×10^{-3}	Dall'Acqua et al. (1974b)
4,5'-Dimethylangelicin	4.0×10^{-2}	Rodighiero et al. (1981b)	0	Rodighiero et al. (1981b)
4,5'-Dimethylpsoralen	14.0×10^{-2}	Rodighiero et al. (1981b)	a	Rodighiero et al. (1981b)

[a]Reported by the authors to be twice that of psoralen [details not given]

Under certain experimental conditions, angelicin plus UVA appeared to induce cross-linking in λ DNA (Lown & Sim, 1978), in phage λ (Kittler et al., 1980) and, as reported in an abstract, in human cell DNA (Gruenert, 1983).

The repair of DNA lesions induced by angelicin plus UVA has been shown in phage λ (Lichtenberg & Yasui, 1983), in E. coli (Bordin et al., 1976; Venturini et al., 1980; Bridges & von Wright, 1981; Grossweiner & Smith, 1981), in S. cerevisiae (Chandra et al., 1973, 1974; Averbeck et al., 1975; Averbeck, 1976; Averbeck et al., 1976; Grant et al., 1979; Jachymczyk et al., 1981), in Aspergillus nidulans (Muronetz et al., 1980), in green monkey kidney cells (Nocentini, 1978; Coppey et al., 1979), in normal human fibroblasts and in xeroderma pigmentosum cells (Coppey et al., 1979; Cleaver & Gruenert, 1984).

In the dark, angelicin was not mutagenic to Salmonella typhimurium TA98 (Venturini et al., 1981) or to repair-proficient (Averbeck & Moustacchi, 1979) or repair-deficient S. cerevisiae (Jachymczyk et al., 1981); it did not induce micronuclei in Chinese hamster ovary cells (Ashwood-Smith et al., 1977) or increase the incidence of chromosomal aberrations or sister chromatid exchanges in normal human fibroblasts, ataxia telangiectasia cells or xeroderma pigmentosum cells (Natarajan et al., 1981). However, angelicin was active in the dark as a frameshift mutagen in E. coli lac⁻z strain ND160 (Ashwood-Smith, 1978; Ashwood-Smith et al., 1980).

Mutations were induced by angelicin and UVA in phage λ in E. coli K12 uvrA (Zavilgelsky et al., 1982) and in a wild-type host E. coli K12 pre-irradiated with 254 nm ultraviolet light (Belogurov & Zavilgelsky, 1979), in E. coli WP2 and WP2 uvrA (Ashwood-Smith et al., 1980; Venturini et al., 1980; Ashwood-Smith et al., 1982), in S. typhimurium

TA100 (Venturini *et al.*, 1981) and TA102 (Levin *et al.*, 1982), in *A. nidulans* (Muronetz *et al.*, 1980) and in *S. cerevisiae* (Averbeck *et al.*, 1975, 1976; Averbeck & Moustacchi, 1979; Grant *et al.*, 1979; Averbeck & Moustacchi, 1980; Averbeck *et al.*, 1981a,b).

Angelicin plus UVA also induced mitotic recombination (Averbeck & Moustacchi, 1979) and cytoplasmic 'petite' mutations in *S. cerevisiae* (Averbeck *et al.*, 1975, 1976; Averbeck & Moustacchi, 1979; Averbeck *et al.*, 1979).

UVA dose-dependent increases in the incidence of micronuclei (Ashwood-Smith *et al.*, 1977) and of sister chromatid exchanges (Ashwood-Smith *et al.*, 1981, 1982; Linnainmaa & Wolff, 1982) were induced in Chinese hamster ovary cells after treatment with angelicin and UVA *in vitro*.

Induction of chromosomal aberrations and sister chromatid exchanges by angelicin plus UVA was observed in normal human foreskin fibroblasts, and in ataxia telangiectasia and xeroderma pigmentosum cells *in vitro* (Ashwood-Smith *et al.*, 1981; Natarajan *et al.*, 1981; Ashwood-Smith *et al.*, 1982).

5-Methylangelicin

5-Methylangelicin formed a noncovalently-bound complex with DNA *in vitro* in the dark. In the presence of UVA, it showed strong covalent photobinding to DNA *in vitro* (Dall'Acqua *et al.*, 1981; Isaacs *et al.*, 1984) but did not form DNA interstrand cross-links (Dall'Acqua *et al.*, 1981).

5-Methylangelicin plus UVA induced prophage in *S. typhimurium* TA1535 and TA1538 (Connor *et al.*, 1983). It was mutagenic to *S. typhimurium* TA98 and TA100 in the dark, in the absence of an exogenous metabolic system; addition of a metabolic system from rats had no potentiating effect (Monti-Bragadin *et al.*, 1981; Venturini *et al.*, 1981). 5-Methylangelicin was not mutagenic to strain TA98 in the presence of UVA (Venturini *et al.*, 1981) but was mutagenic to strain TA100, to *E. coli* excision-deficient strain TM9 (WP2 *uvrA*/R46) and to excision repair-proficient strain TM6 (Pani *et al.*, 1981).

5-Methylangelicin in combination with UVA induced a UVA dose-dependent increase in 6-thioguanine-resistant mutants in Chinese hamster V79 (Pani *et al.*, 1981) and ovary (Loveday & Donahue, 1984) cells.

In combination with UVA, it induced sister chromatid exchanges in Chinese hamster ovary cells (Loveday & Donahue, 1984).

4,4'-Dimethylangelicin

4,4'-Dimethylangelicin formed a complex with DNA *in vitro* in the dark. It photobound covalently to DNA, forming monoadducts but not DNA interstrand cross-links in isolated DNA (Dall'Acqua *et al.*, 1983) and in *E. coli* B$_{48}$ (Baccichetti *et al.*, 1981a,b).

In the dark, 4,4'-dimethylangelicin was not mutagenic to *S. typhimurium* TA98 in the presence or absence of an exogenous metabolic system (Monti-Bragadin *et al.*, 1981). In the presence of UVA, this compound was mutagenic to repair-proficient *E. coli* WP2 *trp⁻* (Baccichetti *et al.*, 1981b).

In haploid *S. cerevisiae*, 4,4′-dimethylangelicin plus UVA induced cytoplasmic 'petite' mutations (Averbeck *et al.*, 1984a).

4,5′-Dimethylangelicin

4,5′-Dimethylangelicin formed a noncovalently-bound complex with DNA *in vitro* in the dark. It showed strong covalent photobinding, but not interstrand cross-links, with DNA *in vitro* (Rodighiero & Dall'Acqua, 1984) and also photobound covalently with the DNA of Ehrlich ascites tumour cells (Bordin *et al.*, 1978, 1979).

In the presence of UVA, it induced prophage λ from lysogenic *E. coli* K12 (Baccichetti *et al.*, 1979).

4,5′-Dimethylangelicin was mutagenic to *S. typhimurium* TA100, but not TA98, in the presence of UVA (Venturini *et al.*, 1981). It did not photoinduce mutations in *E. coli* WP2 or CM561, but was mutagenic to *E. coli* WP2 *uvrA* (Venturini *et al.*, 1980), WP2/R46 and WP2 *uvrA*/R46 (Pani *et al.*, 1981). In *S. cerevisiae*, 4,5′-dimethylangelicin photoinduced nuclear reversions, forward mutations and cytoplasmic 'petite' mutations (Averbeck *et al.*, 1981a,b, 1984a,b).

After treatment with 4,5′-dimethylangelicin and UVA, a UVA dose-dependent increase in 6-thioguanine-resistant mutants was observed in Chinese hamster V79 cells (Pani *et al.*, 1981; Swart *et al.*, 1983).

4,4′,6-Trimethylangelicin

4,4′,6-Trimethylangelicin formed a complex with DNA *in vitro* in the dark (Guiotto *et al.*, 1984). It photobound covalently to DNA *in vitro* in the presence of UVA but did not form DNA interstrand cross-links (Baccichetti *et al.*, 1984; Guiotto *et al.*, 1984).

In the dark, 4,4′,6-trimethylangelicin was not mutagenic to *S. typhimurium* TA98 or TA100 (Guiotto *et al.*, 1984). In the presence of UVA, it was mutagenic to *E. coli* WP2 *uvrA* (Baccichetti *et al.*, 1984; Guiotto *et al.*, 1984).

(b) Humans

Toxic effects

Treatment with *angelicin* [purity unspecified] and irradiation with sunlight or UVA at 365 nm produced slight 'phototoxic' erythema in human skin (Musajo *et al.*, 1954; Musajo & Rodighiero, 1962). Kavli *et al.* (1983b) reported that *angelicin* with subsequent UVA irradiation produced erythema in the depigmented skin of a patient with vitiligo.

Erythema appeared in two patients treated topically on two different areas of damaged skin with 10 μg/cm^2 *4,4′-dimethylangelicin* three and 12 times, respectively, and irradiated with UVA. In the patient treated 12 times, pigmentation was seen in the exposed areas (Recchia *et al.*, 1983a,b).

Pathak *et al.* (1984) described slight melanogenic stimulating activity of *5-methylangelicin* and *4,5′-dimethylangelicin* when applied to normal human skin at 50-500 μg/6 cm^2 (8.3-83 μg/cm^2), followed by UVA exposure of 12 J/cm^2.

Pigmentation, but not erythema, was induced in five psoriatic patients treated topically with 5 μg/cm² *4,4',6-trimethylangelicin* and irradiated with 2.5-13 J/cm² UVA five times a week for two to three weeks (Guiotto *et al.*, 1984).

Effects on reproduction and prenatal toxicity

No data were available to the Working Group.

Absorption, distribution, excretion and metabolism

No data were available to the Working Group.

Mutagenicity and chromosomal effects

No data were available to the Working Group.

3.3 Case reports and epidemiological studies of carcinogenicity to humans

No data were available to the Working Group.

4. Summary of Data Reported and Evaluation

4.1 Exposure data

Angelicin and its methoxy derivatives occur in a number of plants belonging to the *Umbelliferae* family. These compounds have been tested clinically in combination with ultraviolet A radiation for use in the treatment of psoriasis. Human exposure occurs through contact with or ingestion of the plants in which these compounds occur.

4.2 Experimental data

Angelicin, 5-methylangelicin and 4,5'-dimethylangelicin, with and without ultraviolet A radiation, were tested for skin carcinogenicity in mice by skin application. All compounds produced skin cancers when administered with ultraviolet A radiation but not when given alone. The presence of some linear psoralen impurities in the methylangelicins cannot be excluded and may have influenced the results obtained. The studies were inadequate to evaluate the systemic carcinogenicity of these compounds. No data were available to evaluate the carcinogenicity to experimental animals of 4,4'-dimethylangelicin or 4,4',6-trimethylangelicin.

No data were available to evaluate the reproductive effects or prenatal toxicity of angelicin or its methyl derivatives.

Angelicin, in the presence of ultraviolet A radiation, bound covalently to isolated DNA and to DNA in bacteria, yeast and cultured mammalian cells. In the dark, both positive and negative findings were observed for mutagenicity in bacteria, but angelicin was not mutagenic to yeast. In the presence of ultraviolet A radiation, it was mutagenic to phage, bacteria and yeast. In the presence of ultraviolet A radiation, but not in the dark, it induced sister chromatid exchanges, chromosomal aberrations and micronuclei in mammalian cells *in vitro*.

5-Methylangelicin bound covalently to isolated DNA in the presence of ultraviolet A radiation. It was mutagenic to bacteria both in the dark and in the presence of ultraviolet A radiation. In combination with ultraviolet A radiation, it induced mutations and sister chromatid exchanges in mammalian cells *in vitro*.

4,4'-Dimethylangelicin, in the presence of ultraviolet A radiation, bound covalently to isolated DNA and to DNA in bacteria. In the dark, it was not mutagenic to *Salmonella typhimurium*. In the presence of ultraviolet A radiation, it was mutagenic to *Escherichia coli* and induced cytoplasmic petite mutations in *Saccharomyces cerevisiae*.

4,5'-Dimethylangelicin, in the presence of ultraviolet A radiation, bound covalently to isolated DNA and to DNA in cultured mouse tumour cells and was mutagenic to bacteria, yeast and cultured Chinese hamster cells.

4,4',6-Trimethylangelicin, in the presence of ultraviolet A radiation, bound covalently to isolated DNA. In the dark, it was not mutagenic to *Salmonella typhimurium*. In the presence of ultraviolet A radiation, it was mutagenic to *Escherichia coli*.

Overall assessment of data from short-term tests: Angelicin[a]

	Genetic activity			Cell transformation
	DNA damage	Mutation	Chromosomal effects	
Prokaryotes	+*	? +*		
Fungi/Green plants	+*	— +*		
Insects				
Mammalian cells (*in vitro*)	+*		— +*	
Mammals (*in vivo*)				
Humans (*in vivo*)				
Degree of evidence in short-term tests for genetic activity: **Inadequate** (in the dark) **Sufficient** (in combination with UVA)				Cell transformation: No data

*In combination with UVA

[a]The groups into which the table is divided and the symbols used are defined on pp. 19-20 of the Preamble; the degrees of evidence are defined on pp. 20-21.

Overall assessment of data from short-term tests: 5-Methylangelicin[a]

	Genetic activity			Cell transformation
	DNA damage	Mutation	Chromosomal effects	
Prokaryotes	+*	+ +*		
Fungi/Green plants				
Insects				
Mammalian cells (*in vitro*)		+*	+*	
Mammals (*in vivo*)				
Humans (*in vivo*)				
Degree of evidence in short-term tests for genetic activity: **Inadequate** (in the dark) **Sufficient** (in combination with UVA)				Cell transformation: No data

*In combination with UVA

[a]The groups into which the table is divided and the symbols used are defined on pp. 19-20 of the Preamble; the degrees of evidence are defined on pp. 20-21.

Overall assessment of data from short-term tests: 4,4′-Dimethylangelicin[a]

	Genetic activity			Cell transformation
	DNA damage	Mutation	Chromosomal effects	
Prokaryotes	+*	− +*		
Fungi/Green plants		+*		
Insects				
Mammalian cells (*in vitro*)				
Mammals (*in vivo*)				
Humans (*in vivo*)				
Degree of evidence in short-term tests for genetic activity: **Inadequate** (in the dark) **Limited** (in combination with UVA)				Cell transformation: No data

*In combination with UVA

[a]The groups into which the table is divided and the symbols used are defined on pp. 19-20 of the Preamble; the degrees of evidence are defined on pp. 20-21.

Overall assessment of data from short-term tests: 4,5′-Dimethylangelicin[a]

	Genetic activity			Cell transformation
	DNA damage	Mutation	Chromosomal effects	
Prokaryotes	+*	+*		
Fungi/Green plants		+*		
Insects				
Mammalian cells (*in vitro*)	+*	+*		
Mammals (*in vivo*)				
Humans (*in vivo*)				
Degree of evidence in short-term tests for genetic activity: **Inadequate** (in the dark) **Sufficient** (in combination with UVA)				Cell transformation: No data

*In combination with UVA

[a]The groups into which the table is divided and the symbols used are defined on pp. 19-20 of the Preamble; the degrees of evidence are defined on pp. 20-21.

Overall assessment of data from short-term tests: 4,4′,6-Trimethylangelicin[a]

	Genetic activity			Cell transformation
	DNA damage	Mutation	Chromosomal effects	
Prokaryotes	+*	− +*		
Fungi/Green plants				
Insects				
Mammalian cells (*in vitro*)				
Mammals (*in vivo*)				
Humans (*in vivo*)				
Degree of evidence in short-term tests for genetic activity: **Inadequate** (in the dark) **Inadequate** (in combination with UVA)				Cell transformation: No data

*In combination with UVA

[a]The groups into which the table is divided and the symbols used are defined on pp. 19-20 of the Preamble; the degrees of evidence are defined on pp. 20-21.

4.3 Human data

No case report or epidemiological study of the carcinogenicity of angelicin or its synthetic methyl derivatives was available to the Working Group.

4.4 Evaluation[1]

There is *limited evidence* for the carcinogenicity to experimental animals of angelicin, 5-methylangelicin and 4,5'-dimethylangelicin in combination with ultraviolet A radiation. There is *inadequate evidence* for the carcinogenicity of these compounds to experimental animals in the absence of ultraviolet A radiation.

No data were available to evaluate the carcinogenicity to experimental animals of 4,4'-dimethylangelicin or 4,4',6-trimethylangelicin.

No evaluation could be made of the carcinogenicity of angelicin or its methyl derivatives to humans.

5. References

Ashwood-Smith, M.J. (1978) Frameshift mutations in bacteria produced in the dark by several furocoumarins; absence of activity of 4,5',8-trimethylpsoralen. *Mutat. Res., 58*, 23-27

Ashwood-Smith, M.J., Grant, E.L., Heddle, J.A. & Friedmann, G.B. (1977) Chromosome damage in Chinese hamster cells sensitized to near-ultraviolet light by psoralen and angelicin. *Mutat. Res., 43*, 377-385

Ashwood-Smith, M.J., Poulton, G.A., Barker, M. & Mildenberger, M. (1980) 5-Methoxypsoralen, an ingredient in several suntan preparations, has lethal, mutagenic and clastogenic properties. *Nature, 285*, 407-409

Ashwood-Smith, M.J., Natarajan, A.T. & Poulton, G.A. (1981) *Comparative photobiology of psoralens*. In: Cahn, J., Forlot, P., Grupper, C., Meybeck, A. & Urbach, F., eds, *Psoralens in Cosmetics and Dermatology*, New York, Pergamon Press, pp. 117-131

Ashwood-Smith, M.J., Natarajan, A.T. & Poulton, G.A. (1982) Comparative photobiology of psoralens, *J. natl Cancer Inst., 69*, 189-197

Ashwood-Smith, M.J., Poulton, G.A., Ceska, O., Liu, M. & Furniss, E. (1983) An ultrasensitive bioassay for the detection of furocoumarins and other photosensitizing molecules. *Photochem. Photobiol., 38*, 113-118

Averbeck, D. (1976) *Repair of damage induced by near ultraviolet light plus furocoumarin in* Saccharomyces cerevisiae. In: Kiefer, J., ed., *Radiation and Cellular Control Processes*, Berlin (West), Springer-Verlag, pp. 139-146

---

[1]For definition of the italicized term, see Preamble, p. 18.

Averbeck, D. (1984) Photochemistry and photobiology of psoralens. *Proc. Jpn. Soc. invest. Dermatol.*, *8*, 52-73

Averbeck, D. & Moustacchi, E. (1979) Genetic effect of 3-carbethoxyposralen, angelicin, psoralen and 8-methoxypsoralen plus 365 nm irradiation in *Saccharomyces cerevisiae*. Induction of reversions, mitotic crossing-over, gene conversion and cytoplasmic 'petite' mutations. *Mutat. Res.*, *68*, 133-148

Averbeck, D. & Moustacchi, E. (1980) Decreased photo-induced mutagenicity of mono-functional as opposed to bi-functional furocoumarins in yeast. *Photochem. Photobiol.*, *31*, 475-478

Averbeck, D., Chandra, P. & Biswas, R.K. (1975) Structural specificity in the lethal and mutagenic activity of furocoumarins in yeast cells. *Radiat. environ. Biophys.*, *12*, 241-252

Averbeck, D., Biswas, R.K. & Chandra, P. (1976) *Photoinduced mutations by psoralens in yeast cells*. In: Jung, E.G., ed., *Photochemotherapy. Basic Technique and Side Effects*, Stuttgart, Schattauer-Verlag, pp. 97-104

Averbeck, D., Bisagni, E., Marquet, J.P., Vigny, P. & Gaboriau, F. (1979) Photobiological activity in yeast of derivatives of psoralen substituted at the 3,4 and/or the 4',5' reaction site. *Photochem. Photobiol.*, *30*, 547-555

Averbeck, D., Averbeck, S. & Dall'Acqua, F. (1981a) Mutagenic activity of three monofunctional and three bifunctional furocoumarins in yeast (*Saccharomyces cerevisiae*). *Farm. Ed. Sci.*, *36*, 492-505

Averbeck, D., Magana-Schwencke, N. & Moustacchi, E. (1981b) *Genetic effects and repair in yeast of DNA lesions induced by 3-carbethoxy-psoralen and other photoreactive furocoumarins of therapeutic interest*. In: Cahn, J., Forlot, B.P., Grupper, C., Meybeck, A.E. & Urbach, F., eds, *Psoralens in Cosmetics and Dermatology*, New York, Pergamon Press, pp. 143-153

Averbeck, D., Dubertret, L., Craw, M., Truscott, T.G., Dall'Acqua, F., Rodighiero, P., Vedaldi, D. & Land, E.J. (1984a) Photophysical, photochemical and photobiological studies of 4'-methylangelicins, potential agents for photochemotherapy. *Farm. Ed. Sci.*, *39*, 57-69

Averbeck, D., Papadopoulo, D. & Quinto, I. (1984b) Mutagenic effects of psoralens in yeast and V79 Chinese hamster cells. *Natl Cancer Inst. Monogr.*, *66*, 127-136

Baccichetti, F., Bordin, F. & Carlassare, F. (1979) λ-Prophage induction by furocoumarin photosensitization. *Experientia*, *35*, 183-184

Baccichetti, F., Bordin, F., Carlassare, F., Rodighiero, P., Guiotto, A., Peron, M., Capozzi, A. & Dall'Acqua, F. (1981a) 4'-Methylangelicin derivatives: a new group of highly photosensitizing monofunctional furocoumarins. *Farm. Ed. Sci.*, *36*, 585-597

Baccichetti, F., Bordin, F., Carlassare, F., Peron, M., Guiotto, A., Rodighiero, P., Dall'Acqua, F. & Tamaro, M. (1981b) 4,4'-Dimethylangelicin, a monofunctional furocoumarin showing high photosensitizing activity. *Photochem. Photobiol.*, *34*, 649-651

Baccichetti, F., Bordin, F., Carlassare, F., Dall'Acqua, F., Guiotto, A., Pastorini, G., Rodighiero, G., Rodighiero, P. & Vedaldi, D. (1982) *Furocoumarin for the Photochemotherapy of Psoriasis and Related Skin Diseases* (Consiglio Nazionale del Richerche, Italy), *US Patent 4,312,883*

Baccichetti, F., Carlassare, F., Bordin, F., Guiotto, A., Rodighiero, P., Vedaldi, D., Tamaro, M. & Dall' Acqua, F. (1984) 4,4',6-Trimethylangelicin, a new very photoreactive and non skin-phototoxic monofunctional furocoumarin. *Photochem. Photobiol.*, *39*, 525-529

Barth, J., Gast, W., Rytter, M., Hofmann, C. & Young, A.R. (1983) Lethal lymphocyte damage by angular psoralens (Ger.). *Dermatol. Monatschr.*, *169*, 525-528

Belogurov, A.A. & Zavilgelsky, G.B. (1979) Induction of bacteriophage lambda clear mutation during repair of cross-linked DNA. *Stud. biophys.*, *76*, 75-76

Belogurov, A.A. & Zavilgelsky, G.B. (1981) Mutagenic effect of furocoumarin monoadducts and cross-links on bacteriophage lambda. *Mutat. Res.*, *84*, 11-15

Ben-Hur, E. & Song, P.-S. (1984) The photochemistry and photobiology of furocoumarins (psoralens). *Adv. Radiat. Biol.*, *11*, 131-171

Berenbaum, M. (1981) Patterns of furanocoumarin distribution and insect herbivory in the Umbelliferae: plant chemistry and community structure. *Ecology*, *62*, 1254-1266

Beyrich, T. (1968) Comparative study on the occurrence of furocoumarins in some *Heracleum* species. 13. Furocoumarins. *Pharmazie*, *23*, 336-339

Bickers, D.R. & Pathak, M.A. (1984) Psoralen pharmacology: studies on metabolism and enzyme induction. *Natl Cancer Inst. Monogr.*, *66*, 77-84

Bordin, F., Marciani, S., Baccichetti, F.R., Dall'Acqua, F. & Rodighiero, G. (1975) Studies on the photosensitizing properties of angelicin, an angular furocoumarin forming only monofunctional adducts with the pyrimidine bases of DNA. *Ital. J. Biochem.*, *24*, 258-267

Bordin, F., Carlassare, F., Baccichetti, F. & Anselmo, L. (1976) DNA repair and recovery in *Escherichia coli* after psoralen and angelicin photosensitization. *Biochim. biophys. Acta*, *447*, 249-259

Bordin, F., Baccichetti, F. & Carlassare, F. (1978) 4,5'-Dimethylangelicin, a new very active monofunctional furocoumarin, *Z. Naturforsch.*, *33c*, 296-298

Bordin, F., Carlassare, F., Baccichetti, F., Guiotto, A., Rodighiero, P., Vedaldi, D. & Dall'Acqua, F. (1979) 4,5'-Dimethylangelicin: a new DNA-photobinding monofunctional agent. *Photochem. Photobiol.*, *29*, 1063-1070

Bordin, F., Baccichetti, F., Carlassare, F., Peron, M., Dall' Acqua, F., Vedaldi, D., Guiotto A., Rodighiero, P. & Pathak, M.A. (1981) Pre-clinical evaluation of new antiproliferative agents for the photochemotherapy of psoriasis: angelicin derivatives. *Farm. Ed. Sci.*, *36*, 506-518

Bose, A.K., Fujiwara, H., Kamat, V.S., Trivedi, G.K. & Bhattacharyya, S.C. (1979) ^{13}C NMR spectra of some furocoumarins. *Tetrahedron*, *35*, 13-16

Bridges, B.A. & von Wright, A. (1981) Influence of mutations at the rep gene on survival of *Escherichia coli* following ultraviolet light irradiation or 8-methoxypsoralen photosensitization. Evidence for a recA$^+$/rep$^+$-dependent pathway for repair of DNA crosslinks. *Mutat. Res.*, *82*, 229-238

Carlassare, F., Baccichetti, F., Guiotto, A., Rodighiero, P. & Bordin, F. (1984) A comparative study on the phototoxic and antiproliferative responses of various 6-methylangelicins on the animal skin *in vivo*. *Med. Biol. Environ.*, *12*, 459-462

Chandhoke, N. & Ghatak, B.J.R. (1975) Pharmacological investigations of angelicin — a tranquillosedative and anticonvulsant agent. *Indian J. med. Res.*, *63*, 833-841

Chandra, P., Biswas, R.K., Dall'Acqua, F., Marciani, S., Baccichetti, F., Vedaldi, D. & Rodighiero, C. (1973) Post-irradiation dark recovery of photodamage to DNA induced by furocoumarins. *Biophysik*, *9*, 113-119

Chandra, P., Dall'Acqua, F., Marciani, S. & Rodighiero, G. (1974) *Studies on the repair of DNA photodamaged by furocoumarins*. In: Fitzpatrick, T.B., Pathak, M.A., Harber, L.C., Seiji, M. & Kukita, A., eds, *Sunlight and Man. Normal and Abnormal Photobiologic Responses*, Tokyo, University of Tokyo Press, pp. 411-417

Cleaver, J.E. & Gruenert, D.C. (1984) Repair of psoralen adducts in human DNA: differences among xeroderma pigmentosum complementation groups. *J. invest. Dermatol.*, *82*, 311-315

Connor, M.J., Wheeler, L.A. & Lowe, N.J. (1983) The induction of prophage expression in different *Salmonella typhimurium* strains by DNA cross-linking and monoadduct forming psoralens and longwave ultraviolet irradiation. *Carcinogenesis*, *4*, 1451-1454

Coppey, J., Averbeck, D. & Moreno, G. (1979) Herpes virus production in monkey kidney and human skin cells treated with angelicin or 8-methoxypsoralen plus 365 nm light. *Photochem. Photobiol.*, *29*, 797-801

Dall'Acqua, F., Marciani, S., Ciavatta, L. & Rodighiero, G. (1971a) Formation of interstrand cross-linkings in the photoreactions between furocoumarins and DNA. *Z. Naturforsch.*, *26b*, 561-569

Dall'Acqua, F., Marciani, S., Ciavatta, L. & Rodighiero, G. (1971b) Formation of interstrand cross-linkings in the photoreactions between furocoumarins and DNA. *Stud. biophys.*, *29*, 63-70

Dall'Acqua, F., Marciani, S., Vedaldi, D. & Rodighiero, G. (1974a) Studies of the photoreactions (365 nm) between DNA and some methylpsoralens. *Biochim. biophys. Acta*, *353*, 267-273

Dall'Acqua, F., Marciani, S., Vedaldi, D. & Rodighiero, G. (1974b) Skin photosensitization and cross-linkings formation in native DNA by furocoumarins. *Z. Naturforsch.*, *29c*, 635-636

Dall'Acqua, F., Terbojevich, M., Marciani, S., Vedaldi, D. & Recher, M. (1978) Investigation on the dark interaction between furocoumarins and DNA. *Chem.-biol. Interactions*, *21*, 103-115

Dall'Acqua, F., Vedaldi, D., Guiotto, A., Rodighiero, P., Carlassare, F., Baccichetti, F. & Bordin, F. (1981) Methylangelicins: new potential agents for the photochemotherapy of psoriasis. Structure-activity study on the dark and photochemical interactions with DNA. *J. med. Chem.*, *24*, 806-811

Dall'Acqua, F., Vedaldi, D., Bordin, F., Baccichetti, F., Carlassare, F., Tamaro, M., Rodighiero, P., Pastorini, G., Guiotto, A., Recchia, G. & Cristofolini, M. (1983) 4'-Methylangelicins: new potential agents for the photochemotherapy of psoriasis. *J. med. Chem.*, *26*, 870-876

Dall'Acqua, F., Vedaldi, D ., Caffieri, S., Guiotto, A., Bordin, F. & Rodighiero, G. (1984) Chemical basis of the photosensitizing activity of angelicins. *Natl Cancer Inst. Monogr.*, *66*, 55-60

Dall'Acqua, F., Bordin, F., Guiotto, A. & Cristofolini, M. (1985) 4,6,4'-Trimethylangelicin. *Drugs Future*, *10*, 307-308

Grant, E.L., von Borstel, R.C. & Ashwood-Smith, M.J. (1979) Mutagenicity of cross-links and monoadducts of furocoumarins (psoralen and angelicin) induced by 360-nm radiation in excision-repair-defective and radiation-insensitive strains of *Saccharomyces cerevisiae*. *Environ. Mutagenesis*, *1*, 55-63

Grossweiner, L.I. & Smith, K.C. (1981) Sensitivity of DNA repair-deficient strains of *Escherichia coli* K-12 to various furocoumarins and near-ultraviolet radiation. *Photochem. Photobiol.*, *33*, 317-323

Gruenert, D.C. (1983) Psoralen damage in human cells: DNA repair and effects on replication. *Diss. Abstr. int.*, *B 43*, 2469B

Guiotto, A., Rodighiero, P., Pastorini, G., Manzini, P., Bordin, F., Baccichetti, F., Carlassare, F., Vedaldi, D. & Dall'Acqua, F. (1981) Synthesis of some photosensitizing methylangelicins, as monofunctional reagents for DNA. *Eur. J. med. Chem. chim. Ther.*, *16*, 489-494

Guiotto, A., Rodighiero, P., Manzini, P., Pastorini, G., Bordin, F., Baccichetti, F., Carlassare, F., Vedaldi, D., Dall'Acqua, F., Tamaro, M., Recchia, G. & Cristofolini, M. (1984) 6-Methylangelicins: a new series of potential photochemotherapeutic agents for the treatment of psoriasis. *J. med. Chem.*, *27*, 959-967

Hanawalt, P.C., Kaye, J., Smith, C.A. & Zolan, M. (1981) *Cellular responses to psoralen adducts in DNA*. In: Cahn, J., Forlot, B.P., Grupper, C., Meybeck, A. & Urbach, F., eds, *Psoralens in Cosmetics and Dermatology*, New York, Pergamon Press, pp. 133-142

IARC (1980) *IARC Monographs on the Evaluation of the Carcinogenic Risk of Chemicals to Humans*, Vol. 24, *Some Pharmaceutical Drugs*, Lyon, pp. 101-124

ICIS Chemical Information System (1984) *Carbon-13 NMR Spectral Search System* (CNMR), *Mass Spectral Search System* (MSSS), *Infrared Spectral Search System* (IRSS), *Information System for Hazardous Organics in Water* (ISHOW) and *Environmental Fate* (ENVIROFATE), Washington DC, Information Consultants, Inc.

Isaacs, S.T., Wiesehahn, G. & Hallick, L.M. (1984) In vitro characterization of the reaction of four psoralen derivatives with DNA. *Natl Cancer Inst. Monogr.*, *66*, 21-30

Jachymczyk, W.J., von Borstel, R.C., Mowat, M.R.A. & Hastings, P.J. (1981) Repair of interstrand cross-links in DNA of *Saccharomyces cerevisiae* requires two systems for DNA repair: the RAD 3 system and the RAD 51 system. *Mol. gen. Genet.*, *182*, 196-205

Kaufman, K.D. (1961) Synthetic furocoumarins. I. A new synthesis of methyl-substituted psoralenes and isopsoralenes. *J. org. Chem.*, *26*, 117-121

Kavli, G., Krokan, H., Midelfart, K., Volden, G. & Raa, J. (1983a) Extraction, separation, quantification and evaluation of the phototoxic potency of furocoumarins in different parts of *Heracleum laciniatum*. *Photochem. Photobiophys.*, *5*, 159-168

Kavli, G., Midelfart, K., Raa, J. & Volden, G. (1983b) Phototoxicity from furocoumarins (psoralens) of *Heracleum laciniatum* in a patient with vitiligo. Action spectrum studies on bergapten, pimpinellin, angelicin and sphondin. *Contact Derm.*, *9*, 364-366

Kavli, G., Krokan, H., Myrnes, B. & Volden, G. (1984) High pressure liquid chromatographic separation of furocoumarins in *Heracleum laciniatum*. *Photodermatology*, *1*, 85-86

Kaye, J., Smith, C.A. & Hanawalt, P.C. (1980) DNA repair in human cells containing photoadducts of 8-methoxypsoralen or angelicin. *Cancer Res.*, *40*, 696-702

Kittler, L., Hradečná, Z. & Sühnel, J. (1980) Cross-link formation of phage lambda DNA in situ photochemically induced by the furocoumarin derivative angelicin. *Biochim. biophys. Acta*, *607*, 215-220

Levin, D.E., Hollstein, M., Christman, M.F., Schwiers, E.A. & Ames, B.N. (1982) A new *Salmonella* tester strain (TA102) with A:T base pairs at the site of mutation detects oxidative mutagens. *Proc. natl Acad. Sci. USA*, *79*, 7445-7449

Lichtenberg, B. & Yasui, A. (1983) Effects of *rec*B, *rec*F and *uvr*A mutations on Weigle reactivation of λ phages in *Escherichia coli* K12 treated with 8-methoxypsoralen or angelicin and 365-nm light. *Mutat. Res.*, *112*, 253-260

Linnainmaa, K. & Wolff, S. (1982) Sister chromatid exchange induced by short-lived monoadducts produced by the bifunctional agents mitomycin C and 8-methoxypsoralen. *Environ. Mutagenesis*, *4*, 239-247

Loveday, K.S. & Donahue, B.A. (1984) Induction of sister chromatid exchanges and gene mutations in Chinese hamster ovary cells by psoralens. *Natl Cancer Inst. Monogr.*, *66*, 149-155

Lown, J.W & Sim, S.-K. (1978) Photoreaction of psoralen and other furocoumarins with nucleic acids. *Bioorg. Chem.*, *7*, 85-95

Mantulin, W.W. & Song, P.-S. (1973) Excited states of skin-sensitizing coumarins and psoralens. Spectroscopic studies. *J. Am. chem. Soc.*, *95*, 5122-5129

Monti-Bragadin, C., Tamaro, M., Venturini, S., Pani, B., Babudri, N. & Baccichetti, F. (1981) Mutation in bacteria produced in the dark by furocoumarins activated by rat liver microsomes. *Farm. Ed. Sci.*, *36*, 551-556

Mullen, M.P., Pathak, M.A., West, J.D., Harrist, T.J. & Dall'Acqua, F. (1984) Carcinogenic effects of monofunctional and bifunctional furocoumarins. *Natl Cancer Inst. Monogr.*, *66*, 205-210

Muronetz, E.M., Kovtunenko, L.V. & Kameneva, S.V. (1980) The mutagenic effect of near ultraviolet light on the uvs strains of *Aspergillus nidulans* in the presence of 8-methoxypsoralen or angelicin. *Genetika*, *16*, 1168-1175

Musajo, L. & Rodighiero, G. (1962) The skin-photosensitizing furocoumarins. *Experientia*, *18*, 153-161

Musajo, L., Rodighiero, G. & Caporale, G. (1954) Photodynamic activity of natural coumarins (Fr.). *Bull. Soc. Chim. biol.*, *36*, 1213-1224

Musajo, L., Rodighiero, G., Caporale, G., Dall'Acqua, F., Marciani, S., Bordin, F., Baccichetti, F. & Bevilacqua, R. (1974) *Photoreactions between skin-photosensitizing furocoumarins and nucleic acids.* In: Fitzpatrick, T.B., Pathak, M.A., Harber, L.C., Seiji, M. & Kukita, A., eds, *Sunlight and Man. Normal and Abnormal Photobiologic Responses*, Tokyo, University of Tokyo Press, pp. 369-387

Natarajan, A.T., Verdegaal-Immerzeel, E.A.M., Ashwood-Smith, M.J. & Poulton, G.A. (1981) Chromosomal damage induced by furocoumarins and UVA in hamster and human cells including cells from patients with ataxia telangiectasia and xeroderma pigmentosum. *Mutat. Res.*, *84*, 113-124

Nocentini, S. (1978) Impairment of RNA synthesis and its recovery in angelicin photosensitized mammalian cells. A probe for DNA damage and repair. *Biochim. biophys. Acta*, *521*, 160-168

Pani, B., Babudri, N., Venturini, S., Tamaro, M., Bordin, F. & Monti-Bragadin (1981) Mutation induction and killing of prokaryotic and eukaryotic cells by 8-methoxypsoralen, 4,5'-dimethylangelicin, 5-methylangelicin, 4'-hydroxymethyl-4,5'-dimethylangelicin. *Teratog. Carcinog. Mutagenesis*, *1*, 407-415

Pathak, M.A., ed. (1984) *Photobiologic, Toxicologic, and Pharmacologic Aspects of Psoralens* (*Natl Cancer Inst Monogr. No. 66; NIH Publ. No. 84-2692*), Washington DC, US Government Printing Office

Pathak, M.A., Mosher, D.B. & Fitzpatrick, T.B. (1984) Safety and therapeutic effectiveness of 8-methoxypsoralen, 4,5',8-trimethylpsoralen, and psoralen in vitiligo. *Natl Cancer Inst. Monogr.*, *66*, 165-173

Perel'son, M.E. & Sheinker, Y.N. (1967) Structure and properties of α-pyrones, coumarins, and furocoumarins. Part II. UV spectra of coumarins and furocoumarins. *Teor. eksp. Khim.*, *3*, 428-432

Recchia, G., Cristofolini, M., Bordin, F., Dall'Acqua, F. & Rodighiero, P. (1983a) 4'-Methylangelicin, a new photochemotherapeutic agent: Preliminary results (Ital.). *Chron. Dermatol.*, *14*, 651-657

Recchia, G., Cristogolini, M., Bordin, F., Dall'Acqua, F. & Rodighiero, P. (1983b) Methylangelicins in the topical photochemotherapy of psoriasis: preliminary report. *Med. Biol. Environ.*, *11*, 471-474

Reisch, J. & Mester, I. (1979) Psoralen and angelicin by reaction of 7-hydroxycoumarin with 4-chloro-1,3-dioxolan-2-one (Ger.). *Chem. Ber.*, *112*, 1491-1492

Rodighiero, G. & Dall'Acqua, F. (1984) In vitro photoreactions of selected psoralens and methylangelicins with DNA, RNA and proteins. *Natl Cancer Inst. Monogr.*, *66*, 31-40

Rodighiero, G., Musajo, L., Dall'Acqua, F., Marciani, S., Caporale, G. & Ciavatta, M.L. (1969) A comparison between the photoreactivity of some furocoumarins with native DNA and their skin-photosensitizing activity. *Experientia*, *25*, 479-481

Rodighiero, G., Musajo, L., Dall'Acqua, F., Marciani, S., Caporale, G. & Ciavatta, L. (1970) Mechanism of skin photosensitization by furocoumarins. Photoreactivity of various furocoumarins with native DNA and with ribosomal RNA. *Biochim. biophys. Acta*, *217*, 40-49

Rodighiero, G., Dall'Acqua, F., Marciani, S., Chandra, P., Feller, H., Götz, A. & Wacker, A. (1971) Studies on the reactivation of bacteria photodamaged by an angular furocoumarin: angelicin. *Biophysik*, *8*, 1-8

Rodighiero, P., Guiotto, A., Pastorini, G., Dall'Acqua, F., Bordin, F. & Rodighiero, G. (1981a) *Synthesis of methylangelicins: purity problems connected with the presence of psoralens*. In: Cahn, J., Forlot, P., Grupper, P., Meybeck, A. & Urbach, F., eds, *Psoralens in Cosmetics and Dermatology*, New York, Pergamon Press, p. 189

Rodighiero, P., Guiotto, A., Pastorini, G., Manzini, P., Bordin, F., Baccichetti, F., Carlassare, F., Vedaldi, D. & Dall'Acqua, F. (1981b) Photochemical and photo-biological properties of 4,5'-dimethylpsoralen, a bifunctional [impurity] of synthetic 4,5'-dimethylangelicin. *Farm. Ed. Sci.*, *36*, 648-662

Rodighiero, P., Manzini, P., Pastorini, G. & Guiotto, A. (1984a) ^{13}C-NMR spectra and carbon-proton coupling constants of various methylangelicins. *J. heterocycl. Chem.*, *21*, 235-240

Rodighiero, G., Dall'Acqua, F. & Pathak, M.A. (1984b) *Photobiological properties of monofunctional furocoumarin derivatives*. In: Smith, K.C., ed., *Topics in Photo-medicine*, New York, Plenum Press, pp. 319-398

Royer, R., René, L., Buisson, J.-P., Demerseman, P. & Averbeck, D. (1978) Synthesis, spectroscopic characterization and photobiological activities of angelicin and three other angular furocoumarins (Fr.). *Eur. J. med. Chem. chim. Ther.*, *13*, 213-218

van der Sluis, W.G., Van Arkel, J., Fischer, F.C. & Labadie, R.P. (1981) Thin-layer chromatographic assay of photoactive compounds (furocoumarins) using the fungus *Penicillium expansum* as a test organism. *J. Chromatogr.*, *214*, 349-359

Song, P.-S., Shim, S.C. & Mantulin, W.W. (1981) The electronic spectra of psoralens in their ground and triplet excited states. *Bull. chem. Soc. Jpn*, *54*, 315-316

Swart, R.N.J., Beckers, M.A.N. & Schothorst, A.A. (1983) Phototoxicity and mutagenicity of 4,5'-dimethylangelicin and long-wave ultraviolet irradiation in Chinese hamster cells and human skin fibroblasts. *Mutat. Res., 124*, 271-279

Szafarz, D., Zajdela, F., Bornecque, C. & Barat, N. (1983) Evaluation of DNA crosslinks and monoadducts in mouse embryo fibroblasts after treatment with mono- and bifunctional furocoumarins and 365 nm (UVA) irradiation. Possible relationship to carcinogenicity. *Photochem. Photobiol., 38*, 557-562

Thompson, H.J. & Brown, S.A. (1984) Separations of some coumarins of higher plants by liquid chromatography. *J. Chromatogr., 314*, 323-326

Vande Casteele, K., Geiger, H. & Van Sumere, C.F. (1983) Separation of phenolics (benzoic acids, cinnamic acids, phenylacetic acids, quinic acid esters, benzaldehydes and acetophenones, miscellaneous phenolics) and coumarins by reversed-phase high-performance liquid chromatography. *J. Chromatogr., 258*, 111-124

Venturini, S., Tamaro, M., Monti-Bragadin, C., Bordin, F., Baccichetti, F. & Carlassare, F. (1980) Comparative mutagenicity of linear and angular furocoumarins in *Escherichia coli* strains deficient in known repair functions. *Chem.-biol. Interactions, 30*, 203-207

Venturini, S., Tamaro, M., Monti-Bragadin, C. & Carlassare, F. (1981) Mutagenicity in *Salmonella typhimurium* of some angelicin derivatives proposed as new mono-functional agents for the photochemotherapy of psoriasis. *Mutat. Res., 88*, 17-22

Zavilgelsky, G.B., Belogurov, A.A. & Krüger, D.H. (1982) ω-Reactivation and ω-muta-genesis in bacteriophages λ and T7: comparison of action of ultraviolet irradiation (254 nm) and furocoumarin photosensitization (Russ.). *Genetika, 18*, 24-35

3-CARBETHOXYPSORALEN

1. Chemical and Physical Data

1.1 Synonyms and trade names

Chem. Abstr. Services Reg. No.: 20073-24-9
Chem. Abstr. Name: 7-Oxo-7*H*-furo[3,2-*g*][1]benzopyran-6-carboxylic acid, ethyl ester
IUPAC Systematic Name: Ethyl 7-oxo-7*H*-furo[3,2-*g*][1]benzopyran-6-carboxylate;
[(6-hydroxy-5-benzofuranyl)methylene]malonic acid, δ-lactone, ethyl ester
Synonyms: 3-CPs; 3-ethoxycarbonylpsoralen; ethyl 3-psoralencarboxylate

1.2 Structural and molecular formulae and molecular weight

$C_{14}H_{10}O_5$ Mol. wt: 258.23

1.3 Chemical and physical properties of the pure substance

(a) *Description*: Orange needles (Worden *et al.*, 1969)

(b) *Melting-point*: 153-154°C (Worden *et al.*, 1969)

(c) *Spectroscopy data*: Ultraviolet (Averbeck *et al.*, 1979; Vigny *et al.*, 1979; Gaboriau *et al.*, 1981), infrared and nuclear magnetic resonance (Jameson *et al.*, 1984), fluorescence (Vigny *et al.*, 1979; Gaboriau *et al.*, 1981) and triplet and radical anion and cation absorption spectral data (Craw *et al.*, 1983; Bensasson *et al.*, 1984) have been reported.

(d) *Solubility*: Very slightly soluble in water (13 mg/l) (Dall'Acqua *et al.*, 1981);
soluble in acetone (Dubertret *et al.*, 1979) and ethanol (Mullen *et al.*, 1984)

(e) *Stability*: Water-ethanol solutions of 3-carbethoxypsoralen under 365 nm irradiation showed degradation (Vigny *et al.*, 1979; Dubertret *et al.*, 1981)

1.4 Technical products and impurities

No data were available to the Working Group.

2. Production, Use, Occurrence and Analysis

2.1 Production and use

(a) *Production*

3-Carbethoxypsoralen is not currently produced in commercial quantities. Queval and
Bisagni (1974) and Worden *et al.* (1969) described laboratory-scale synthesis of this
compound utilizing 5-formyl 6-hydroxybenzofuran as the immediate precursor.

(b) *Use*

3-Carbethoxypsoralen has been investigated for potential use in the photochemotherapy of psoriasis and other dermatological conditions (Dubertret *et al.*, 1979, 1981).

2.2 Occurrence

3-Carbethoxypsoralen is not known to occur as a natural product.

2.3 Analysis

3-Carbethoxypsoralen can be separated from its thymidine adducts using reverse-phase
high-performance liquid chromatography (Cadet *et al.*, 1983).

3. Biological Data Relevant to the Evaluation
of Carcinogenic Risk to Humans

3.1 Carcinogenicity studies in animals

(a) *Skin application*

Mouse: Groups of 20 male and 20 female XVIInc/Z mice, 12-14 weeks old, received skin
applications of 40 μl of an acetone solution of 3-carbethoxypsoralen on each ear (15

$\mu g/cm^2$) on five days per week for 21 or 39 weeks (106 or 196 treatments). The mice were each irradiated 15 min after the skin application (using four Philips HPW 125 lamps, wavelength mostly 365 nm; <340 nm eliminated by running-water filter using two Pyrex glass slides) to give a dose of 365 nm light at the level of the ears of 28 J/m²/sec (dose of 1.68 × 10⁴ J/m² as a 10-min irradiation each time). No skin tumour or other skin lesion was observed. One control group of 20 males and 20 females received 115 applications on each ear of 15 $\mu g/cm^2$ methoxsalen (because of the photocarcinogenic potential of this chemical [see IARC, 1980]) followed by a radiation dose of 1.68 × 10⁴ J/m²; 37/40 animals were alive when the first skin carcinoma appeared, and 92% of them developed tumours at the site of application (mostly squamous-cell carcinomas). Two other control groups of ten males and ten females each received either 106 applications of 3-carbethoxypsoralen without irradiation or 106 UVA radiation doses of 1.68 × 10⁴ J/m² without 3-carbethoxypsoralen; no skin tumour or other skin lesion was observed in animals in either of these groups. The experiment was terminated when the animals were 22 months old, at which time >85% mice were alive in all groups (Dubertret et al., 1979).

A group of 40 male Skh:hairless-1 albino mice, six weeks old, was given thrice-weekly applications of 0.05 ml of a 0.1% ethanol solution of crystalline 3-carbethoxypsoralen on the skin of the back for 50 weeks. The experiment was terminated at 12-15 months [time unspecified]. The animals were then immobilized for 45 min and irradiated with UVA light (six FR 40T12/PUVA Sylvania Lifeline bulbs emitting radiation of 320-400 nm, with a maximum wavelength of 355 nm; wavelengths <320 nm were eliminated with a Mylar filter [irradiance unspecified]). The radiation dose per treatment was 1 × 10⁴ J/m² (total dose, 120 × 10⁴ J/m²). Four groups of 20 mice each were treated with 3-carbethoxypsoralen alone or with UVA irradiation only (total doses, 148, 250 and 751.5 × 10⁴ J/m²). No skin tumour was observed in any of these groups. In a fifth control group of 20 animals treated with a 0.1% ethanol solution of methoxsalen followed by 1.0 × 10⁴ J/m² UVA irradiation (total dose, 220 × 10⁴ J/m²), the tumour yield was 70% [mortality rate unspecified] with time required to produce a tumour incidence of 50% in surviving animals of 60 weeks (Mullen et al., 1984).

(b) Intraperitoneal administration

Mouse: A group of 20 male and 20 female XVIInc/Z mice, 12-14 weeks of age, received 36 intraperitoneal injections of 20 mg/kg bw (0.4 mg/mouse) 3-carbethoxypsoralen in olive oil, each of which was followed 60 min later by 1.68 × 10⁴ J/m² UVA irradiation (four Philips HPW 125 lamps, 365 nm; <340 nm eliminated by filters). The experiment was terminated when animals were 22 months old, at which time 38/40 animals in the treated group were still alive; no tumour was observed. A control group of 20 male and 20 female Swiss mice received intraperitoneal injections of methoxsalen followed by irradiation at the same dose levels. In this group, 37/40 animals were alive when the first tumours appeared; 90% of them developed tumours, which were mostly sarcomas of the ears but also occurred on other hairless areas (paws) (Dubertret et al., 1979).

3.2 Other relevant biological data

(a) Experimental systems

The photochemical and photobiological properties of 3-carbethoxypsoralen have been reviewed (Dubertret *et al.*, 1981; Averbeck, 1982).

Toxic effects

Administration of 10-1000 $\mu g/2.5$ cm^2 3-carbethoxypsoralen and subsequent irradiation with UVA (>320 nm) did not induce any visible change in the dorsal shaved skin of albino guinea-pigs (Pathak *et al.*, 1967).

3-Carbethoxypsoralen administered topically (4 mg/mouse) in acetone or orally (25 mg/kg bw) in corn oil followed by irradiation with UVA (50 kJ/m^2) 1 or 2 h later, respectively, did not significantly increase epidermal ornithine decarboxylase activity or S-adenosyl-L-methionine decarboxylase activity in hairless mice (Connor & Lowe, 1984). Groups of female Skh:hairless-1 mice received a single dose of 25 mg/kg bw 3-carbethoxypsoralen in corn oil by gavage and were irradiated with UVA 2 h later (5 J/cm^2), or a single topical application of 200 μl of a 2% solution of 3-carbethoxypsoralen in acetone on the back with UVA irradiation 1 h later (5 J/cm^2). 3-Carbethoxypsoralen failed to induce epidermal ornithine decarboxylase activity; topical application of 50 μl of a 1% 3-carbethoxypsoralen solution plus UVA stimulated rather than suppressed DNA synthesis (Lowe *et al.*, 1984). In contrast, Dall'Acqua *et al.* (1981) reported that topical application of 3-carbethoxypsoralen to mice, followed by irradiation with 365 nm light inhibited epidermal DNA synthesis.

Various enzymes (glutamate dehydrogenase, 6-phosphogluconate dehydrogenase, lysozyme, enolase and ribonuclease) were inactivated by irradiation for 3 h at 365 nm in the presence of 3-carbethoxypsoralen. Inactivation appeared to be mediated by singlet oxygen (Veronese *et al.*, 1982).

Effects on reproduction and prenatal toxicity

No data were available to the Working Group.

Absorption, distribution, excretion and metabolism

^{14}C-Labelled 3-carboxypsoralen rapidly penetrated mouse epidermis (Dubertret *et al.*, 1979).

Mutagenicity and other short-term tests

3-Carbethoxypsoralen was reported to form a complex with DNA *in vitro* in the dark in several studies (Vigny *et al.*, 1979; Dall'Acqua *et al.*, 1981; Gaboriau *et al.*, 1981; Ronfard-Haret *et al.*, 1982; Rodighiero & Dall'Acqua, 1984) but not in another (Isaacs *et al.*, 1984). It photobound covalently to DNA *in vitro* (Averbeck *et al.*, 1978; Vigny *et al.*, 1979; Magaña-Schwencke *et al.*, 1980; Dall'Acqua *et al.*, 1981; Gaboriau *et al.*, 1981; Cadet *et al.*, 1983; Rodighiero & Dall'Acqua, 1984) and in *Saccharomyces cerevisiae* (Averbeck *et al.*, 1978; Averbeck, 1985), but did not produce DNA interstrand cross-links in either system (Averbeck *et al.*, 1978; Gaboriau *et al.*, 1981).

In the presence of UVA, 3-carbethoxypsoralen induced prophage in *Salmonella typhimurium* TA1535 but not in TA1538 (Connor *et al.*, 1983). In a DNA repair test in *Escherichia coli*, the *recA* strain was more sensitive to 3-carbethoxypsoralen plus UVA than the wild-type strain (Grossweiner & Smith, 1981).

DNA damage induced by 3-carbethoxypsoralen plus UVA was repaired in *S. cerevisiae*, as observed by an increase in the sensitivity of repair-defective mutants as compared to wild types (Averbeck *et al.*, 1978; Averbeck & Averbeck, 1979; Henriques & Moustacchi, 1980a,b).

In the dark, this compound was not mutagenic to *S. typhimurium* TA1535, TA1537, TA1538, TA98 or TA100 when tested in the absence of an exogenous metabolic system at concentrations of up to 900 μg/plate (Quinto *et al.*, 1984). 3-Carbethoxypsoralen plus UVA induced cytoplasmic 'petite' mutations in *S. cerevisiae* (Juliani *et al.*, 1976; Averbeck & Moustacchi, 1979; Averbeck *et al.*, 1981; Averbeck, 1985). It photoinduced reverse (Averbeck & Moustachi, 1980; Cassier *et al.*, 1980; Averbeck *et al.*, 1981) and forward mutations in haploid *S. cerevisiae* (Cassier *et al.*, 1980; Averbeck *et al.*, 1981) and reverse mutations and mitotic recombination in diploid *S. cerevisiae* (Averbeck & Moustacchi, 1979; Averbeck, 1985).

3-Carbethoxypsoralen plus UVA increased the number of 6-thioguanine-resistant mutants in cultured Chinese hamster V79 and ovary cells (Papadopoulo *et al.*, 1983; Loveday & Donahue, 1984).

This compound photoinduced sister chromatid exchanges in cultured Chinese hamster ovary cells (Ashwood-Smith *et al.*, 1981; Loveday & Donahue, 1984) and increased the incidence of sister chromatid exchanges in cultured human embryonic fibroblasts (Billardon *et al.*, 1984).

(b)   Humans

Toxic effects

When 2% 3-carbethoxypsoralen in lanolin was applied to the skin of ten psoriatic patients 2 h before UVA irradiation (mean dose of 417 J/cm²), four times per week for an average of 33 treatments, erythema was reported in six patients and pruritus in three of these six. Localized hyperpigmentation was not observed (Dubertret *et al.*, 1979).

Effects on reproduction and prenatal toxicity

No data were available to the Working Group.

Absorption, distribution, excretion and metabolism

No data were available to the Working Group.

Mutagenicity and chromosomal effects

No data were available to the Working Group.

3.3 Case reports and epidemiological studies on carcinogenicity to humans

No data were available to the Working Group.

4. Summary of Data Reported and Evaluation

4.1 Exposure data

There is no known human exposure to 3-carbethoxypsoralen, other than in limited clinical trials for the treatment of psoriasis.

4.2 Experimental data

3-Carbethoxypsoralen was tested for skin carcinogenicity in two experiments in two strains of mice by skin application with and without ultraviolet A radiation and in one study in mice by intraperitoneal administration with subsequent ultraviolet A radiation. No skin tumour was observed in 3-carbethoxypsoralen-treated mice in any of the three studies, with ultraviolet A radiation. The studies were inadequate to evaluate the systemic carcino-genicity of 3-carbethoxypsoralen.

No data were available to evaluate the reproductive effects or prenatal toxicity of 3-carbethoxypsoralen to experimental animals.

In the presence of ultraviolet A radiation, 3-carbethoxypsoralen bound covalently to isolated DNA and induced DNA damage in *Salmonella typhimurium*, *Escherichia coli* and *Saccharomyces cerevisiae*. It was not mutagenic to *Salmonella typhimurium* in the dark in the absence of an exogenous metabolic system. In combination with ultraviolet A radiation, 3-carbethoxypsoralen induced mutations and mitotic recombination in yeast and mutations and sister chromatid exchanges in cultured mammalian cells *in vitro*.

4.3 Human data

No case report or epidemiological study of the carcinogenicity of 3-carbethoxypsoralen was available to the Working Group.

4.4 Evaluation[1]

On the basis of experiments designed to test only the carcinogenicity to mouse skin of 3-carbethoxypsoralen in combination with ultraviolet A radiation, there is *no evidence* of carcinogenicity to experimental animals.

---

[1]For definition of the italicized terms, see Preamble, p. 18.

Overall assessment of data from short-term tests: 3-Carbethoxypsoralen[a]

	Genetic activity			Cell transformation
	DNA damage	Mutation	Chromosomal effects	
Prokaryotes	+*	?		
Fungi/Green plants	+*	+*		
Insects				
Mammalian cells (*in vitro*)		+*	+*	
Mammals (*in vivo*)				
Humans (*in vivo*)				
Degree of evidence in short-term tests for genetic activity: **Inadequate** (in the dark) **Sufficient** (in combination with UVA)				Cell transformation: No data

*In combination with UVA

[a]The groups into which the table is divided and the symbols used are defined on pp. 19-20 of the Preamble; the degrees of evidence are defined on pp. 20-21.

There is *inadequate evidence* for the carcinogenicity to experimental animals of 3-carbethoxypsoralen in the absence of ultraviolet A radiation.

No evaluation could be made of the carcinogenicity of 3-carbethoxypsoralen to humans.

5. References

Ashwood-Smith, M.J., Natarajan, A.T. & Poulton, G.A. (1981) *Comparative photobiology of psoralens*. In: Cahn, J., Forlot, P., Grupper, C., Meybeck, A. & Urbach, F., eds, *Psoralens in Cosmetics and Dermatology*, New York, Pergamon Press, pp. 117-131

Averbeck, D. (1982) *Photobiology of furocoumarins*. In: Hélène, C., Charlier, M., Montenay-Garestier, T. & Laustriat, G., eds, *Trends in Photobiology*, New York, Plenum Press, pp. 295-308

Averbeck, D. (1985) Relationship between lesions photoinduced by mono- and bifunctional furocoumarins in DNA and genotoxic effects in diploid yeast. *Mutat. Res.*, *151*, 217-233

Averbeck, D. & Averbeck, S. (1979) *Dose-rate effects of furocoumarins plus 365-nm radiation on the cytoplasmic and nuclear genetic level in* Saccharomyces cerevisiae. In: Edwards, H.E., Navaratnam, S., Parsons, B.J. & Phillips, G.O., eds, *Radiation Biology and Chemistry, Research Developments*, Amsterdam, Elsevier, pp. 453-466

Averbeck, D. & Moustacchi, E. (1979) Genetic effect of 3-carbethoxypsoralen, angelicin, psoralen and 8-methoxypsoralen plus 365-nm irradiation in *Saccharomyces cerevisiae*. Induction of reversions, mitotic crossing-over, gene conversion and cytoplasmic 'petite' mutations. *Mutat. Res., 68,* 133-148

Averbeck, D. & Moustacchi, E. (1980) Decreased photo-induced mutagenicity of mono-functional as opposed to bi-functional furocoumarins in yeast. *Photochem. Photobiol., 31,* 475-478

Averbeck, D., Moustacchi, E. & Bisagni, E. (1978) Biological effects and repair of damage photoinduced by a derivative of psoralen substituted at the 3,4 reaction site. Photoreactivity of this compound and lethal effect in yeast. *Biochim. biophys. Acta, 518,* 464-481

Averbeck, D., Bisagni, E., Marquet, J.P., Vigny, P. & Gaboriau, F. (1979) Photobiological activity in yeast of derivatives of psoralen substituted at the 3,4 and/or the 4',5' reaction site. *Photochem. Photobiol., 30,* 547-555

Averbeck, D., Averbeck, S. & Dall'Acqua, F. (1981) Mutagenic activity of three monofunctional and three bifunctional furocoumarins in yeast (*Saccharomyces cerevisiae*). *Farm. Ed. Sci., 36,* 492-505

Bensasson, R.V., Chalvet, O., Land, E.J. & Ronfard-Haret, J.C. (1984) Triplet, radical anion and radical cation spectra of furocoumarins. *Photochem. Photobiol., 39,* 287-291

Billardon, C., Levy, S. & Moustacchi, E. (1984) Induction in human skin fibroblasts of sister-chromatid exchanges (SCEs) by photoaddition of two new monofunctional pyridopsoralens in comparison to 3-carbethoxypsoralen and 8-methyoxypsoralen. *Mutat. Res., 138,* 63-70

Cadet, J., Voituriez, L., Gaboriau, F., Vigny, P. & Della Negra, S. (1983) Characterization of photocycloaddition products from reaction between thymidine and the mono-functional 3-carbethoxypsoralen. *Photochem. Photobiol., 37,* 363-371

Cassier, C., Chanet, R., Henriques, J.A.P. & Moustacchi, E. (1980) The effects of three *pso* genes on induced mutagenesis: a novel class of mutationally defective yeast. *Genetics, 96,* 841-857

Connor, M.J. & Lowe, N.J. (1984) The induction of erythema, edema, and the polyamine synthesis enzymes ornithine decarboxylase and *S*-adenosyl-L-methionine decarboxyl-ase in hairless mouse skin by psoralens and longwave ultraviolet light. *Photochem. Photobiol., 39,* 787-792

Connor, M.J., Wheeler, L.A. & Lowe, N.J. (1983) The induction of prophage expression in different *Salmonella typhimurium* strains by DNA cross-linking and monoadduct forming psoralens and longwave ultraviolet radiation. *Carcinogenesis, 4,* 1451-1454

Craw, M., Bensasson, R.V., Ronfard-Haret, J.C., Sa e Melo, M.T. & Truscott, T.G. (1983) Some photophysical properties of 3-carbethoxypsoralen, 8-methoxypsoralen and 5-methoxypsoralen triplet states. *Photochem. Photobiol.*, *37*, 611-615

Dall'Acqua, F., Vedaldi, D., Baccichetti, F., Bordin, F. & Averbeck, D. (1981) Photochemotherapy of skin diseases: comparative studies on the photochemical and photobiological properties of various mono-and bifunctional agents. *Farm. Ed. Sci.*, *36*, 519-535

Dubertret, L., Averbeck, D., Zajdela, F., Bisagni, E., Moustacchi, E., Touraine, R. & Latarjet, R. (1979) Photochemotherapy (PUVA) of psoriasis using 3-carbethoxypsoralen, a non-carcinogenic compound in mice. *Br. J. Dermatol.*, *101*, 379-389

Dubertret, L., Averbeck, D., Bensasson, R., Bisagni, E., Gaboriau, F., Land, E.J., Nocentini, S., Macedo de Sa E Melo, M.T., Moustacchi, E., Morlière, P., Ronfard-Haret, J.C., Santus, R., Vigny, P., Zajdela, F. & Latarjet, R. (1981) *Photophysical, photochemical, photobiological and phototherapeutic properties of 3-carbethoxypsoralen.* In: Cahn, J., Forlot, B.P., Grupper, C., Meybeck, A.E. & Urbach, F., eds, *Psoralens in Cosmetics and Dermatology*, New York, Pergamon Press, pp. 245-256

Gaboriau, F., Vigny, P., Averbeck, D. & Bisagni, E. (1981) Spectroscopic study of the dark interaction and of the photoreaction between a new monofunctional psoralen: 3-carbethoxy psoralen, and DNA. *Biochimie*, *63*, 899-905

Grossweiner, L.I. & Smith, K.C. (1981) Sensitivity of DNA repair-deficient strains of *Escherichia coli* K-12 to various furocoumarins and near-ultraviolet radiation. *Photochem. Photobiol.*, *33*, 317-323

Henriques, J.A.P. & Moustacchi, E. (1980a) Sensitivity to photoaddition of mono- and bifunctional furocoumarins of X-ray sensitive mutants of *Saccharomyces cerevisiae*. *Photochem. Photobiol.*, *31*, 557-563

Henriques, J.A.P. & Moustacchi, E. (1980b) Isolation and characterization of *pso* mutants sensitive to photo-addition of psoralen derivatives in *Saccharomyces cerevisiae*. *Genetics*, *95*, 273-288

IARC (1980) *IARC Monographs on the Evaluation of the Carcinogenic Risk of Chemicals to Humans*, Vol. 24, *Some Pharmaceutical Drugs*, Lyon, pp. 101-124

Isaacs, S.T., Wiesehahn, G. & Hallick, L.M. (1984) In vitro characterization of the reaction of four psoralen derivatives with DNA. *Natl Cancer Inst. Monogr.*, *66*, 21-30

Jameson, C.W., Dunnick, J.K., Brown, R.D. & Murrill, E. (1984) Chemical characterization of psoralens used in the National Toxicology Program research projects. *Natl Cancer Inst. Monogr.*, *66*, 103-113

Juliani, M.H., Hixon, S. & Moustacchi, E. (1976) Mitochondrial genetic damage induced in yeast by a photoactivated furocoumarin in combination with ethidium bromide or ultraviolet light. *Mol. gen. Genet.*, *145*, 249-254

Loveday, K.S. & Donahue, B.A. (1984) Induction of sister chromatid exchanges and gene mutations in Chinese hamster ovary cells by psoralens. *Natl Cancer Inst. Monogr.*, *66*, 149-155

Lowe, N.J., Connor, M.J., Cheong, E.S., Akopiantz, P. & Breeding, J.H. (1984) Psoralen and ultraviolet A effects on epidermal ornithine decarboxylase induction and DNA synthesis in the hairless mouse. *Natl Cancer Inst. Monogr.*, *66*, 73-76

Magaña-Schwencke, N., Averbeck, D., Pegas-Henriques, J.-A. & Moustacchi, E. (1980) Absence of interstrand bridges in DNA treated with 3-carbethoxypsoralen and irradiation at 365 nm. *C.R. Acad. Sci. Paris*, *291*, Serie D, 207-210

Mullen, M.P., Pathak, M.A., West, J.D., Harrist, T.J. & Dall'Acqua, F. (1984) Carcinogenic effects of monofunctional and bifunctional furocoumarins. *Natl. Cancer Inst. Monogr.*, *66*, 205-210

Papadopoulo, D., Sagliocco, F. & Averbeck, D. (1983) Mutagenic effects of 3-carbethoxypsoralen and 8-methoxypsoralen plus 365-nm irradiation in mammalian cells. *Mutat. Res.*, *124*, 287-297

Pathak, M.A., Worden, L.R. & Kaufman, K.D. (1967) Effect of structural alterations on the photosensitizing potency of furocoumarins (psoralens) and related compounds. *J. invest. Dermatol.*, *48*, 103-118

Queval, P. & Bisagni, E. (1974) New synthesis of psoralen and related compounds (Fr.). *Eur. J. med. Chem. chim. Ther.*, *9*, 335-340

Quinto, I., Averbeck, D., Moustacchi, E., Hrisoho, Z. & Moron, J. (1984) Frameshift mutagenicity in *Salmonella typhimurium* of furocoumarins in the dark. *Mutat. Res.*, *136*, 49-54

Rodighiero, G. & Dall'Acqua, F. (1984) In vitro photoreactions of selected psoralens and methylangelicins with DNA, RNA and proteins. *Natl Cancer Inst. Monogr.*, *66*, 31-40

Ronfard-Haret, J.C., Averbeck, D., Bensasson, R.V., Bisagni, E. & Land, E.J. (1982) Some properties of the triplet excited state of the photosentizing furocoumarin: 3-carbethoxypsoralen. *Photochem. Photobiol.*, *35*, 479-489

Veronese, F.M., Schiavon, O., Bevilacqua, R., Bordin, F. & Rodighiero, G. (1982) Photoinactivation of enzymes by linear and angular furocoumarins. *Photochem. Photobiol.*, *36*, 25-30

Vigny, P., Gaboriau, F., Duquesne, M., Bisagni, E. & Averbeck, D. (1979) Spectroscopic properties of psoralen derivatives substituted by carbethoxy groups at the 3,4 and/or 4',5' reaction site. *Photochem. Photobiol.*, *30*, 557-564

Worden, L.R., Kaufman, K.D., Weis, J.A. & Schaaf, T.K. (1969) Synthetic furocoumarins. IX. A new synthetic route to psoralen. *J. org. Chem.*, *34*, 2311-2313

5-METHOXYPSORALEN

1. Chemical and Physical Data

1.1 Synonyms and trade names

Chem. Abstr. Services Reg. No.: 484-20-8

Chem. Abstr. Name: 4-Methoxy-7*H*-furo[3,2-*g*][1]benzopyran-7-one

IUPAC Systematic Names: 6-Hydroxy-4-methoxy-5-benzofuranacrylic acid, δ-lactone; 4-methoxy-7*H*-furo[3,2-*g*][1]benzopyran-7-one

Synonyms: Bergaptan; bergapten; bergaptene; heraclin; majudin; 5-methoxy-6,7-furanocoumarin; 5-MOP

1.2 Structural and molecular formulae and molecular weight

$C_{12}H_8O_4$ Mol. wt: 216.19

1.3 Chemical and physical properties of the pure substance

(*a*)   *Description*: Needles from ethanol (Windholz, 1983)

(*b*)   *Melting-point*: 188°C with sublimation (Windholz, 1983)

(*c*)   *Spectroscopy data*: Ultraviolet (Sadtler Research Laboratories, 1985 [32766[a]]), infrared (Jameson *et al.*, 1984; Sadtler Research Laboratories, 1985; prism/grating [59028]), proton nuclear magnetic resonance (Sadtler Research Laboratories, 1985 [32018]), C-13 nuclear magnetic resonance (Bergenthal *et al.*, 1978; Elgamal *et al.*, 1978; Ivie, 1978; Elgamal *et al.*, 1979; Mitra *et al.*, 1979; Duddeck *et al.*, 1980;

---

[a]Spectrum number in Sadtler compilation

Jameson *et al.*, 1984), fluorescence (Mantulin & Song, 1973; Matsumoto & Isobe, 1981; Song *et al.*, 1981; Bettero & Benassi, 1983; Sa E Melo *et al.*, 1984a) and mass spectral data (ICIS Chemical Information System, 1984 [MSSS]) have been reported.

(*d*) *Solubility*: Practically insoluble in boiling water; slightly soluble in glacial acetic acid, chloroform, benzene and warm phenol; soluble in absolute ethanol (Windholz, 1983)

1.4 Technical products and impurities

One preparation of 5-methoxypsoralen contained 7.3% of a dimethoxypsoralen isomer (Jameson *et al.*, 1984).

2. Production, Use, Occurrence and Analysis

2.1 Production and use

(*a*) *Production*

5-Methoxypsoralen has been isolated from oil of bergamot, which is derived from the Mediterranean fruit *Citrus bergamia* (Cieri, 1969). Kalbrunner first isolated 5-methoxy-psoralen from bergamot oil in 1834 (Fowlks, 1959).

5-Methoxypsoralen was first synthesized in 1937 by Späth *et al.*, by the condensation of 3,4,6-triacetoxycoumaran with ethyl sodium formyl acetate and methylation of the resulting product. Other synthetic routes have been described which use 6-formyl-7-hydroxy-5-methoxycoumarin-7-*O*-acetic acid (Howell & Robertson, 1937), the methyl ester of 2,6-dioxy-4-methoxybenzoic acid (Caporale, 1958) and 5-allyloxy-7-hydroxycoumarin (Ahluwalia *et al.*, 1969) as precursors.

One French manufacturer is currently producing commercial quantities of 5-methoxy-psoralen and first introduced it as a pharmaceutical in 1983 (Paul de Haen International, 1984).

(*b*) *Use*

5-Methoxypsoralen, in combination with UVA, is commonly used as a photochemo-therapeutic agent for the treatment of psoriasis (Hönigsmann *et al.*, 1979).

As a component of bergamot oil, 5-methoxypsoralen is present in some perfumes and fragances, sunscreen preparations and food products (Furia & Bellanca, 1971; Ashwood-Smith, 1979; Anon., 1981; Marks, 1984).

(c)   *Regulatory status and guidelines*

The US Hazardous Substances Act (US Consumer Product Safety Commission, 1973) classifies consumer products containing 2% or more bergamot oil as 'strong sensitizers'. The 1976 Cosmetic Directive of the European Economic Community (1976) excludes the use of furocoumarins in cosmetics except for the normal content of natural essences.

Bergamot oil is not currently listed as a 'generally recognized as safe' (GRAS) food additive or natural flavouring substance by the US Food and Drug Administration (1984).

2.2 Occurrence

(a)   *Natural occurrence*

5-Methoxypsoralen is found in oil of bergamot, which is derived from the rind of the orange-like Mediterranean fruit *Citrus bergamia*. Natural bergamot oil typically contains 3000-3600 μg/g 5-methoxypsoralen. Nearly all bergamot oil sold in the USA for use in consumer products has been steam-distilled, which reportedly removes 5-methoxypsoralen and any other furocoumarins (Ashwood-Smith *et al.*, 1980).

5-Methoxypsoralen can not only be isolated from bergamot oil (Suzuki *et al.*, 1979; Croud *et al.*, 1983) but has also been found in expressed oil of lime (*Citrus aurantifolia*) (Cieri, 1969), oils of grapefruit (*C. paradisi*) and sour orange (*C. aurantium*) (Fisher & Trama, 1979), leaves of the fig tree (*Ficus carica*) (Innocenti *et al.*, 1982), parsley (*Petroselinum crispum*) (Rodighiero & Allegri, 1959) and parsnip (*Pastinaca sativa*) (Berenbaum, 1981; Ivie *et al.*, 1981), celery (*Apium graveolens*) (Beier *et al.*, 1983), *Bolanites aegyptiaca*, an Egyptian bark (Seida *et al.*, 1981) and numerous Umbelliferae, including *Ammi majus* from US and Egyptian sources (Balbaa *et al.*, 1975; Haggag & Hilal, 1977; Ivie, 1978; Hilal *et al.*, 1982), *Angelica atropurpurea*, *Cicuta maculata* and *C. bulbifera*, *Conium maculatum* and *Sium suave* (Berenbaum, 1981) and in numerous species of *Heracleum* (Beyrich, 1968; Berenbaum, 1981; Kavli *et al.*, 1983a,b, 1984). Elevated levels (10 μg/g) were found in diseased celery (Ashwood-Smith *et al.*, 1985).

Measured levels in various plants and plant extracts are listed in Table 1.

(b)   *Foods*

Bergamot oil has been reported as an additive in nonalcoholic beverages (8.9 μg/g), ice cream (7.9 μg/g), sweets (27 μg/g), baked goods (29 μg/g), gelatins and puddings (5.3-90 μg/g), chewing-gum (43 μg/g) and icings (1.0-130 μg/g) (Furia & Bellanca, 1971).

(c)   *Other*

Concentrations of 5-methoxypsoralen in perfumes have been reported to range from 0-100 μg/ml (Zaynoun, 1978), while sunscreen preparations with bergamot oil contain 10-50 μg/ml 5-methoxypsoralen (Ashwood-Smith & Poulton, 1981; Cartwright & Walter, 1983). An early sample of a perfume, produced in 1964, contained 1000 μg/ml (Marzulli & Maibach, 1970).

Table 1. Natural occurrence of 5-methoxypsoralen in plants and plant extracts

Sample source	Concentration (μg/g)	Reference
Angelica (seed)	400	Cieri (1969)
Angelica (root)	1000	Ding & Zhang (1981)
Ammi majus	1100-1500	Balbaa *et al.* (1975); Ivie (1978)
Bergamot (*Citrus bergamia*) oil	0-1130	Susuki *et al.* (1979)
	3700	Marzulli & Maibach (1970); Croud *et al.* (1983)
	3000-3600	Cieri (1969)
	3900	Opdyke (1973)
Celery (*Apium graveolens*)	0.04-0.69	Beier *et al.* (1983); Ashwood-Smith *et al.* (1985)
Lime (*C. aurantifolia*) oil	1700-3300	Cieri (1969)
Parsnip (*Pastinaca sativa*)	3-4	Ivie *et al.* (1981)

2.3 Analysis

Selected methods for the analysis of 5-methoxypsoralen in various matrices are identified in Table 2. 5-Methoxypsoralen has been measured in various media using thin-layer chromatography (TLC), fluorimetry, gas chromatography, high-performance liquid chromatography, ultraviolet spectroscopy and mass spectrometry, alone or in combination with other methods.

Bioassays using microorganisms have also been used, on the basis of the light-induced phototoxicity of 5-methoxypsoralen toward several species *in vitro*. These assays involve growing *Candida albicans*, *Penicillium expansum* or a DNA repair-deficient strain of *Escherichia coli* on agar plates to confluence and spotting furocoumarin solutions onto the plates. The plates are irradiated with long-wave ultraviolet (UVA) light, and the presence and size of the clear (killed zones) surrounding the sample are measured. The sensitivity of such bioassays is in the ng to μg range, depending on the microorganisms used as the detector species (Zaynoun, 1978; van der Sluis *et al.*, 1981; Ashwood-Smith *et al.*, 1983; Kavli *et al.*, 1983a,b).

A variety of TLC methods have been used in the analysis of 5-methoxypsoralen. For sample preparation, plant materials have been extracted with methanol, ethyl acetate or chloroform (Balbaa *et al.*, 1975; Hilal *et al.*, 1982; Ashwood-Smith *et al.*, 1983; Kavli *et al.*, 1983a,b); 5-methoxypsoralen has been isolated from fragrance preparations by chemical modification (using the opening and reclosure of the lactone ring) and ether extractions.

Table 2. Methods for the analysis of 5-methoxypsoralen

Sample matrix	Sample preparation	Assay procedure[a]	Limit of detection	Reference
Bergamot oil	Saponify; wash with diethyl ether; acidify to recyclize lactone; extract with chloroform	GC/FID GC/MS	1 μg/g	Suzuki et al. (1979)
Fragrances	Saponify; wash with diethyl ether; acidify to recyclize lactone; extract with diethyl ether	TLC/FL	10 μg/g	Wisneski (1976)
Parsnip root	Extract with ethyl acetate; isolate by TLC; extract from TLC gel with diethyl ether	GC/FID	0.3 μg/g	Ivie et al. (1981)
Perfume and sunscreen products	Extract with dichloromethane	HPLC/UV	1 μg/g	Bettero & Benassi (1981)
	Inject directly or (for emulsions) dilute with tetrahydrofuran and pass through 0.45-μm filter	HPLC/FL	5 ng/g	Bettero & Benassi (1983)

[a]Abbreviations: GC, gas chromatography; FID, flame-ionization detection; MS, mass spectrometry; TLC, thin-layer chromatography; FL, fluorimetric detection; HPLC, high-performance liquid chromatography; UV, ultraviolet detection

One- and two-dimensional TLC have been used to separate 5-methoxypsoralen from other furocoumarins. TLC plate fractions have been quantified by fluorimetry directly on the plate, with a sensitivity of 0.2 μg and a linear response of 10-1000 μg/g (Wisneski, 1976); by fluorimetry on eluted TLC samples, with a reported sensitivity of 0.5 μg/g (Hilal et al., 1982); and by measuring phototoxicity in microorganisms (van der Sluis et al., 1981; Ashwood-Smith et al., 1983).

High-performance liquid chromatography has been used by several research groups to separate and quantify 5-methoxypsoralen in plant extracts and essential oils, using both normal and reverse-phase columns (Berenbaum, 1981; Verger, 1981; Thompson & Brown, 1984). Ultraviolet detection is reported to provide sensitivity in the μg/g range (Bettero & Benassi, 1981; Beier et al., 1983; Vande Casteele et al., 1983), while fluorescence detection provided sensitivity in the ng/g range (Fisher & Trama, 1979; Bettero & Benassi, 1983).

Exposure of humans to 5-methoxypsoralen can be monitored by measuring concentrations of 5-methoxypsoralen in plasma using high-performance liquid chromatography and gas chromatography, with a limit of detection of approximately 5 ng/ml (Schmid et al., 1981).

3. Biological Data Relevant to the Evaluation of Carcinogenic Risk to Humans

3.1 Carcinogenicity studies in animals

Skin application

Mouse: Groups of 20 male and 20 female hairless albino mice (an outbred strain from the Institute of Dermatology, London), eight to ten weeks old, received topical applications of 0.01% or 0.03% solutions of crystalline 5-methoxypsoralen or methoxsalen (purity, 100%; confirmed by absorption spectroscopy, thin-layer chromatography and mass spectrometry) in 70:30 (v/v) BP-grade arachis oil and isopropyl myristate on both flanks on five days per week for up to 37 weeks. After each application, the animals were immobilized for 30 min and then received simulated solar irradiation (vertically-mounted, water-cooled 6 KW Xenon arc simulating solar radiation with 2-mm Schott glass WG320 filter) for 50 min. The estimated daily dose of irradiation was 1.7×10^4 J/m², of which approximately 400 J/m² were UVB radiation. Seven control groups were either left untreated or were treated with vehicle alone, arachis oil alone, simulated solar irradiation alone, vehicle plus irradiation, or applications of 0.03% 5-methoxypsoralen or 0.03% methoxsalen without irradiation. The groups treated with methoxsalen and irradiation served as controls (because of the photocarcinogenic potential of this chemical [see IARC, 1980]). Mortality rates and mean numbers of skin tumours >1 mm in diameter per surviving animal after 26 weeks of treatment are summarized in Table 3. A random sample of tumours was examined histologically, and 83% of the skin tumours in the group treated with 5-methoxypsoralen and irradiation were found to be papillomas. Trend tests using life-table methods indicated a positive dose-related trend in incidence for treatment with either 5-methoxypsoralen ($p <$ 0.01) or methoxsalen ($p < 0.01$) in combination with simulated solar radiation. A dose-adjusted life-table test comparing the relative tumour incidences in these two groups showed no statistically significant difference at the 5% level (Young *et al.*, 1983). [The Working Group noted that the duration of the studies with 5-methoxypsoralen was too short to evaluate the carcinogenicity of this chemical alone.]

A group of 20 male and 20 female XVIInc/Z albino mice, 12-14 weeks old, received topical applications of 40 μl of a 0.025% solution of 5-methoxypsoralen (purity, 100%; confirmed by high-performance liquid chromatography and mass spectrometry) in acetone on each ear (≃ 10 μg/cm²) on five days per week for 23 weeks (115 treatments). Fifteen minutes after each application, mice were immobilized and irradiated for 10 min (four Philips, HPW 125 lamps, 365 nm; wavelengths <340 nm were eliminated by running-water filter of two 6-mm Pyrex glass slides; irradiance at ear level, 28 J/m²/sec), corresponding to a dose of 1.68×10^4 J/m². Eight months after the last 5-methoxypsoralen application, the 20 females received thrice-weekly promoting applications of 1 μg 12-*O*-tetradecanoylphorbol 13-acetate (TPA; 40 applications). Two control groups of 40 mice each received 115 applications of psoralen or methoxsalen plus UVA irradiation. Further control groups of 21 mice [sex unspecified] received applications of acetone followed by chronic radiation treatment or skin applications of psoralen without irradiation and were followed for 21

Table 3. Total and mean numbers of skin tumours per mouse surviving at 26 weeks[a]

Treatment[b]	Total no. of tumours No. of surviving mice	Mean no. of tumours/mouse
No treatment	2/40	0.05
Vehicle alone	1/31	0.03
Arachis oil alone	8/39	0.2
SSR alone	18/33	0.5
Vehicle plus SSR	14/39	0.4
Methoxsalen (0.03%) alone	6/26	0.2
5-MOP (0.03%) alone	5/31	0.2
Methoxsalen (0.03%) + SSR	372/38	9.8
5-MOP (0.03%) + SSR	179/31	5.8
Methoxsalen (0.01%) + SSR	69/36	1.9
5-MOP (0.01%) + SSR	84/34	2.5

[a]From Young et al. (1983)

[b]SSR, simulated solar radiation; 5-MOP, 5-methoxypsoralen

months. After 16 months, 19/20 males treated with 5-methoxypsoralen plus UVA were alive; 17/20 (85%) surviving the minimal latency developed skin carcinomas, and 25% had multiple tumours. After 15 months, 18/20 females treated with 5-methoxypsoralen plus UVA plus TPA were alive; all developed tumours, and 66% had multiple tumours (see also Table 4). In the first two control groups, 37/38 (97%) mice receiving psoralen treatment plus irradiation developed tumours, and 20/38 (52%) had multiple tumours; 34/37 (92%) of mice receiving methoxsalen plus irradiation developed tumours, and 16/37 (45%) had multiple tumours. Mean latent periods for tumour development were 16 months for treatment with 5-methoxypsoralen plus irradiation, 13.5 months for treatment with methoxsalen plus irradiation and 9.3 months for treatment with psoralen plus irradiation. Most of the tumours were squamous-cell carcinomas invading the dermis and cartilage. Metastases in the regional cervical lymph nodes occurred in 20% of tumour-bearing animals. At 22 months of age, 20/21 and 19/21 mice receiving treatment with acetone plus irradiation and treatment with psoralen alone, respectively, were still alive; no tumour was observed in either group (Zajdela & Bisagni, 1981). [The Working Group noted that a control group receiving 5-methoxypsoralen without UVA was not included in this study.]

Groups of 15 female HRS/J hairless albino mice, eight weeks old, received skin application of 4 μl/cm^2 Sun System III oil (containing 25 mg/kg 5-methoxypsoralen and ethyl hexyl-*para*-methoxycinnamate, a UVB screen) on their backs on five days per week for 20 weeks. The mice were immobilized for 60 min after each application and were irradiated (1000-watt Xenon arc solar-simulator with dichroic mirror, 335-nm long pass filter and

Table 4. Skin tumour incidences in mice treated with psoralens with and without irradiation, or with irradiation alone[a]

Treatment[b]	No. of animals	No. of animals at risk	% of animals with tumour
(5-MOP + UVA) × 115	20M	20[c]	85
(5-MOP + UVA) × 115 + TPA	20F	18[c]	100
(Methoxsalen + UVA) × 115	40 (20M+20F)	37[c]	92
(Psoralen + UVA) × 115	40 (20M+20F)	38[c]	97.3
Psoralen × 140	21	19[d]	0
UVA × 196	21	20[d]	0

[a]From Zajdela and Bisagni (1981)

[b]5-MOP, 5-methoxypsoralen; TPA, 12-O-tetradecanoylphorbol 13-acetate; UVA, 1.8 J/cm² 365 nm; psoralen, topical applications of 10 μg/cm²

[c]Number of animals alive when the first carcinoma was observed in each group

[d]Number of animals at the age of 22 months

water filter; UVA flux, 13 mW/cm²; UVB flux, 19 μW/cm²). Groups received 2.5×10^4, 5×10^4 or 10×10^4 J/m² UVA radiation. One control group of 15 mice received applications of Sun System III oil only, and another group of six mice received UVA irradiation only (10×10^4 J/m²). The number of tumours >1 mm in diameter per surviving mouse at 44 weeks of observation was dependent on the dose of radiation: 0.8 tumours at 2.5, 3.5 tumours at 5 and 8 tumours at 10×10^4 J/m²; the percentages of animals with two or more tumours at that time were 13 at 2.5, 86 at 5 and 100 at 10×10^4 J/m². At 44 weeks, 15/15, 14/15 and 9/15 animals were still alive in the three groups, respectively. By 52 weeks, some of the tumours had developed into large invasive tumours fixed to underlying tissue, especially in the group receiving the highest dose of radiation. Histological examination showed that atypical squamous-cell papillomas had progressed to invasive squamous-cell carcinomas (Cartwright & Walter, 1983). [The Working Group noted the lack of controls given vehicle plus UVA and the inadequate number of animals in the group receiving UV radiation alone, and that the duration of the studies with 5-methoxypsoralen (Sun-System III) alone was too short to evaluate the carcinogenicity of this compound itself.]

3.2 Other relevant biological data

(a) Experimental systems

The photochemistry and photobiology of psoralens, including 5-methoxypsoralen, have been reviewed (Musajo & Rodighiero, 1962; Scott *et al.*, 1976; Song & Tapley, 1979; Pathak, 1984).

Toxic effects

The oral LD_{50} for 5-methoxypsoralen has been reported to be 8100 mg/kg bw in NMRI Hanover mice, >30 000 mg/kg bw in Wistar AF rats and 9000 mg/kg bw in Hartley guinea-pigs (Herold *et al.*, 1981).

When 5-methoxypsoralen was given orally to beagle dogs at daily doses of 100 or 400 mg/kg (eight days), 60 mg/kg (28 days) or 48 mg/kg (26 weeks) [bw presumed], at the highest doses tested there were delayed signs of behavioural toxicity, bullous dermatitis, bilateral keratitis, decreased food consumption and decreased weight gain. The cutaneous lesions were reversible, whereas the ocular lesions were not. Hepatomegaly, necrosis and hepatic inflammation occurred in the 48-mg/kg dose group. In the group receiving 60 mg/kg per day, polycythemia was present 24 h after administration of the last dose. At doses lower than those specified there was no marked change (Herold *et al.*, 1981). [The Working Group noted the inadequate reporting of the data.]

When daily doses of 70, 280 or 560 mg/kg 5-methoxypsoralen were given orally to Wistar AF rats for one year, several slight changes were observed at the highest dose, such as increased water consumption, decreased weight gain, reduced blood urea and increased liver weight. Thyroid hypofunction occurred early and persisted. Epidermoid cysts of the thyroid (in males) were present in approximately one-third of slides examined from all three treated groups [the numbers for controls were not given]. A dose-dependent perimedullary connective tissue proliferation of the adrenals was observed in females (Herold *et al.*, 1981). [The Working Group noted the inadequate reporting of the data.]

Application of 5-methoxypsoralen to guinea-pig skin (50 or 100 μg/2.5 cm^2) and exposure to UV radiation or administration of an oral dose of 8.6 mg/kg bw 5-methoxypsoralen and exposure to UV radiation induced marked erythema (Pathak & Fitzpatrick, 1959).

5-Methoxypsoralen and UVA irradiation (306-428 nm; maximum, 345 nm) killed cultured human lymphocytes. Blast transformation stimulated by phytohaemagglutinin did not alter this effect (Barth *et al.*, 1983). In studies of phytohaemagglutinin-stimulated blast transformation of cultured human lymphocytes, combined exposure to various concentrations of 5-methoxypsoralen and UVA irradiation (345 nm) produced no inhibition when exposure occurred 24 h before stimulation, but there was inhibition when exposure occurred 36 h after stimulation (Gast *et al.*, 1983).

5-Methoxypsoralen plus UVA inhibited DNA synthesis in Chinese hamster ovary cells (Weniger, 1981), in Ehrlich ascites tumour cells (Musajo *et al.*, 1974) and in the epidermis of Skh:hairless-1 mice after topical application (Lowe *et al.*, 1984).

5-Methoxypsoralen, applied topically (2 mg/mouse) or administered orally (25 mg/kg bw) and followed by UVA irradiation (50 kJ/m^2) to Skh/hrl female hairless mice, markedly increased epidermal ornithine decarboxylase activity (Connor & Lowe, 1984). A commercial sunscreen preparation (Sun-System III) containing unspecified amounts of 5-methoxy-psoralen and ethylhexyl-*para*-methoxycinnamate also induced ornithine decarboxylase in female albino HRS/J mice after UVA irradiation (335 nm) (Walter *et al.*, 1982).

Effects on reproduction and prenatal toxicity

Groups of 26 pregnant female Sprague-Dawley rats were given 5-methoxypsoralen orally at daily doses of 0, 70 or 560 mg/kg bw on days 6-15 of gestation. With 560 mg/kg, there was maternal toxicity (decreased weight gain, fewer litters), but no significant increase in anomalies in surviving fetuses (Herold *et al.*, 1981).

Groups of 15 pregnant female New Zealand rabbits were given 5-methoxypsoralen orally at daily doses of 0, 70 or 560 mg/kg bw on days 7-18 of gestation. With 560 mg/kg, there was maternal toxicity (decreased weight gain; only 50% of dams gave birth to living pups). There was a dose-dependent increase in fetal abnormalities: 15.4% in controls, 41.7% with 70 mg/kg and 57.1% with 560 mg/kg (Herold *et al.*, 1981). [The Working Group noted that the types, frequencies and distribution of fetal anomalies were not specified.]

Absorption, distribution, excretion and metabolism

In young adult Hartley guinea-pigs, a linear relation was found between serum and epidermal concentrations of 5-methoxypsoralen, and the observed skin phototoxicity correlated with the serum 5-methoxypsoralen concentration (Kornhauser *et al.*, 1982).

Mutagenicity and other short-term tests

5-Methoxypsoralen formed a noncovalently-bound complex with DNA *in vitro* in the dark (Dall'Acqua & Rodighiero, 1966; Dall'Acqua *et al.*, 1978; Isaacs *et al.*, 1984). It photobound covalently to DNA *in vitro* (Musajo *et al.*, 1966a,b; Musajo & Rodighiero, 1970; Rodighiero *et al.*, 1970; Sa È Melo *et al.*, 1984a), in *Saccharomyces cerevisiae* (Averbeck, 1985) and in Chinese hamster V79 cells (Papadopoulo & Averbeck, 1985). It photoinduced interstrand cross-links in DNA *in vitro* (Dall'Acqua *et al.*, 1971) and in Chinese hamster V79 cells (Papadopoulo & Averbeck, 1985). DNA photobinding *in vitro* was dependent on UVA dose (Isaacs *et al.*, 1984; Rodighiero & Dall'Acqua, 1984).

In a DNA repair test, 5-methoxypsoralen with UVA inhibited semiconservative DNA synthesis and induced unscheduled DNA synthesis in human embryonic skin and muscle fibroblasts (Wottawa & Viernstein, 1982).

5-Methoxypsoralen alone was reported to be mutagenic to *Salmonella typhimurium* TA100 in the presence or absence of an exogenous metabolic system (S9) (Pool & Deutsch-Wenzel, 1979) and to *Escherichia coli lac⁻* z (ND160) (Ashwood-Smith *et al.*, 1980).

5-Methoxypsoralen plus UVA reduced survival of repair-deficient mutants of *Bacillus subtilis* and *E. coli* (Song *et al.*, 1975; Pool *et al.*, 1982); addition of S9 inhibited the lethal activity (Pool *et al.*, 1982). 5-Methoxypsoralen photoinduced prophage expression in *S. typhimurium* TA1535 and TA1538 (Connor *et al.*, 1983).

In combination with UVA, 5-methoxypsoralen induced mutations in *S. typhimurium* TA100 in the absence of an exogenous metabolic system (Pool & Deutsch-Wenzel, 1979). It was not mutagenic to *B. subtillis* (Song *et al.*, 1975) but induced a UVA dose-dependent increase in mutations in *E. coli* WP2 *try⁻* (Ashwood-Smith *et al.*, 1980, 1981).

5-Methoxypsoralen plus UVA induced revertants and forward mutations in haploid *S. cerevisiae* (Averbeck *et al.*, 1981a,b, 1984) and cytoplasmic 'petite' mutations in haploid and diploid *S. cerevisiae* (Averbeck *et al.*, 1984; Averbeck, 1985). In diploid *S. cerevisiae*, 5-methoxypsoralen plus UVA induced nuclear mutations and mitotic recombination (Averbeck, 1985).

The compound induced mutations in the green algae, *Chlamydomonas reinhardii*, in the presence of UVA (Schimmer *et al.*, 1980; Schimmer, 1981).

5-Methoxypsoralen with UVA induced an increase in 6-thioguanine-resistant mutants in Chinese hamster V79 (Papadopoulo & Averbeck, 1985; Averbeck & Papadopoulo, 1986) and cultured ovary cells (Loveday & Donahue, 1984). The response was dependent on UVA dose (Loveday & Donahue, 1984; Papadopoulo & Averbeck, 1985).

5-Methoxypsoralen plus UVA induced an increase in the incidence of sister chromatid exchanges, which was dependent on UVA dose, in Chinese hamster ovary cells (Ashwood-Smith *et al.*, 1980, 1981, 1982; Loveday & Donahue, 1984) and also in cultured normal human foreskin fibroblasts and in ataxia telangiectasia and xeroderma pigmentosum cells. The increase was greater in ataxia telangiectasia and xeroderma pigmentosum cells than in normal cells (Natarajan *et al.*, 1981; Ashwood-Smith *et al.*, 1982).

5-Methoxypsoralen plus UVA induced chromosomal aberrations in normal human foreskin fibroblasts and in ataxia telangiectasia and xeroderma pigmentosum cells in culture; these effects were more frequent in ataxia telangiectasia and xeroderma pigmentosum cells (Natarajan *et al.*, 1981). As reported in an abstract, an increase in chromosomal aberrations was also found in human lymphocytes after treatment *in vitro* with 5-methoxypsoralen in combination with UVA (Abel & Muth, 1985).

(b)   Humans

Toxic effects

Application of 4-200 μg/2.5 cm^2 5-methoxypsoralen to human skin and irradiation with UVA induced erythema 22 min to 36 h after irradiation, followed by marked pigmentation seven to 15 days later (Musajo *et al.*, 1954; Pathak & Fitzpatrick, 1959; Zaynoun *et al.*, 1977; Walter *et al.*, 1982).

5-Methoxypsoralen has been reported to be the single active agent in berloque dermatitis, causing patchy hyperpigmentation of the face and neck (Opdyke, 1973; Zaynoun *et al.*, 1977).

Kavli *et al.* (1983b) performed photoepicutaneous tests with psoralens isolated from the umbelliferous plant *Heracleum laciniatum* on normal volunteers. 5-Methoxypsoralen was the most strongly phototoxic, being active at 0.001% in ethanol. Reactions reached their maximum 72 h after exposure. The action spectrum of 5-methoxypsoralen was determined, and maximum photosensitivity was seen at 330-335 nm. Phototoxicity could also be produced in a patient with vitiligo (Kavli *et al.*, 1983c).

Effects on reproduction and prenatal toxicity

No data were available to the Working Group.

Absorption, distribution, excretion and metabolism

Following oral administration of 40 mg 5-methoxypsoralen to healthy male volunteers, absorption was documented by measurement of plasma levels. The plasma concentrations peaked 2-4 h after administration and declined to low levels by 8 h. Distribution to the skin after topical application of 0.15 and 0.0015% 5-methoxypsoralen was evident from photosensitization, persisting up to 8 h, to 366 nm UV light with an irradiance of 22 mW/cm^2 2 h after administration. Minute amounts of 5-methoxypsoralen were excreted in urine and bile (Schmid *et al.*, 1981).

5-Methoxypsoralen binds to human serum proteins, principally albumin (Artuc *et al.*, 1979; Veronese *et al.*, 1979). Data on 5-methoxypsoralen binding to low-density lipoproteins suggest that these are the primary vehicle for intracellular transport of 5-methoxypsoralen (Sa E Melo *et al.*, 1984b).

Mutagenicity and chromosomal effects

No data were available to the Working Group.

3.3 Case reports and epidemiological studies of carcinogenicity to humans

Mezzadra *et al.* (1981) surveyed 87 employees in the bergamot oil production industry in southern Italy, 42 of whom had direct contact with bergamot essence and 45 who were involved in the cultivation, harvesting and transportation of bergamot fruit, and 31 people resident in the same area. 'Keratomas' or 'epitheliomas' of the skin were found in 15 (19%) of 79 exposed workers and in five (16%) of the comparison group. The bergamot-exposed group was older, on average (47 years), than the comparison group (39 years). [The Working Group noted that the possible confounding effects of age, sex and outdoor employment were not considered.]

4. Summary of Data Reported and Evaluation

4.1 Exposure data

5-Methoxypsoralen is found in a variety of plant species, including parsnips and celery, in bergamot and lime oils, and in derivative products. Use of foods, beverages, perfumes and sunscreen preparations containing these products results in human exposure. Exposure also occurs when 5-methoxypsoralen is used as a drug, in conjunction with ultraviolet A radiation, for the treatment of skin disorders. Occupational exposure occurs during the extraction of this compound from bergamot oil and its preparation into foods and consumer goods.

4.2 Experimental data

5-Methoxypsoralen was tested in combination with ultraviolet A or solar-simulated radiation for skin carcinogenicity in two experiments in two strains of mice by skin application. It produced papillomas and squamous-cell carcinomas of the skin.

The studies were inadequate to evaluate the systemic carcinogenicity of 5-methoxypsoralen.

Maternally toxic doses of 5-methoxypsoralen did not increase the number of anomalies in surviving fetuses of treated rats.

5-Methoxypsoralen in the presence of ultraviolet A radiation bound covalently to isolated DNA and to DNA in yeast and cultured mammalian cells, and induced prophage expression in bacteria. In the presence of ultraviolet A radiation, it was mutagenic to bacteria, green algae and yeast and induced mutations, sister chromatid exchanges and chromosomal aberrations in mammalian cells *in vitro*. Studies of 5-methoxypsoralen in the absence of ultraviolet A radiation were inadequate for evaluation.

Overall assessment of data from short-term tests: 5-Methoxypsoralen[a]

	Genetic activity			Cell transformation
	DNA damage	Mutation	Chromosomal effects	
Prokaryotes	+*	+*		
Fungi/Green plants	+*	+*		
Insects				
Mammalian cells (*in vitro*)	+*	+*	+*	
Mammals (*in vivo*)				
Humans (*in vivo*)				
Degree of evidence in short-term tests for genetic activity: **Sufficient** (in combination with UVA)				Cell transformation: No data

*In combination with UVA

[a]The groups into which the table is divided and the symbols used are defined on pp. 19-20 of the Preamble; the degrees of evidence are defined on pp. 20-21.

4.3 Human data

One small survey showed no excess prevalence of skin tumours in workers in the bergamot oil production industry, but this study had methodological weaknesses.

4.4 Evaluation[1]

On the basis of experiments designed to test only the carcinogenicity to mouse skin of 5-methoxypsoralen in combination with ultraviolet A radiation or solar-simulated radiation, there is *sufficient evidence*[2] of carcinogenicity to experimental animals.

There is *inadequate evidence* for the carcinogenicity of 5-methoxypsoralen to experimental animals in the absence of ultraviolet A radiation.

There is *inadequate evidence* for the carcinogenicity of 5-methoxypsoralen to humans.

5. References

Abel, G. & Muth, A. (1985) Modification of the clastogenicity of 5-MOP plus UV-A by the anticlastogen AET dependent on treatment conditions (Abstract No. 12). *Mutat. Res.*, *147*, 130

Ahluwalia, V.K., Seshadri, T.R. & Venkateswarlu, P. (1969) A convenient synthesis of bergapten. *Indian J. Chem.*, *7*, 831-832

Anon. (1981) Sunscreens, photocarcinogenesis, melanogenesis, and psoralens. *Br. med. J.*, *283*, 335-336

Artuc, M., Stuettgen, G., Schalla, W., Schaefer, H. & Gazith, J. (1979) Reversible binding of 5- and 8-methoxypsoralen to human serum protein (albumin) and to epidermis *in vitro*. *Br. J. Dermatol.*, *101*, 669-677

Ashwood-Smith, M.J. (1979) Possible cancer hazard associated with 5-methoxypsoralen in suntan preparations. *Br. med. J.*, *218*, 1144

Ashwood-Smith, M.J. & Poulton, G.A. (1981) Inappropriate regulations governing the use of oil of bergamot in suntan preparations. *Mutat. Res.*, *85*, 389-390

Ashwood-Smith, M.J., Poulton, G.A., Barker, M. & Mildenberger, M. (1980) 5-Methoxypsoralen, an ingredient in several suntan preparations, has lethal, mutagenic and clastogenic properties. *Nature*, *285*, 407-409

Ashwood-Smith, M.J., Natarajan, A.T. & Poulton, G.A. (1981) *Comparative photobiology of psoralens*. In: Cahn, J., Forlot, P., Grupper, C., Meybeck, A. & Urbach, F., eds, *Psoralens in Cosmetics and Dermatology*, New York, Pergamon Press, pp. 117-131

Ashwood-Smith, M.J., Natarajan, A.T. & Poulton, G.A. (1982) Comparative photobiology of psoralens. *J. natl Cancer Inst.*, *69*, 189-197

---

[1]For definitions of the italicized terms, see Preamble, pp. 18 and 22.

[2]In the absence of adequate data on humans, it is reasonable, for practical purposes, to regard chemicals or exposures for which there is *sufficient evidence* of carcinogenicity in animals as if they represented a carcinogenic risk to humans.

Ashwood-Smith, M.J., Poulton, G.A., Ceska, O., Liu, M. & Furniss, E. (1983) An ultrasensitive bioassay for the detection of furocoumarins and other photosensitizing molecules. *Photochem. Photobiol.*, *38*, 113-118

Ashwood-Smith, M.J., Ceska, O. & Chaudhary, S.K. (1985) Mechanisms of photosensitizing reactions to diseased celery. *Br. med. J.*, *290*, 1249

Averbeck, D. (1985) Relationship between lesions photoinduced by mono-and bifunctional furocoumarins in DNA and genotoxic effects in diploid yeast. *Mutat. Res.*, *151*, 217-233

Averbeck, D. & Papadopoulo, D. (1986) *Genetic effects of DNA mono- and diadducts photoinduced by furocoumarins in eukaryotic cells*. In: Singer, B. & Bartsch, H., eds, *The Role of Cyclic Nucleic Acid Adducts in Carcinogenesis and Mutagenesis* (*IARC Scientific Publications No. 70*), Lyon, International Agency for Research on Cancer, pp. 299-312

Averbeck, D., Averbeck, S. & Dall'Acqua, F. (1981a) Mutagenic activity of three monofunctional and three bifunctional furocoumarins in yeast (*Saccharomyces cerevisiae*). *Farm. Ed. Sci.*, *36*, 492-505

Averbeck, D., Magaña-Schwencke, N. & Moustacchi, E. (1981b) *Genetic effects and repair in yeast of DNA lesions induced by 3-carbethoxypsoralen and other photoreactive furocoumarins of therapeutic interest*. In: Cahn, J., Forlot, B.P., Grupper, C., Meybeck, A.E. & Urbach, F., eds, *Psoralens in Cosmetics and Dermatology*, New York, Pergamon Press, pp. 143-153

Averbeck, D., Papadopoulo, D. & Quinto, I. (1984) Mutagenic effects of psoralens in yeast and V79 Chinese hamster cells. *Natl Cancer Inst. Monogr.*, *66*, 127-136

Balbaa, S.I., Hilal, S.H. & Haggag, M.Y. (1975) A preliminary study of the effect of phosphorus fertilizers on the yield of fruits of *Ammi majus* L. grown in Egypt and their content of furocoumarins. *Egypt. J. pharm. Sci.*, *16*, 351-358

Barth, J., Gast, W., Rytter, M., Hofmann, C. & Young, A.R. (1983) Lethal lymphocyte damage by angular psoralens (Ger.). *Dermatol. Monatsschr.*, *169*, 525-528

Beier, R.C., Ivie, G.W., Oertli, E.H. & Holt, D.L. (1983) HPLC analysis of linear furocoumarins (psoralens) in healthy celery (*Apium graveolens*). *Food Chem. Toxicol.*, *21*, 163-165

Berenbaum, M. (1981) Patterns of furanocoumarin distribution and insect herbivory in the Umbelliferae: plant chemistry and community structure. *Ecology*, *62*, 1254-1266

Bergenthal, D., Rözsa, Z., Mester, I. & Reisch, J. (1978) On the ^{13}C-NMR spectroscopy of coumarins from Rutaceae (Ger.). *Arch. Pharm.*, *311*, 1026-1029

Bettero, A. & Benassi, C.A. (1981) Determination of bergapten in suntan cosmetics. *Farm. Ed. Prat.*, *36*, 140-147

Bettero, A. & Benassi, C.A. (1983) Determination of bergapten and citropten in perfumes and suntan cosmetics by high-performance liquid chromatography and fluorescence. *J. Chromatogr.*, *280*, 167-171

Beyrich, T. (1968) Comparative study on the occurrence of furocoumarins in some *Heracleum* species. 13. Furocoumarins (Ger.). *Pharmazie, 23*, 336-339

Caporale, G. (1958) New synthesis of bergapten (Ital.). *Ann. Chim., 48*, 650-656

Cartwright, L.E. & Walter, J.F. (1983) Psoralen-containing sunscreen is tumorigenic in hairless mice. *J. Am. Acad. Dermatol., 8*, 830-836

Cieri, U.R. (1969) Characterization of the steam nonvolatile residue of bergamot oil and some other essential oils. *J. Am. off. anal. Chem., 52*, 719-728

Connor, M.J. & Lowe, N.J. (1984) The induction of erythema, edema, and the polyamine synthesis enzymes ornithine decarboxylase and S-adenosyl-L-methionine decarboxylase in hairless mouse skin by psoralens and longwave ultraviolet light. *Photochem. Photobiol., 39*, 787-792

Connor, M.J., Wheeler, L.A. & Lowe, N.J. (1983) The induction of prophage expression in different *Salmonella typhimurium* strains by DNA cross-linking and monoadduct forming psoralens and longwave ultraviolet radiation. *Carcinogenesis, 4*, 1451-1454

Croud, V.B., Michaelis, J.R. & Pindar, A.G. (1983) Isolation of bergapten and limettin from bergamot oil. *Analyst, 108*, 1532-1534

Dall'Acqua, F. & Rodighiero, G. (1966) The dark-interaction between furocoumarins and nucleic acids. *Rend. Sci. fis. mat. nat. Lincei (Rome), 40*, 411-422

Dall'Acqua, F., Marciani, S., Ciavatta, L. & Rodighiero, G. (1971) Formation of inter-strand cross-linkings in the photoreactions between furocoumarins and DNA. *Z. Naturforsch., 26b*, 561-569

Dall'Acqua, F., Terbojevich, M., Marciani, S. & Recher, M. (1978) Investigation on the dark interaction between furocoumarins and DNA. *Chem.-biol. Interactions, 21*, 103-115

Ding, Y. & Zhang, H. (1981) Determination of coumarins in *Angelica dahurica* var. *formosana* by thin-layer chromatography and UV spectrophotometry (Chin.). *Yaoxue Tongbao, 16*, 16-17 [*Chem. Abstr., 96*, 91709j]

Duddeck, H., Elgamal, M.H.A., Abd Elhady, F.K. & Shalaby, N.M.M. (1980) A novel assignment method in the ^{13}C NMR spectroscopy of coumarins and furocoumarins. *Org. magn. Reson., 14*, 256-257

Elgamal, M.H.A, Elewa, N.H., Elkhirsy, E.A.M. & Duddeck, H. (1978) *^{13}C NMR spectroscopy as a tool for structural elucidation of furocoumarins and furochromones.* In: Marekov, N., Ognyanov, I. & Orahovats, A., eds, *11th International IUPAC Symposium on the Chemistry of Natural Products, Sofia, Bulgaria*, Sofia, Bulgarian Academy of Science, pp. 271-274

Elgamal, M.H.A, Elewa, N.H., Elkhrisy, E.A.M. & Duddeck, H. (1979) ^{13}C NMR chemical shifts and carbon-proton coupling constants of some furocoumarins and furochromones. *Phytochemistry, 18*, 139-143

European Economic Community (1976) Directive of the Council of 27 July 1976 concerning the comparing of legislations of member states connected with cosmetic products. *Eur. Commun. off. J., L262*, 169-200

Fisher, J.F. & Trama, L.A. (1979) High-performance liquid chromatographic determination of some coumarins and psoralens found in citrus peel oils. *J. agric. Food Chem.*, *27*, 1334-1337

Fowlks, W.L. (1959) The chemistry of the psoralens. *J. invest. Dermatol.*, *32*, 249-254

Furia, T.E. & Bellanca, N. (1971) *Fenaroli's Handbook of Flavor Ingredients*, Cleveland, OH, Chemical Rubber Co., pp. 48-49

Gast, W., Rytter, M. & Barth, J. (1983) Action of 5-methoxypsoralen on phyto-haemagglutinin-stimulated lymphocyte transformation *in vitro* (Ger.). *Dermatol. Monatsschr.*, *169*, 195-199

Haggag, M.Y. & Hilal, S.H. (1977) Gas chromatography of furocoumarins. *Egypt. J. pharm. Sci.*, *18*, 71-76

Herold, H., Berbey, B., Angignard, D. & Le Duc, R. (1981) *Toxicological study of the compound 5-methoxy-psoralen (5-MOP)*. In: Cahn, J., Forlot, P., Grupper, C., Maybeck, A. & Urbach, F., eds, *Psoralens in Cosmetics and Dermatology*, New York, Pergamon Press, pp. 303-309

Hilal, S.H., Radwan, A.S., Haggag, M.Y, Melek, F.R. & Abdel Khalek, S.M. (1982) Fluorimetric analysis of furocoumarins. *Egypt. J. pharm. Sci.*, *23*, 365-370

Hönigsmann, H., Jaschke, E., Gschnait, F., Brenner, W., Fritsch, P. & Wolff, K. (1979) 5-Methoxypsoralen (bergapten) in photochemotherapy of psorasis. *Br. J. Dermatol.*, *101*, 369-378

Howell, W.N. & Robertson, A. (1937) Furano-compounds. Part I. A synthesis of bergapten. *J. chem. Soc.*, 293-294

IARC (1980) *IARC Monographs on the Evaluation of the Carcinogenic Risk of Chemicals to Humans*, Vol. 24, *Some Pharmaceutical Drugs*, Lyon, pp. 101-124

ICIS Chemical Information System (1984) *Carbon-13 NMR Spectral Search System (CNMR)*, *Mass Spectral Search System (MSSS)*, *Infrared Spectral Search System (IRSS)*, *Information System for Hazardous Organics in Water* (ISHOW) and *Environmental Fate* (ENVIROFATE), Washington DC, Information Consultants, Inc.

Innocenti, G., Bettero, A. & Caporale, G. (1982) HPLC determination of coumarinic constituents in leaves of *Ficus carica* (Ital.). *Farm. Ed. Sci.*, *37*, 475-485

Isaacs, S.T., Wiesehahn, G. & Hallick, L.M. (1984) In vitro characterization of the reaction of four psoralen derivatives with DNA. *Natl Cancer Inst. Monogr.*, *66*, 21-30

Ivie, G.W. (1978) Linear furocoumarins (psoralens) from the seed of Texas *Ammi majus* L. (Bishop's weed). *J. agric. Food Chem.*, *26*, 1394-1403

Ivie, G.W., Holt, D.L. & Ivey, M.C. (1981) Natural toxicants in human foods: psoralens in raw and cooked parsnip root. *Science*, *213*, 909-910

Jameson, C.W., Dunnick, J.K., Brown, R.D. & Murrill, E. (1984) Chemical characterization of psoralens used in the National Toxicology Program research projects. *Natl Cancer Inst. Monogr.*, *66*, 103-113

Kavli, G., Krokan, H., Midelfart, K., Volden, G. & Raa, J. (1983a) Extraction, separation, quantification and evaluation of the phototoxic potency of furocoumarins in different parts of *Heracleum laciniatum*. *Photobiochem. Photobiophys.*, *5*, 159-168

Kavli, G., Raa, J., Johnson, B.E., Volden, G. & Haugsbø, S. (1983b) Furocoumarins of *Heracleum laciniatum*: isolation, phototoxicity, absorption and action spectra studies. *Contact Dermatol.*, *9*, 257-262

Kavli, G., Midelfart, K., Raa, J. & Volden, G. (1983c) Phototoxicity from furocoumarin (psoralens) of *Heracleum laciniatum* in a patient with vitiligo. Action spectrum studies on bergapten, pimpinellin, angelicin and sphondin. *Contact Dermatol.*, *9*, 364-366

Kavli, G., Krokan, H., Myrnes, B. & Volden, G. (1984) High pressure liquid chromatographic separation of furocoumarins in *Heracleum laciniatum*. *Photodermatology*, *1*, 85-86

Kornhauser, A., Wamer, W.G. & Giles, A.L., Jr (1982) Psoralen phototoxicity: correlation with serum and epidermal 8-methoxypsoralen and 5-methoxypsoralen in the guinea pig. *Science*, *217*, 733-735

Loveday, K.S. & Donahue, B.A. (1984) Induction of sister chromatid exchanges and gene mutations in Chinese hamster ovary cells by psoralens. *Natl Cancer Inst. Monogr.*, *66*, 149-155

Lowe, N.J., Connor, M.J., Cheong, E.S., Akopiantz, P. & Breeding, J.H. (1984) Psoralen and ultraviolet A effects on epidermal ornithine decarboxylase induction and DNA synthesis in the hairless mouse. *Natl Cancer Inst. Monogr.*, *66*, 73-76

Mantulin, W.W. & Song, P.-S. (1973) Excited states of skin-sensitizing coumarins and psoralens. Spectroscopic studies. *J. Am. chem. Soc.*, *95*, 5122-5129

Marks, R. (1984) Sunscreens. *Prescrib. J.*, *24*, 32-37

Marzulli, F.N. & Maibach, H.I. (1970) Perfume phototoxicity. *J. Soc. cosmet. Chem.*, *21*, 695-715

Matsumoto, H. & Isobe, A. (1981) Solvent effect on the emmission spectra and the fluorescence quantum yields of psoralens. *Chem. pharm. Bull.*, *29*, 603-608

Mezzadra, G., Guarneri, B., Grupper, C. & Forlot, P. (1981) *Effects of chronic field exposure of humans to bergapten*. In: Cahn, J., Forlot, P., Grupper, C., Maybeck, A. & Urbach, F., eds, *Psoralens in Cosmetics and Dermatology*, New York, Pergamon Press, pp. 383-386

Mitra, A.K., Patra, A. & Ghosh, A. (1979) Carbon-13 NMR spectra of some furocoumarins. *Indian J. Chem.*, *17B*, 385

Musajo, L. & Rodighiero, G. (1962) The skin-photosensitizing furocoumarins. *Experientia*, *18*, 153-161

Musajo, L. & Rodighiero, G. (1970) Studies on the photo-C_4-cyclo-addition reactions between skin-photosensitizing furocoumarins and nucleic acids. *Photochem. Photobiol.*, *11*, 27-35

Musajo, L., Rodighiero, G. & Caporale, G. (1954) Photodynamic activity of natural coumarins (Fr.). *Bull. Soc. Chim. biol.*, *36*, 1213-1224

Musajo, L., Rodighiero, G., Breccia, A., Dall'Acqua, F. & Malesani, G. (1966a) The photoreaction between DNA and the skin-photosensitizing furocoumarins studied using labelled bergapten. *Experentia, 22,* 75

Musajo, L., Rodighiero, G., Breccia, A., Dall'Acqua, F. & Malesani, G. (1966b) Skin-photosensitizing furocoumarins: photochemical interaction between DNA and - $O^{14}CH_3$-bergapten (5-methoxy-psoralen). *Photochem. Photobiol., 5,* 739-745

Musajo, L., Rodighiero, G., Caporale, G., Dall'Acqua, F., Marciani, S., Bordin, F., Baccichetti, F. & Bevilacqua, R. (1974) *Photoreactions between skin-photosensitizing furocoumarins and nucleic acids.* In: Fitzpatrick, T.B., Pathak, M.A., Harber, L.C., Seiji, M. & Kukita, A., eds, *Sunlight and Man. Normal and Abnormal Photobiologic Responses,* Tokyo, University of Tokyo Press, pp. 369-387

Natarajan, A.T., Verdegaal-Immerzeel, E.A.M., Ashwood-Smith, M.J. & Poulton, G.A. (1981) Chromosomal damage induced by furocoumarins and UVA in hamster and human cells including cells from patients with ataxia telangiectasia and xeroderma pigmentosum. *Mutat. Res., 84,* 113-124

Opdyke, D. (1973) Bergamot oil expressed. *Food Cosmet. Toxicol., 11,* 1031-1032

Papadopoulo, D. & Averbeck, D. (1985) Genotoxic effects and DNA photoadducts induced in Chinese hamster V79 cells by 5-methoxypsoralen and 8-methoxypsoralen. *Mutat. Res., 151,* 281-291

Pathak, M.A. (1984) Mechanisms of psoralen photosensitization reactions. *Natl Cancer Inst. Monogr., 66,* 41-46

Pathak, M.A. & Fitzpatrick, T.B. (1959) Bioassay of natural and synthetic furocoumarins (psoralens). *J. invest. Dermatol., 32,* 509-518

Paul de Haen International (1984) *de Haen Nonproprietary Name Index,* Vol. XV, *1941-1983,* Englewood, CO, p. 8

Pool, B.L. & Deutsch-Wenzel, R.P. (1979) Evidence of the mutagenic effect of 5-methoxypsoralen (bergapten) (Ger.). *Arztl. Kosmetol., 9,* 349-355

Pool, B.L., Klein, R. & Deutsch-Wenzel, R.P. (1982) Genotoxicity of 5-methoxypsoralen and near ultraviolet light in repair-deficient strains of *Escherichia coli* WP2. *Food Chem. Toxicol., 20,* 177-181

Rodighiero, G. & Allegri, G. (1959) Research on the content of bergapten in celery and parsley (Ital.). *Farmaco, 14,* 727-733

Rodighiero, G. & Dall'Acqua, F. (1984) In vitro photoreactions of selected psoralens and methylangelicins with DNA, RNA and proteins. *Natl Cancer Inst. Monogr., 66,* 31-40

Rodighiero, G., Musajo, L., Dall'Acqua, F., Marciani, S., Caporale, G. & Ciavatta, L. (1970) Mechanism of skin photosensitization by furocoumarins. Photoreactivity of various furocoumarins with native DNA and ribosomal RNA. *Biochim. biophys. Acta, 217,* 40-49

Sadtler Research Laboratories (1985) *The Sadtler Standard Spectra, Supplementary Index,* Philadelphia, PA

Sa E Melo, T., Morlière, P., Santus, R. & Dubertret, L. (1984a) Photoreactivity of 5-methoxypsoralen with calf thymus DNA upon excitation in the UVA. *Photochem. Photobiol.*, *7*, 121-131

Sa E Melo, T. de, Morlière, P., Goldstein, S., Santus, R., Dubertret, L. & Lagrange, D. (1984b) Binding of 5-methoxypsoralen to human serum low density lipoproteins. *Biochem. biophys. Res. Commun.*, *120*, 670-676

Schimmer, O. (1981) Comparison of photomutagenic activities of 5-MOP (bergapten) and 8-MOP (xanthotoxin) in *Chlamydomonas reinhardii* (Ger.). *Mutat. Res.*, *89*, 283-296

Schimmer, O., Beck, R. & Dietz, U. (1980) Phototoxicity and photomutagenicity of furocoumarins and furocoumarins from medicinal plants in *Chlamydomonas reinhardii*. Comparison of biological activities as a basis of risk evaluation (Ger.). *J. med. Plant Res.*, *40*, 68-76

Schmid, J., Brickl, R., Busch, U. & Koss, F.W. (1981) *Comparison of pharmacokinetics pharmacodynamics and metabolism of 8-MOP, 5-MOP and TMP*. In: Cahn, J., Forlot, P., Grupper, C., Maybeck, A. & Urbach, F., eds, *Psoralens in Cosmetics and Dermatology*, New York, Pergamon Press, pp. 109-116

Scott, B.R., Pathak, M.A. & Mohn, G.R. (1976) Molecular and genetic basis of furocoumarin reactions. *Mutat. Res.*, *39*, 29-74

Seida, A.A., Kinghorn, A.D., Cordell, G.A. & Farnsworth, N.R. (1981) Isolation of bergapten and marmesin from *Balanites aegyptiaca*. *J. med. Plant Res.*, *43*, 92-103

van der Sluis, W.G., van Arkel, J., Fischer, F.C. & Labadie, R.P. (1981) Thin-layer chromatographic assay of photoactive compounds (furocoumarins) using the fungus *Penicillium expansum* as a test organism. *J. Chromatogr.*, *214*, 349-359

Song, P.-S. & Tapley, K.J., Jr (1979) Photochemistry and photobiology of psoralens. *Photochem. Photobiol.*, *29*, 1177-1197

Song, P.-S., Mantulin, W.W., McInturff, D., Felkner, I.C. & Harter, M.L. (1975) Photoreactivity of hydroxypsoralens and their photobiological effects in *Bacillus subtilis*. *Photochem. Photobiol.*, *21*, 317-324

Song, P.-S., Shim, S.C. & Mantulin, W.W. (1981) The electronic spectra of psoralens in their ground and triplet excited states. *Bull. chem. Soc. Jpn*, *54*, 315-316

Späth, E., Wessely, F. & Kubiczek, G. (1937) Synthesis of bergaptens. (XXIV. On natural coumarins) (Ger.). *Chem. Ber.*, *70*, 478-479

Suzuki, H., Nakamura, K. & Iwaida, M. (1979) Detection and determination of bergapten in bergamot oil and in cosmetics. *J. Soc. cosmet. Chem.*, *30*, 393-400

Thompson, H.J. & Brown, S.A. (1984) Separations of some coumarins of higher plants by liquid chromatography. *J. Chromatogr.*, *314*, 323-336

US Consumer Product Safety Commission (1973) Hazardous substances and articles; administration and enforcement regulations. *Fed. Regist.*, *38*, 27012-27032

US Food and Drug Administration (1984) Food and drugs. Natural flavoring substances and natural substances used in conjunction with flavors. *US Code fed. Regul.*, *Title 21*, Part 172.510, 44-47

Vande Casteele, K., Geiger, H. & Van Sumere, C.F. (1983) Separation of phenolics (benzoic acids, cinnamic acids, phenylacetic acids, quinic acid esters, benzaldehydes and acetophenones, miscellaneous phenolics) and coumarins by reversed-phase high-performance liquid chromatography. *J. Chromatogr.*, *258*, 111-124

Verger, G. (1981) *Control and dosage of 5-methoxypsoralen in raw material and finished products in cosmetics by high performance liquid chromatography*. In: Cahn, J., Forlot, P., Grupper, C., Maybeck, A. & Urbach, F., eds, *Psoralens in Cosmetics and Dermatology*, New York, Pergamon Press, pp. 337-346

Veronese, F.M., Bevilacqua, R., Schiavon, O. & Rodighiero, G. (1979) Drug-protein interaction: plasma protein binding of furocoumarins. *Farm. Ed. Sci.*, *34*, 716-725

Walter, J.F., Gange, R.W. & Mendelson, I.R. (1982) Psoralen-containing sunscreen induces phototoxicity and epidermal ornithine decarboxylase activity. *J. Am. Acad. Dermatol.*, *6*, 1022-1027

Weniger, P. (1981) A comparison of the photochemical actions of 5- and 8-methoxy-psoralen on CHO cells. *Toxicology*, *22*, 53-58

Windholz, M., ed. (1983) *The Merck Index*, 10th ed., Rahway, NJ, Merck & Co., p. 165

Wisneski, H.H. (1976) Determination of bergapten in fragrance preparations by thin layer chromatography and spectrophotofluorometry. *J. Assoc. off. anal. Chem.*, *59*, 547-551

Wottawa, A. & Viernstein, H. (1982) *Screening of furocoumarins under PUVA conditions with a short-term DNA-repair tests*. In: Natarajan, A.J., Obe, G. & Altmann, H., eds, *Progress in Mutation Research*, Vol. 4, *DNA Repair, Chromosome Alterations and Chromatin Structure*, Amsterdam, Elsevier, pp. 279-284

Young, A.R., Magnus, I.A., Davies, A.C. & Smith, N.P. (1983) A comparison of the phototumorigenic potential of 8-MOP and 5-MOP in hairless albino mice exposed to solar simulated radiation. *Br. J. Dermatol.*, *108*, 507-518

Zajdela, E. & Bisagni, E. (1981) 5-Methoxypsoralen, the melanogenic additive in sun-tan preparations, is tumorigenic in mice exposed to 365 nm u.v. radiation. *Carcinogenesis*, *2*, 121-127

Zaynoun, S.T. (1978) The quantitative analysis of bergapten in perfumes. *J. Soc. cosmet. Chem.*, *29*, 247-263

Zaynoun, S.T., Johnson, B.E. & Frain-Bell, W. (1977) A study of oil of bergamot and its importance as a phototoxic agent. *Br. J. Dermatol.*, *96*, 475-482

PYRIDO[3,4-*c*]PSORALEN AND
7-METHYLPYRIDO[3,4-*c*]PSORALEN

1. Chemical and Physical Data

Pyrido[3,4-c]psoralen

1.1 Synonyms and trade names

Chem. Abstr. Services Reg. No.: 85878-62-2

Chem. Abstr. Name: 5*H*-Furo[3′,2′:6,7][1]benzopyrano[3,4-*c*]pyridin-5-one

IUPAC Systematic Names: 5*H*-Furo[3′,2′:6,7][1]benzopyrano[3,4-*c*]pyridin-5-one; 4-(6-hydroxy-5-benzofuranyl)nicotinic acid, δ-lactone

1.2 Structural and molecular formulae and molecular weight

$C_{14}H_7NO_3$

Mol. wt: 237.21

1.3 Chemical and physical properties of the pure substance

(*a*)   *Description*: White needles in dichloromethane-ethanol (Moron *et al.*, 1983)

(*b*)   *Melting-point*: 284-288°C (Moron *et al.*, 1983)

(*c*)   *Spectroscopy data*: Ultraviolet (Moron *et al.*, 1983; Blais *et al.*, 1984), proton nuclear magnetic resonance (Moron *et al.*, 1983) and fluorescence spectral data (Blais *et al.*, 1984) have been reported.

(*d*)   *Solubility*: Very slightly soluble in water (0.8 mg/l) (Blais *et al.*, 1984)

7-Methylpyrido[3,4-c]psoralen

1.1 Synonyms and trade names

Chem. Abstr. Services Reg. No.: 85878-63-3

Chem. Abstr. Name: 7-Methyl-5*H*-furo[3',2':6,7][1]benzopyrano[3,4-c]pyridin-5-one

IUPAC Systematic Names: 4-(6-Hydroxy-7-methyl-5-benzofuranyl)nicotinic acid, δ-lactone; 7-methyl-5*H*-furo[3',2':6,7][1]benzopyrano[3,4-c]pyridin-5-one

1.2 Structural and molecular formulae and molecular weight

$C_{15}H_9NO_3$ Mol. wt: 251.24

1.3 Chemical and physical properties of the pure substance

(a) *Description*: White crystals in dichloromethane-ethanol (Moron *et al.*, 1983)

(b) *Melting-point*: 272-274°C (Moron *et al.*, 1983)

(c) *Spectroscopy data*: Ultraviolet (Moron *et al.*, 1983; Blais *et al.*, 1984), proton nuclear magnetic resonance (Moron *et al.*, 1983) and fluorescence spectral data (Blais *et al.*, 1984) have been reported.

(d) *Solubility*: Very slightly soluble in water (0.8 mg/l) (Blais *et al.*, 1984)

1.4 Technical products and impurities

No data were available to the Working Group.

2. Production, Use, Occurrence and Analysis

2.1 Production and use

(a) *Production*

Moron *et al.* (1983) described the synthesis of pyrido[3,4-c]psoralen and 7-methylpyrido-[3,4-c]psoralen *via* the von Pechmann reaction in which 1-benzyl-3-ethoxycarbonylpiperidin-4-one undergoes condensation with 6-hydroxycoumarin or 6-hydroxy-7-methyl-coumarin acetates. The final product is produced by aromatization with palladium on charcoal in boiling diphenyl ether.

These compounds are currently produced only for research purposes.

(b)   Use

Clinical trials of pyrido[3,4-c]psoralen and 7-methylpyrido[3,4-c]psoralen and long-wave radiation (UVA) for psoriasis have been reported (Dubertret et al., 1985).

2.2 Occurrence

Pyrido[3,4-c]psoralen and 7-methylpyrido[3,4-c]psoralen are not known to occur as natural products.

2.3 Analysis

No specific analytical method for detecting or quantifying pyrido[3,4-c]psoralens has been reported.

3. Biological Data Relevant to the Evaluation of Carcinogenic Risk to Humans

3.1 Carcinogenicity studies in animals

Skin application

Mouse: In a preliminary report, 17NCZ albino mice received topical applications of 15 μg/cm^2 pyrido[3,4-c]psoralen or 7-methylpyrido[3,4-c]psoralen followed by irradiation with 1.18 J/cm^2 UVA light; a total of 115 treaments were given. The skin tumour incidences were reported to be 39% and 56% after 21 months compared with 80% with methoxsalen (Dubertret et al., 1985). [The Working Group noted the incomplete reporting of this study.]

3.2 Other relevant biological data

(a)   Experimental systems

Toxic effects

In combination with UVA, both pyrido[3,4-c]psoralen and its 7-methyl derivative exhibited strong inhibitory effects on DNA synthesis in cultured human fibroblasts (Nocentini, 1986).

No visible change was seen in ears of 17NCZ albino mice following topical application of either compound (15 μg/cm^2) plus UVA irradiation (1.18 J/cm^2) (Dubertret et al., 1985).

Effects on reproduction and prenatal toxicity

No data were available to the Working Group.

Absorption, distribution, excretion and metabolism

No data were available to the Working Group.

Mutagenicity and other short-term tests

Pyrido[3,4-*c*]psoralen and 7-methylpyrido[3,4-*c*]psoralen formed noncovalently-bound complexes with DNA *in vitro* in the dark, and both photobound covalently to isolated DNA *in vitro*, forming monoadducts only (Blais *et al.*, 1984).

7-Methylpyrido[3,4-*c*]psoralen photobound covalently to the DNA in *Saccharomyces cerevisiae* (Magaña-Schwencke & Moustacchi, 1985; Averbeck, 1985); no DNA interstrand cross-link was formed (Moustacchi *et al.*, 1983; Magaña-Schwencke & Moustacchi, 1985). It photobound covalently to DNA in cultured normal human fibroblasts (Nocentini, 1986) and, as reported in an abstract, in cultured simian cells (Nocentini, 1984).

The removal of 7-methylpyrido[3,4-*c*]psoralen-photoinduced monoadducts was more efficient in wild-type than in DNA repair-deficient *S. cerevisiae* (Moustacchi *et al.*, 1983; Magaña-Schwencke & Moustacchi, 1985). Exposure of *S. cerevisiae* to this compound plus UVA resulted in DNA single strand-breaks (Magaña-Schwencke & Moustacchi, 1985).

In cultured normal human fibroblasts, unscheduled DNA synthesis and DNA strand breaks were induced by treatment with 7-methylpyrido[3,4-*c*]psoralen in combination with UVA (Nocentini, 1986).

In the dark, both pyrido[3,4-*c*]psoralen and 7-methylpyrido[3,4-*c*]psoralen were mutagenic to *Salmonella typhimurium* TA1537 in the absence of a metabolic system (Quinto *et al.*, 1984).

Both pyridopsoralens photoinduced cytoplasmic 'petite' mutations in haploid (Averbeck *et al.*, 1985) and diploid (Averbeck, 1985) *S. cerevisiae*. In haploid *S. cerevisiae*, these two compounds plus UVA induced nuclear reverse and forward mutations (Averbeck *et al.*, 1985). In diploid *S. cerevisiae*, in the presence of UVA, they induced nuclear reversions and mitotic recombination (Averbeck, 1985).

It was reported in an abstract that, in combination with UVA, both compounds induced 6-thioguanine-resistant mutants in Chinese hamster V79 cells (Papadopoulo *et al.*, 1984).

In the dark, the 7-methyl derivative, but not pyrido[3,4-*c*]psoralen, induced an increase in the incidence of sister chromatid exchanges in cultured human fibroblasts. In combination with UVA, both compounds induced an increase in sister chromatid exchanges as a function of UVA dose (Billardon *et al.*, 1984).

It was reported in an abstract that both compounds plus UVA induced cell transformation in mouse embryo C3H 10T1/2 cells (Papadopoulo *et al.*, 1984).

(b)   Humans

Toxic effects

Slight erythema was produced in normal skin after application of either pyrido[3,4-c]-psoralen or 7-methylpyrido[3,4-c]psoralen (10 μg/cm^2) followed by irradiation with 20 J/cm^2 UVA (Dubertret *et al.*, 1985).

Effects on reproduction and prenatal toxicity

No data were available to the Working Group.

Absorption, distribution, excretion and metabolism

No data were available to the Working Group.

Mutagenicity and chromosomal effects

No data were available to the Working Group.

3.3 Case reports and epidemiological studies of carcinogenicity to humans

No data were available to the Working Group.

4. Summary of Data Reported and Evaluation

4.1 Exposure data

There is no known human exposure to pyrido[3,4-c]psoralen or 7-methylpyrido[3,4-c]-psoralen, other than in limited clinical trials for the treatment of psoriasis.

4.2 Experimental data

In one incompletely reported study of pyrido[3,4-c]psoralen and 7-methylpyrido[3,4-c]-psoralen in combination with ultraviolet A radiation in mice, skin tumours were observed. No data were available to evaluate the carcinogenicity to experimental animals of pyrido[3,4-c]psoralen or 7-methylpyrido[3,4-c]psoralen in the absence of ultraviolet A radiation.

No data were available to evaluate the reproductive effects or prenatal toxicity of pyrido[3,4-c]psoralen or 7-methylpyrido[3,4-c]psoralen to experimental animals.

In the presence of ultraviolet A radiation, pyrido[3,4-c]psoralen and 7-methylpyrido[3,4-c]-psoralen bound covalently to isolated DNA. In combination with ultraviolet A radiation, 7-methylpyrido[3,4-c]psoralen induced DNA damage in yeast and human fibroblasts *in vitro*. Both compounds were mutagenic to *Salmonella typhimurium* in the dark. In the presence of ultraviolet A radiation, pyrido[3,4-c]psoralen and 7-methylpyrido[3,4-c]-psoralen induced mutations and mitotic recombination in yeast. In the dark, 7-methyl-pyrido[3,4-c]psoralen, but not pyrido[3,4-d]psoralen, induced sister chromatid exchanges in mammalian cells *in vitro*; and, in combination with ultraviolet A irradiation, both compounds induced sister chromatid exchanges in cultured mammalian cells.

Overall assessment of data from short-term tests: Pyrido[3,4-c]psoralen[a]

	Genetic activity			Cell transformation
	DNA damage	Mutation	Chromosomal effects	
Prokaryotes	+*	+		
Fungi/Green plants		+*		
Insects				
Mammalian cells (*in vitro*)			− +*	
Mammals (*in vivo*)				
Humans (*in vivo*)				
Degree of evidence in short-term tests for genetic activity: **Inadequate** (in the dark) **Sufficient** (in combination with UVA)				Cell transformation: No data

*In combination with UVA

[a]The groups into which the table is divided and the symbols used are defined on pp. 19-20 of the Preamble; the degrees of evidence are defined on pp. 20-21.

Overall assessment of data from short-term tests: 7-Methylpyrido[3,4-c]psoralen[a]

	Genetic activity			Cell transformation
	DNA damage	Mutation	Chromosomal effects	
Prokaryotes	+*	+		
Fungi/Green plants	+*	+*		
Insects				
Mammalian cells (*in vitro*)	+*		+ +*	
Mammals (*in vivo*)				
Humans (*in vivo*)				
Degree of evidence in short-term tests for genetic activity: **Limited** (in the dark) **Sufficient** (in combination with UVA)				Cell transformation: No data

*In combination with UVA

[a]The groups into which the table is divided and the symbols used are defined on pp. 19-20 of the Preamble; the degrees of evidence are defined on pp. 20-21.

4.3 Human data

No case report or epidemiological study of the carcinogenicity of pyrido[3,4-c]psoralen or 7-methylpyrido[3,4-c]psoralen was available to the Working Group.

4.4 Evaluation[1]

There is *inadequate evidence* that pyrido[3,4-c]psoralen or 7-methylpyrido[3,4-c]-psoralen in combination with ultraviolet A radiation is carcinogenic to experimental animals. No data were available to evaluate the carcinogenicity of pyrido[3,4-c]psoralen or 7-methylpyrido[3,4-c]psoralen to experimental animals in the absence of ultraviolet A radiation.

No evaluation could be made of the carcinogenicity of pyrido[3,4-c]psoralen or 7-methyl-pyrido[3,4-c]psoralen to humans.

5. References

Averbeck, D. (1985) Relationship between lesions photoinduced by mono-and bi-functional furocoumarins in DNA and genotoxic effects in diploid yeast. *Mutat. Res.*, *151*, 217-233

Averbeck, D., Averbeck, S., Bisagni, E. & Moron, L. (1985) Lethal and mutagenic effects photoinduced in haploid yeast (*Saccharomyces cerevisiae*) by two new monofunctional pyridopsoralens compared to 3-carbethoxypsoralen and 8-methoxypsoralen. *Mutat. Res.*, *148*, 47-57

Billardon, C., Levy, S. & Moustacchi, E. (1984) Induction in human skin fibroblasts of sister-chromatid exchanges (SCEs) by photoaddition of two new monofunctional pyridopsoralens in comparison to 3-carbethoxypsoralen and 8-methoxypsoralen. *Mutat. Res.*, *138*, 63-70

Blais, J., Vigny, P., Moron, J. & Bisagni, E. (1984) Spectroscopic properties and photoreactivity with DNA of new monofunctional pyridopsoralens. *Photochem. Photobiol.*, *39*, 145-156

Dubertret, L., Averbeck, D., Bisagni, E., Moron, J., Moustacchi, E., Billardon, C., Papadopoulo, D., Nocentini, S., Vigny, P., Blais, J., Bensasson, R.V., Ronfard-Haret, J.C., Land, E.J., Zajdela, F. & Latarjet, R. (1985) Photochemotherapy using pyridopsoralens. *Biochimie*, *67*, 417-422

Magaña-Schwencke, N. & Moustacchi, E. (1985) A new monofunctional pyridopsoralen: photoreactivity and repair in yeast. *Photochem. Photobiol.*, *42*, 43-49

Moron, J., Nguyen, C.H. & Bisagni, E. (1983) Synthesis of 5*H*-furo[3',2':6,7][1]benzo-pyrano[3,4-c]pyridin-5-ones and 8*H*-pyrano[3',2':5,6]benzofuro[3,2-c]pyridin-8-ones (pyridopsoralens). *J. chem. Soc. Perkin Trans.*, *1*, 225-229

---

[1]For definition of the italicized term, see Preamble, p. 18.

Moustacchi, E., Cassier, C., Chanet, R., Magaña-Schwencke, N., Saeki, T. & Henriques, J.A.P. (1983) *Biological role of photoinduced cross-links and monoadducts in yeast DNA: genetic control and steps involved in their repair*. In: Bridges, B.A. & Friedberg, E.C., eds, *Cellular Responses to DNA Damage*, New York, Alan R. Liss, pp. 37-106

Nocentini, S. (1984) DNA photobinding of 7-methyl (3,4-*c*) psoralen and 8-methoxy-psoralen, removal of lesions and biological effects in cultured human and simian cells (Abstract No. TPM-C16). *Photochem. Photobiol.*, *39* (Suppl.), 55S

Nocentini, S. (1986) DNA photobinding of 7-methylpyrido(3,4-*c*)psoralen and 8-methoxy-psoralen. Effects on macromolecular synthesis, repair and survival in cultured human cells. *Mutat. Res.*, *161*, 181-192

Papadopoulo, D., Averbeck, D., Moron, J. & Bisagni, E. (1984) Genotoxic effects photoinduced in mammalian cells in vitro by two new synthetized monofunctional furocoumarins (Abstract No. TPM-C12). *Photochem. Photobiol.*, *39* (Suppl.), 54S

Quinto, I., Averbeck, D., Moustacchi, E., Hrisoho, Z. & Moron, J. (1984) Frameshift mutagenicity in *Salmonella typhimurium* of furocoumarins in the dark. *Mutat. Res.*, *136*, 49-54

4,5',8-TRIMETHYLPSORALEN

1. Chemical and Physical Data

1.1 Synonyms and trade names

Chem. Abstr. Services Reg. No.: 3902-71-4

Chem. Abstr. Name: 2,5,9-Trimethyl-7*H*-furo[3,2-*g*][1]benzopyran-7-one

IUPAC Systematic Names: 6-Hydroxy-β,2,7-trimethyl-5-benzofuranacrylic acid, δ-lactone; 2,5,9-trimethyl-7*H*-furo[3,2-*g*][1]benzopyran-7-one

Synonyms: NSC-71047; TMP; Trimethylpsoralen; 2',4,8-trimethylpsoralen; trioxalen; trioxsalen; trioxysalen; trisoralen

1.2 Structural and molecular formulae and molecular weight

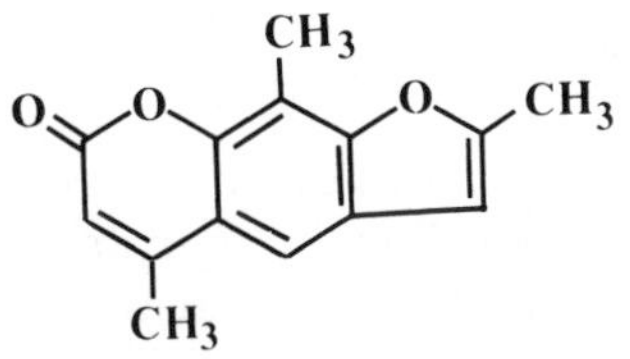

$C_{14}H_{12}O_3$

Mol. wt: 228.25

1.3 Chemical and physical properties of the pure substance

(*a*) *Description*: White to off-white or greyish, tasteless, odourless crystalline solid or prisms (Hassan & Loutfy, 1981); colourless prisms from chloroform (Kaufman, 1961; Windholz, 1983)

(*b*) *Melting-point*: 234.5-235°C (Kaufman, 1961; Windholz, 1983)

(*c*) *Spectroscopy data*: Ultraviolet (Sadtler Research Laboratories, 1985 [32768[a]]), infrared (Sadtler Research Laboratories, 1985; prism/grating [59030]), proton

---

[a]Spectrum number in Sadtler compilation

nuclear magnetic resonance (Sadtler Research Laboratories, 1985 [32020]), C-13 nuclear magnetic resonance (Elgamal *et al.*, 1979; Hassan & Loutfy, 1981), fluorescence (Mantulin & Song, 1973; Song *et al.*, 1981; Lai *et al.*, 1982) and mass spectral data (ICIS Chemical Information System, 1984 [MSSS]) have been reported.

(*d*)   *Solubility*: Soluble in dichloromethane; slightly soluble in ethanol and chloroform; practically insoluble in water (Windholz, 1983)

1.4 Technical products and impurities

4,5',8-Trimethylpsoralen is available as a USP grade containing not less than 97.0% and not more than 103.0% active ingredient, calculated on a dried basis (US Pharmacopeial Convention, 1985).

The primary US, European and Australian manufacturers supply trimethylpsoralen in 5-mg tablets.

2. Production, Use, Occurrence and Analysis

2.1 Production and use

(*a*)   *Production*

Synthesis of 4,5',8-trimethylpsoralen was described by Kaufman (1961); it involves a Claisen rearrangement of 7-allyloxy-4,8-dimethylcoumarin to give 6-allyl-4,8-dimethyl-7-hydroxy coumarin, which is acetylated, brominated and cyclized to 4,5',8-trimethylpsoralen.

An improved method has been reported which involves the addition of a furan ring to 6-allyl-4,8-dimethyl-7-hydroxycoumarin, reaction of this intermediate with concentrated sulphuric acid, and subsequent dehydrogenation to yield the final product (Hassan & Loutfy, 1981).

4,5',8-Trimethylpsoralen was first introduced onto the US market in 1965 (Sittig, 1979). Currently, one US manufacturer produces this compound in commercial quantities, and several firms make available research quantities.

One Italian pharmaceutical firm is known to manufacture 4,5',8-trimethylpsoralen (Marini, 1985) and has made it available commercially since 1970. A Swiss firm began marketing this product in 1981 (Paul de Haen International, 1984). It is also currently produced by two manufacturers in Finland and one in the UK.

In Japan, the sole manufacturer made 4,5',8-trimethylpsoralen available in 1969 (Paul de Haen International, 1984). It is also produced by one pharmaceutical firm in India (Pathak *et al.*, 1984) and one company in Australia (James, 1981).

(b)   Use

4,5′,8-Trimethylpsoralen has been used in combination with UVA or sunlight for the treatment of vitiligo, psoriasis and certain other conditions.

This compound, in conjunction with UV light, was introduced to facilitate repigmentation in vitiligo (Sehgal, 1971; Pathak et al., 1984). It has also been administered orally and by skin baths with UVA irradiation for the treatment of psoriasis and other skin disorders (Fischer & Alsins, 1976; Hannuksela & Karvonen, 1978; Väätäinen et al., 1979; Gilman et al., 1980; Väätäinen et al., 1981a) and has been administered orally to enhance pigmentation and increase tolerance to sunlight (McEvoy, 1985).

2.2 Occurrence

4,5′,8-Trimethylpsoralen has been isolated from celery infected with the pink-rot fungus, *Sclerotinia sclerotiorum*. It has not been detected in uninfected celery (Scheel et al., 1963; Floss et al., 1969).

2.3 Analysis

4,5′,8-Trimethylpsoralen has been determined in human plasma by extraction with dichloromethane, toluene or n-hexane:isopropanol and analysis by reverse-phase high-performance liquid chromatography (HPLC) or gas chromatography/mass spectrometry with a sensitivity of 2 ng/ml (Fischer et al., 1980; Chakrabarti et al., 1982). A lower detection limit of 25 pg/ml was obtained by using a glass capillary column with gas chromatography/mass spectrometry (Taskinen et al., 1980). Calibration curves were linear up to 1200 ng/ml with HPLC (Chakrabarti et al., 1982).

4,5′,8-Trimethylpsoralen can be separated from other furocoumarins by thin-layer chromatography, and this is the official method of identification of the US Pharmacopeia (US Pharmacopeial Convention, 1985). Quantification is performed by ultraviolet spectroscopy. As for other compounds that can be activated by light, thin-layer chromatography fractions can be identified by the combined effects of light and chemicals on several microorganisms. These bioassay methods can detect as little as 1 ng (van der Sluis et al., 1981; Ashwood-Smith et al., 1983).

3. Biological Data Relevant to the Evaluation of Carcinogenic Risk to Humans

3.1   Carcinogenicity studies in animals

Skin application

Mouse: It was reported in an abstract that two groups of 30 female mice [strain unspecified] were given thrice-weekly applications on the shaved back skin of 100 μg

4,5',8-trimethylpsoralen or 600 μg methoxsalen dissolved in 0.2 ml acetone for nine months (110 treatments). A control group received 0.2 ml acetone alone. Immediately after each skin application, the mice were irradiated with UVA light [characteristics of irradiation source unspecified]: 4,5',8-trimethylpsoralen group, single dose — 0.3×10^4 J/m², total dose — 33 J/cm²; methoxsalen group and controls, single dose — 1.1 J/cm², total dose — 123.1 J/cm². The concentrations of psoralens and irradiation doses were chosen by analogy with topical treatment of psoriasis in humans using methoxsalen plus UVA (PUVA). One squamous-cell carcinoma developed in 30 survivors in the methoxsalen group after 11 months, when two-thirds of the mice were killed; at 18 months, all the remaining mice were killed and 5/10 animals in that group had malignant tumours. Neither 4,5',8-trimethylpsoralen with UVA nor acetone alone induced a neoplastic lesion (Hannuksela *et al.*, 1985). [The Working Group noted that the study was reported as an abstract and that the radiation dose used was low.]

3.2 Other relevant biological data

(a) Experimental systems

The photobiological and photochemical properties of 4,5',8-trimethylpsoralen have been reviewed (Scott *et al.*, 1976; Hearst, 1981a).

Toxic effects

Female mice given thrice-weekly applications on the shaved back skin of 100 μg 4,5',8-trimethylpsoralen dissolved in 0.2 ml acetone showed alopecia and atrophy of the skin (Hannuksela *et al.*, 1985). Application of 4,5',8-trimethylpsoralen (2.5 μg/cm²) to guinea-pig skin and exposure to UVA irradiation induced erythema (Pathak *et al.*, 1967).

4,5',8-Trimethylpsoralen plus UVA caused severe inhibition of DNA synthesis in XD cells of tobacco (Heimer *et al.*, 1978), in Erlich ascites tumour cells (Baccichetti *et al.*, 1976; Dall'Acqua *et al.*, 1981), in human amnion (AV$_3$) cells (Trosko & Isoun, 1970, 1971), in human lymphocytes (Bohr & Nielsen, 1984) and in epidermal cells of mice *in vivo* after topical application (Dall'Acqua *et al.*, 1981).

Effects on reproduction and prenatal toxicity

No data were available to the Working Group.

Absorption, distribution, excretion and metabolism

Two hours after administration of a single oral dose of 10 mg 4,5',8-trimethylpsoralen to guinea-pigs, concentrations (in ng per g of tissue) were: epidermis, 226 ± 15; dermis 25 ± 6; and whole skin 176 ± 12; levels of 244 ± 17 and 63 ± 6 ng/ml were found in aqueous and vitreous humours, respectively (Chakrabarti *et al.*, 1982).

It was reported in an abstract that, following oral or intraperitoneal administration of ³H-4,5',8-trimethylpsoralen to mice, over 88% of the radioactivity was excreted in urine within 8 h; 4,5',8-trimethylpsoralen was present in liver, skin and blood (Pathak *et al.*, 1974a).

After oral administration of 150 mg/kg bw 4,5′,8-trimethylpsoralen to male CD-1 mice, it was metabolized to 4,8-dimethyl-5′-carboxypsoralen (Mandula et al., 1976). Other metabolites appear to be present but have not been characterized (Bickers & Pathak, 1984).

Oral administration to male CD-1 mice of 0.8 mg/kg bw per day for six days had no effect on cytochrome P450-dependent oxidations (Bickers et al., 1982).

Mutagenicity and other short-term tests

4,5′,8-Trimethylpsoralen formed molecular complexes with isolated DNA in the dark (Dall'Acqua et al., 1981). It photobound covalently, with formation of monoadducts and/or interstrand cross-links reported in isolated DNA *in vitro* (Cole, 1970, 1971a; Musajo & Rodighiero, 1972a,b; Dall'Acqua et al., 1974a,b; Musajo et al., 1974; Pathak et al., 1974a,b; Dall'Acqua et al., 1981; Hearst, 1981a,b; Kanne et al., 1982; Rodighiero & Dall'Acqua, 1984), and in DNA of *Escherichia coli* (Cole, 1970, 1971a; Sinden & Cole, 1981), *Saccharomyces cerevisiae* (Miller et al., 1984), phage λ (Cole, 1970, 1971a,b; Cassuto et al., 1977; Lin et al., 1977; Kondoleon et al., 1982), Chinese hamster V79 cells (Ben-Hur & Elkind, 1973), mouse L1210 (Cohen et al., 1980) and L5178Y (Cole, 1970) leukaemia cells and in cultured human lymphocytes (Bohr & Nielsen, 1984). It also photobound covalently to DNA in guinea-pig skin *in vivo* (Pathak & Krämer, 1969).

Repair of interstrand cross-links induced by 4,5′,8-trimethylpsoralen plus UVA has been shown in *E. coli* (Cole, 1973; Cole et al., 1976, 1978; Sinden & Cole, 1978). During this process, no double-strand break appears to occur (Cole et al., 1976, 1978). The repair of DNA monoadducts and DNA interstrand cross-links induced by this compound plus UVA has also been observed in *S. cerevisiae* (Miller et al., 1984).

In mouse L1210 leukaemia cells (Cohen et al., 1980), DNA breaks were not induced and no protein-DNA cross-link was formed after treatment with 4,5′,8-trimethylpsoralen in combination with UVA. Following treatment of guinea-pig skin *in vivo*, a progressive elimination of the photoproducts from DNA was observed (Baden et al., 1972). In cultured human lymphocytes, alkaline elution appears to indicate the induction of single-strand breaks at sites of cross-links formed by 4,5′,8-trimethylpsoralen and UVA (Bohr & Nielsen, 1984).

In the plasmid pBR322 (growing in *E. coli* K12 RR1F⁻), this compound plus UVA induced mutagenicity (Yoon, 1982). The same treatment induced an increase in mutations in bacteriophage T_4 plated on *E. coli* (Yarosh et al., 1980).

4,5′,8-Trimethylpsoralen induced the expression of the damage-inducible SFIA in the dark in *E. coli* K12 in the SOS-Chromotest. In the presence of a metabolic system, the activity was decreased (Lecointe, 1984).

In the dark, 4,5′,8-trimethylpsoralen was not mutagenic in *E. coli lac⁻* z (ND160) (Ashwood-Smith, 1978).; however, it was mutagenic to *E. coli* WP2 *uvrA⁻* (pKM101) in the presence of a metabolic system both in the dark and with UVA (Kirkland et al., 1983). In the dark, it was mutagenic to *S. typhimurium* TA1537, in the absence of metabolic activation, but not to other strains (TA1535, TA1538, TA98 and TA100) (Quinto et al., 1984). It was not mutagenic to TA100 or TA98 either in the dark or in combination with UVA, in the presence or absence of a metabolic system (Kirkland *et al.*, 1983).

In the presence of UVA, 4,5',8-trimethylpsoralen induced DNA cross-links and was mutagenic in the bacterium *Deinococcus radiodurans* (Yatagai & Kitayama, 1983).

In *S. cerevisiae*, it has been shown to photoinduce cytoplasmic 'petite' mutations (Swanbeck & Thyresson, 1974; Averbeck *et al.*, 1981a,b, 1984) and nuclear reverse (Averbeck *et al.*, 1981a,b; Averbeck, 1982; Averbeck *et al.*, 1984) and forward mutations (Averbeck *et al.*, 1981a,b, 1984).

Seedlings of barley (*Hordeum vulgare*, variety Iyoti) grown under normal daylight from seeds treated with 4,5',8-trimethylpsoralen showed a concentration-dependent induction of chromosomal aberrations (Kak & Kaul, 1981).

In cultured normal human lymphocytes, 4,5',8-trimethylpsoralen plus UVA induced an increase in the incidence of sister chromatid exchanges (Gaynor & Carter, 1978; Carter *et al.*, 1982) and of chromosomal aberrations (Waksvik *et al.*, 1977). The increase in the incidence of sister chromatid exchanges was proportional to the UVA dose (Gaynor & Carter, 1978). Cultured fibroblasts from patients with dyskeratosis congenita exhibited the same sensitivity to sister chromatid exchange induction by 4,5',8-trimethylpsoralen plus UVA as normal diploid human fibroblasts (Kano & Fujiwara, 1982a). The frequency of induction of sister chromatid exchanges was higher in cultured fibroblasts from a Fanconi's anaemia patient than in those from a normal human subject (Kano & Fujiwara, 1982b).

A metabolite of 4,5',8-trimethylpsoralen, 4,8-dimethyl-5'-carboxypsoralen, and its methyl ester photobound to isolated DNA, forming DNA interstrand cross-links (Pathak *et al.*, 1983). In haploid yeast, it was less mutagenic than 4,5',8-trimethylpsoralen as a function of UVA dose, but as mutagenic as a function of survival (Averbeck, 1982).

(b)   Humans

Toxic effects

Application of 5-25 μg/2.5 cm² 4,5',8-trimethylpsoralen to human skin followed by irradiation with UVA induced marked erythema within 36 h and marked pigmentation within 15 days (Pathak & Fitzpatrick, 1959).

Application of 0.2-1.0 μg/cm² 4,5',8-trimethylpsoralen to skin followed by UVA irradiation produced photosensitization, manifested by erythema, oedema, desquamation and hyperpigmentation. In contrast, oral administration of 0.3-1.2 mg/kg bw followed by UVA produced little photosensitization. This difference was attributed to the rapid biotransformation of 4,5',8-trimethylpsoralen when administered orally (Mandula *et al.*, 1976).

It was reported in an abstract that the maximal response to 4,5',8-trimethylpsoralen for delayed skin erythema occurred with 320-335 nm (Cripps & Lowe, 1978).

Dose-related side effects, including nausea, pruritus and dizziness, have been noted during treatment with 4,5',8-trimethylpsoralen (Pathak *et al.*, 1984).

Effects on reproduction and prenatal toxicity

No data were available to the Working Group.

Absorption, distribution, excretion and metabolism

4,5',8-Trimethylpsoralen and its metabolite, 4,8-dimethyl-5'-carboxypsoralen, were detected in the urine of humans following oral administration of the parent compound (Mandula *et al.*, 1976; Pathak *et al.*, 1983). A correlation has been reported between the concentration of 4,5',8-trimethylpsoralen in the plasma and skin phototoxicity (Brickl *et al.*, 1984a,b).

Salo *et al.* (1981) determined the plasma concentrations of 4,5',8-trimethylpsoralen 1 h after a bath of 50 mg in 150 l water, and 2 h after ingestion of 0.6 mg/kg bw. Wide variations were observed among patients and at different stages of the treatment. Plasma levels found following ingestion were approximately 10-100 times those after the bath treatment.

In vitiligo patients who received 30 mg 4,5',8-trimethylpsoralen orally, blood levels were 30-800 ng/ml after 2 h and 27-120 ng/ml after 24 h (Chakrabarti *et al.*, 1982).

Mutagenicity and chromosomal effects

No data were available to the Working Group.

3.3 Case reports and epidemiological studies of carcinogenicity to humans

During the third week of daily oral treatment with 10 mg 4,5',8-trimethylpsoralen before sunbathing, a 30-year-old patient with vitiligo developed a pigmented lesion on his back, at which time treatment was discontinued. The lesion grew slowly and, several months later, was removed and diagnosed as a malignant melanoma (Forrest & Forrest, 1980).

Of a series of 139 psoriatic patients treated with 4,5',8-trimethylpsoralen baths and UVA radiation for one to 23 months (mean, ten months), 57 were followed after treatment for periods varying from two to 14 months. No skin malignancy was seen (Väätäinen *et al.*, 1981b).

4. Summary of Data Reported and Evaluation

4.1 Exposure data

4,5',8-Trimethylpsoralen (trioxsalen) has been used in conjunction with ultraviolet A radiation in the treatment of vitiligo, psoriasis and other skin disorders. Human exposure occurs through the oral administration or skin application of these products.

4.2 Experimental data

In one incompletely reported study of the skin carcinogenicity of 4,5',8-trimethyl-psoralen in combination with ultraviolet A radiation in mice, no skin tumour was described. No data were available to evaluate the carcinogenicity to experimental animals of 4,5',8-trimethylpsoralen in the absence of ultraviolet A radiation.

No data were available to evaluate the reproductive effects or prenatal toxicity of 4,5′,8-trimethylpsoralen to experimental animals.

In the presence of ultraviolet A radiation, 4,5′,8-trimethylpsoralen bound covalently to isolated DNA and to DNA in bacteria, yeast and mammalian cells in culture, and in guinea-pig skin *in vivo*. It induced DNA damage in bacteria in the dark. In combination with ultraviolet A radiation, it induced mutation in bacteriophage. The compound was mutagenic to bacteria in the dark and with ultraviolet A radiation, and to yeast in the presence of ultraviolet A radiation. 4,5′,8-Trimethylpsoralen induced chromosomal aberrations in *Hordeum vulgare* grown under normal daylight and in the presence of ultraviolet A radiation induced sister chromatid exchanges and chromosomal aberrations in cultured mammalian cells.

Overall assessment of data from short-term tests: 4,5′,8-Trimethylpsoralen[a]

	Genetic activity			Cell transformation
	DNA damage	Mutation	Chromosomal effects	
Prokaryotes	+ +*	+ +*		
Fungi/Green plants	+*	+*	+*	
Insects				
Mammalian cells (*in vitro*)	+*		+*	
Mammals (*in vivo*)	+*			
Humans (*in vivo*)				
Degree of evidence in short-term tests for genetic activity: **Inadequate** (in the dark) **Sufficient** (in combination with UVA)				Cell transformation: No data

*In combination with UVA

[a]The groups into which the table is divided and the symbols used are defined on pp. 19-20 of the Preamble; the degrees of evidence are defined on pp. 20-21.

4.3 Human data

One case of melanoma was reported in a patient treated orally with 4,5′,8-trimethylpsoralen. In a small series of patients treated topically with 4,5′,8-trimethylpsoralen and ultraviolet radiation, no skin malignancy was seen after short-term follow-up.

4.4 Evaluation[1]

There is *inadequate evidence* for the carcinogenicity of 4,5′,8-trimethylpsoralen in combination with ultraviolet A radiation to experimental animals. No data were available to evaluate the carcinogenicity of 4,5′,8-trimethylpsoralen to experimental animals in the absence of ultraviolet A radiation.

There is *inadequate evidence* for the carcinogenicity of 4,5′,8-trimethylpsoralen to humans.

5. References

Ashwood-Smith, M.J. (1978) Frameshift mutations in bacteria produced in the dark by several furocoumarins: absence of activity of 4,5′,8-trimethylpsoralen. *Mutat. Res., 58,* 23-27

Ashwood-Smith, M.J., Poulton, G.A., Ceska, O., Liu, M. & Furniss, E. (1983) An ultrasensitive bioassay for the detection of furocoumarins and other photosensitizing molecules. *Photochem. Photobiol., 38,* 113-118

Averbeck, D. (1982) *Photobiology of furocoumarins.* In: Helene, M., Charlier, M., Montenay-Garestier, T. & Laustriat, G., eds, *Trends in Photobiology,* New York, Plenum Press, pp. 295-308

Averbeck, D., Averbeck, S. & Dall'Acqua, F. (1981a) Mutagenic activity of three monofunctional and three bifunctional furocoumarins in yeast (*Saccharomyces cerevisiae*). *Farm. Ed. Sci., 36,* 492-505

Averbeck, D., Magaña-Schwencke, N. & Moustacchi, E. (1981b) *Genetic effects and repair in yeast of DNA lesions induced by 3-carbethoxypsoralen and other photoreactive furocoumarins of therapeutic interest.* In: Cahn, J., Forlot, B.P., Grupper, C., Meybeck, A.E. & Urbach, F., eds, *Psoralens in Cosmetics and Dermatology,* New York, Pergamon Press, pp. 143-153

Averbeck, D., Papadopoulo, D. & Quinto, I. (1984) Mutagenic effects of psoralens in yeast and V79 Chinese hamster cells. *Natl Cancer Inst. Monogr., 66,* 127-136

Baccichetti, F., Bordin, F., Marciani, S., Dall'Acqua, F. & Rodighiero, G. (1976) Contribution of monofunctional adducts formed by furocoumarins with DNA to the inhibition of nucleic acids synthesis. *Z. Naturforsch., 31c,* 207-208

Baden, H.P., Parrington, J.M., Delhanty, J.D.A. & Pathak, M.A. (1972) DNA synthesis in normal and xeroderma pigmentosum fibroblasts following treatment with 8-methoxy-psoralen and long wave ultraviolet light. *Biochim. biophys. Acta, 262,* 247-255

Ben-Hur, E. & Elkind, M.M. (1973) DNA cross-linking in Chinese hamster cells exposed to near ultraviolet light in the presence of 4,5′,8-trimethylpsoralen. *Biochim. biophys. Acta, 331,* 181-193

---

[1]For definitions of the italicized terms, see Preamble, pp. 18 and 22.

Bickers, D.R., Mukhtar, H., Molica, S.J., Jr & Pathak, M.A. (1982) The effect of psoralens on hepatic and cutaneous drug metabolizing enzymes and cytochrome P-450. *J. invest. Dermatol.*, *79*, 201-205

Bohr, V. & Nielsen, P.E. (1984) Psoralen-DNA crosslink repair in human lymphocytes. Comparison of alkaline elution with electron microscopy. *Biochim. biophys. Acta*, *783*, 183-186

Brickl, R., Schmid, J. & Koss, F.W. (1984a) Pharmacokinetics and pharmacodynamics of psoralens after oral administration: considerations and conclusions. *Natl Cancer Inst. Monogr.*, *66*, 63-67

Brickl, R., Schmid, J. & Koss, F.W. (1984b) Clinical pharmacology of oral psoralen drugs. *Photodermatology*, *1*, 174-186

Carter, D.M., Lyons, M.F. & Windhorst, D.B. (1982) Photopromotion of sister chromatid exchanges by psoralen derivatives. *Arch. dermatol. Res.*, *272*, 239-244

Cassuto, E., Gross, N., Bardwell, E. & Howard-Flanders, P. (1977) Genetic effects of photoadducts and photocross-links in the DNA of phage λ exposed to 360 nm light and tri-methylpsoralen or khellin. *Biochim. biophys. Acta*, *475*, 589-600

Chakrabarti, S.G., Grimes, P.E., Minus, H.R., Kenney, J.A., Jr & Pradhan, T.K. (1982) Determination of trimethylpsoralen in blood, ophthalmic fluid, and skin. *J. invest. Dermatol.*, *79*, 374-377

Cohen, L.F., Ewig, R.A.G., Kohn, K.W. & Glaubiger, D. (1980) Interstrand DNA crosslinking by 4,5′,8-trimethylpsoralen plus monochromatic ultraviolet light. Studies by alkaline elution in mouse L1210 leukemia cells. *Biochim. biophys. Acta*, *610*, 56-63

Cole, R.S. (1970) Light-induced cross-linking of DNA in the presence of a furocoumarin (psoralen). Studies with phage λ, *Escherichia coli* and mouse leukemia cells. *Biochim. biophys. Acta*, *217*, 30-39

Cole, R.S. (1971a) Psoralen monoadducts and interstrand cross-links in DNA. *Biochim. biophys. Acta*, *254*, 30-39

Cole, R.S. (1971b) Inactivation of *Escherichia coli*, F′ episomes at transfer, and bacteriophage lambda by psoralen plus 360-nm light: significance of deoxyribonucleic acid cross-links. *J. Bacteriol.*, *107*, 846-852

Cole, R.S. (1973) Repair of DNA containing interstrand crosslinks in *Escherichia coli*: sequential excision and recombination. *Proc. natl Acad. Sci. USA*, *70*, 1064-1068

Cole, R.S., Levitan, D. & Sinden, R.R. (1976) Removal of psoralen interstrand cross-links from DNA of *Escherichia coli*: mechanism and genetic control. *J. mol. Biol.*, *103*, 39-59

Cole, R.S., Sinden, R.R., Yoakum, G.H. & Broyles, S. (1978) *On the mechanism for repair of cross-linked DNA in* E. coli *treated with psoralen and light*. In: Hanawalt, P.C., Friedberg, E.C. & Fox, C.F., eds, *DNA Repair Mechanisms*, New York, Academic Press, pp. 287-290

Cripps, D.J. & Lowe, N.J. (1978) Action spectra of topical psoralen. A reevaluation (Abstract). *J. invest. Dermatol.*, *70*, 214

Dall'Acqua, F., Marciani, S., Vedaldi, D. & Rodighiero, G. (1974a) Studies on the photoreactions (365 nm) between DNA and some methylpsoralens. *Biochim. biophys. Acta, 353*, 267-273

Dall'Acqua, F., Marciani, S., Vedaldi, D. & Rodighiero, G. (1974b) Skin photo-sensitization and cross-linkings formation in native DNA by furocoumarins. *Z. Natur-forsch., 29c*, 635-636

Dall'Acqua, F., Vedaldi, D., Baccichetti, F., Bordin, F. & Averbeck, D. (1981) Photochemo-therapy of skin-diseases: comparative studies on the photochemical and photo-biological properties of various mono-and bifunctional agents. *Farm. Ed. Sci., 36*, 519-535

Elgamal, M.H.A., Elewa, N.H., Elkhrisy, E.A.M. & Duddeck, H. (1979) ^{13}C NMR chemical shifts and carbon-proton coupling constants of some furocoumarins and furochromones. *Phytochemistry, 18*, 139-143

Fischer, T. & Alsins, J. (1976) Treatment of psoriasis with trioxsalen baths and dysprosium lamps. *Acta dermatovenerol., 56*, 383-390

Fischer, T., Hartvig, P. & Bondesson, U. (1980) Plasma concentrations after bath treatment and oral administration of trioxsalen. *Acta dermatovenerol., 60*, 177-179

Floss, H.G., Guenther, H. & Hadwiger, L.A. (1969) Biosynthesis of furanocoumarins in diseased celery. *Phytochemistry, 8*, 585-588

Forrest, J.B. & Forrest, H.J. (1980) Case report: malignant melanoma arising during drug therapy for vitiligo. *J. surg. Oncol., 13*, 337-340

Gaynor, A.L. & Carter, D.M. (1978) Greater promotion in sister chromatid exchanges by trimethylpsoralen than by 8-methoxypsoralen in the presence of UV-light. *J. invest. Dermatol., 71*, 257-259

Gilman, A.G., Goodman, L.S. & Gilman, A., eds (1980) *The Pharmacological Basis of Therapeutics*, 6th ed., New York, MacMillan Publishing Co., pp. 957-958

Hannuksela, M. & Karvonen, J. (1978) Trioxsalen bath plus UVA effective and safe in the treatment of psoriasis. *Br. J. Dermatol., 99*, 703-707

Hannuksela, M., Stenbäck, F. & Lahti, A. (1985) Carcinogenicity of topical PUVA treatment. A lifelong study in mice (Abstract). *J. invest. Dermatol., 84*, 433

Hassan, M.M.A. & Loutfy, M.A. (1981) *Trioxsalen*. In: Florey, K., ed., *Analytical Profiles of Drug Substances*, Vol. 10, New York, Academic Press, pp. 705-727

Hearst, J.E. (1981a) Psoralen photochemistry. *Ann. Rev. Biophys. Bioeng., 10*, 69-86

Hearst, J.E. (1981b) Psoralen photochemistry and nucleic acid structure. *J. invest. Dermatol., 77*, 39-44

Heimer, Y.M., Ben-Hur, E. & Riklis, E. (1978) Photosensitized inhibition of nitrate reductase induction by 4,5′,8-trimethylpsoralen and near ultraviolet light. *Biochim. biophys. Acta, 519*, 499-506

ICIS Chemical Information System (1984) *Carbon-13 NMR Spectral Search System* (CNMR), *Mass Spectral Search System* (MSSS), *Infrared Spectral Search System* (IRSS), *Information System for Hazardous Organics in Water* (ISHOW) and *Environmental Fate* (ENVIROFATE), Washington DC, Information Consultants, Inc.

James, R., ed. (1981) *Mims Annual 1981*, 5th Ed., Artarmon, N.S.W., Australia, IMS Publishing, p. 15.43

Kak, S.N. & Kaul, B.L. (1981) Seedling injury and mitotic aberrations induced by psoralens in barley *Hordeum vulgare. Indian J. exp. Biol., 19*, 643-644

Kanne, D., Straub, K., Rapoport, H. & Hearst, J.E. (1982) Psoralen-deoxyribonucleic acid photoreaction. Characterization of the monoaddition products from 8-methoxy-psoralen and 4,5',8-trimethylpsoralen. *Biochemistry, 21*, 861-871

Kano, Y. & Fujiwara, Y. (1982a) Dyskeratosis congenita: survival, sister-chromatid exchange and repair following treatments with crosslinking agents. *Mutat. Res., 103*, 327-332

Kano, Y. & Fujiwara, Y. (1982b) Higher inductions of twin and single sister chromatid exchanges by cross-linking agents in Fanconi's anemia cells. *Human Genet., 60*, 233-238

Kaufman, K.D. (1961) Synthetic furocoumarins. I. A new synthesis of methyl-substituted psoralenes and isopsoralenes. *J. org. Chem., 26*, 117-121

Kirkland, D.J., Creed, K.L. & Mannisto, P. (1983) Comparative bacterial mutagenicity studies with 8-methoxypsoralen and 4,5',8-trimethylpsoralen in the presence of near-ultraviolet light and in the dark. *Mutat. Res., 116*, 73-82

Kondoleon, S.K., Walter, M.A. & Hallick, L.M. (1982) Kinetics of simian virus 40 and lambda inactivation by photoaddition of psoralen derivatives. *Photochem. Photobiol., 36*, 325-331

Lai, T.-I., Lim, B.T. & Lim, E.C. (1982) Photophysical properties of biologically important molecules related to proximity effects: psoralens. *J. Am. chem. Soc., 104*, 7631-7635

Lecointe, P. (1984) Induction of the SFIA SOS repair function by psoralens in the dark. *Mutat. Res., 131*, 111-113

Lin, P.-F., Bardwell, E. & Howard-Flanders, P. (1977) Initiation of genetic exchanges in λ phage-prophage crosses. *Proc. natl Acad. Sci. USA, 74*, 291-295

Mandula, B.B., Pathak, M.A. & Dudek, G. (1976) Photochemotherapy: identification of a metabolite of 4,5',8-trimethylpsoralen. *Science, 193*, 1131-1133

Mantulin, W.W. & Song, P.-S. (1973) Excited states of skin-sensitizing coumarins and psoralens. Spectroscopic studies. *J. Am. chem. Soc., 95*, 5122-5129

Marini, L. (1985) *L'Informatore Farmaceutico*, Milan, Organizzazione Editoriale Medico-Farmaceutica S.R.L., p. 134

McEvoy, G.K., ed. (1985) *Trioxsalen. Drug Information '85*, Washington DC, American Society of Hospital Pharmacists, pp. 1660-1662

Miller, R.D., Prakash, S. & Prakash, L. (1984) Different effects of *RAD* genes of *Saccharomyces cerevisiae* on incisions of interstrand crosslinks and monoadducts in DNA induced by psoralen plus near UV light treatment. *Photochem. Photobiol.*, *39*, 349-352

Musajo, L. & Rodighiero, G. (1972a) *Mode of photosensitizing action of furocoumarins.* In: Giese, A., ed., *Photophysiology*, Vol. 7, New York, Academic Press, pp. 115-147

Musajo, L. & Rodighiero, C. (1972b) Photo-C_4-cyclo-addition reactions to the nucleic acids. *Res. Progr. org. biol. med. Chem.*, *3*, 155-182

Musajo, L., Rodighiero, G., Caporale, G., Dall'Acqua, F., Marciani, S., Bordin, F., Baccichetti, F. & Bevilacqua, R. (1974) *Photoreactions between skin-photosensitizing furocoumarins and nucleic acids.* In: Fitzpatrick, T.B., Pathak, M.A., Harber, L.C., Seiji, M. & Kukita, A., eds, *Sunlight and Man. Normal and Abnormal Photobiologic Responses*, Tokyo, University of Tokyo Press, pp. 369-387

Pathak, M.A. & Fitzpatrick, T.B. (1959) Bioassay of natural and synthetic furocoumarins (psoralens). *J. invest. Dermatol.*, *32*, 509-518

Pathak, M.A. & Krämer, D.M. (1969) Photosensitization of skin *in vivo* by furocoumarins (psoralens). *Biochim. biophys. Acta*, *195*, 197-206

Pathak, M.A., Worden, L.R. & Kaufman, K.D. (1967) Effect of structural alterations on the photosensitizing potency of furocoumarins (psoralens) and related compounds. *J. invest. Dermatol.*, *48*, 103-118

Pathak, M.A., Dall'Acqua, F., Rodighiero, G. & Parrish, J.A. (1974a) Metabolism of psoralens (Abstract No. 8). *J. invest. Dermatol.*, *62*, 347

Pathak, M.A., Krämer, D.M. & Fitzpatrick, T.B. (1974b) *Photobiology and photochemistry of furocoumarins (psoralens).* In: Fitzpatrick, T.B., Pathak, M.A., Harber, L.C., Seiji, M. & Kukita, A., eds, *Sunlight and Man. Normal and Abnormal Photobiologic Responses*, Tokyo, University of Tokyo Press, pp. 335-368

Pathak, M.A., Marciani, M.S., Guiotto, A. & Rodighiero, C. (1983) A study of the relationship between photosensitizing and therapeutic activity of 4,5′,8-trimethylpsoralen and its major metabolite 4,8-dimethyl-5′-carboxypsoralen. *J. invest. Dermatol.*, *81*, 533-539

Pathak, M.A., Mosher, D.B. & Fitzpatrick, T.B. (1984) Safety and therapeutic effectiveness of 8-methoxypsoralen, 4,5′,8-trimethylpsoralen and psoralen in vitiligo. *Natl Cancer Inst. Monogr.*, *66*, 165-173

Paul de Haen International (1984) *de Haen Nonproprietary Name Index*, Vol. XV, *1941-1983*, Englewood, CO, p. 81

Quinto, I., Averbeck, D., Moustacchi, E., Hrisoho, Z. & Moron, J. (1984) Frameshift mutagenicity in *Salmonella typhimurium* of furocoumarins in the dark. *Mutat. Res.*, *136*, 49-54

Rodighiero, G. & Dall'Acqua, F. (1984) In vitro photoreactions of selected psoralens and methylangelicins with DNA, RNA and proteins. *Natl Cancer Inst. Monogr.*, *66*, 31-40

Sadtler Research Laboratories (1985) *The Sadtler Standard Spectra, Supplementary Index*, Philadelphia, PA

Salo, O.P., Lassus, A. & Taskinen, J. (1981) Trioxsalen bath plus UVA treatment of psoriasis. Plasma concentration of the drug and clinical results. *Acta dermatovenerol.*, *61*, 551-554

Scheel, L.D., Perone, V.B., Larkin, R.L. & Kupel, R.E. (1963) The isolation and characterization of two phototoxic furanocoumarins (psoralens) from diseased celery. *Biochemistry*, *2*, 1127-1131

Scott, B.R., Pathak, M.A., Mohn, G.R. (1976) Molecular and genetic basis of furocoumarin reactions. *Mutat. Res.*, *39*, 29-74

Sehgal, V.N. (1971) Oral trimethylpsoralen in vitiligo in children: a preliminary report. *Br. J. Dermatol.*, *95*, 454-456

Sinden, R.R. & Cole, R.S. (1978) Repair of cross-linked DNA and survival of *Escherichia coli* treated with psoralen and light: effects of mutations influencing genetic recombination and DNA metabolism. *J. Bacteriol.*, *136*, 538-547

Sinden, R.R. & Cole, R.S. (1981) *Measurement of cross-links formed by treatment with 4,5',8-trimethylpsoralen and light.* In: Friedberg, E.C. & Hanawalt, P.C., eds, *DNA Repair*, Vol. 1, Part A, New York, Marcel Dekker, pp. 69-81

Sittig, M. (1979) *Pharmaceutical Manufacturing Encyclopedia*, Park Ridge, NJ, Noyes Data Corp., pp. 629-630

van der Sluis, W.G., van Arkel, J., Fischer, F.C. & Labadie, R.P. (1981) Thin-layer chromatographic assay of photoactive compounds (furocoumarins) using the fungus *Penicillium expansum* as a test organism. *J. Chromatogr.*, *214*, 349-359

Song, P.-S., Shim, S.C. & Mantulin, W.W. (1981) The electronic spectra of psoralens in their ground and triplet excited states. *Bull. chem. Soc. Jpn*, *54*, 315-316

Swanbeck, G. & Thyresson, M. (1974) Induction of respiration-deficient mutants in yeast by psoralen and light. *J. invest. Dermatol.*, *63*, 242-244

Taskinen, J., Vahvelainen, N. & Nore, P. (1980) Determination of trioxsalen in human plasma in the picogram range by glass capillary gas chromatography mass spectrometry. *Biomed. mass Spectrom.*, *7*, 556-559

Trosko, J.E. & Isoun, M. (1970) Studies on the photosensitizing effect of trisoralen on human cells *in vitro* (Abstract No. GC-5). *Radiat. Res.*, *43*, 266

Trosko, J.E. & Isoun, M. (1971) Photosensitizing effect of trisoralen on DNA synthesis in human cells grown *in vitro*. *Int. J. Radiat. Biol.*, *19*, 87-92

US Pharmacopeial Convention (1985) *The United States Pharmacopeia*, 21st rev., Rockville, MD, pp. 1096-1097

Väätäinen, N., Hannuksela, M. & Karvonen, J. (1979) Local photochemotherapy in nodular prurigo. *Acta dermatovenerol.*, *59*, 544-547

Väätäinen, N., Hannuksela, M. & Karvonen, J. (1981a) Trioxsalen baths plus UV-A in the treatment of lichen planus and urticaria pigmentosa. *Clin. exp. Dermatol.*, *6*, 133-138

Väätäinen, N., Hannuksela, M. & Karvonen, J. (1981b) Long-term local trioxsalen photochemotherapy in psoriasis. *Dermatologica*, *163*, 229-231

Waksvik, H., Brøgger, A. & Stene, J. (1977) Psoralen/UVA treatment and chromosomes. I. Aberrations and sister chromatid exchange in human lymphocytes *in vitro* and synergism with caffeine. *Human Genet.*, *38*, 195-207

Windholz, M., ed. (1983) *The Merck Index*, 10th ed., Rahway, NJ, Merck & Co., pp. 1390-1391

Yarosh, D.B., Johns, V., Mufti, S., Bernstein, C. & Bernstein, H. (1980) Inhibition of UV and psoralen-plus-light mutagenesis in phage T4 by gene 43 antimutator polymerase alleles. *Photochem. Photobiol.*, *31*, 341-350

Yatagai, F. & Kitayama, S. (1983) Mutation induction by cross-links in DNA of *Deinococcus radiodurans*. *Biochem. biophys. Res. Commun.*, *112*, 458-463

Yoon, K. (1982) Localized mutagenesis of the tetracycline promoter region in pBR322 by 4,5′,8-trimethylpsoralen. *Mutat. Res.*, *93*, 253-262

SUMMARY OF EVALUATIONS

SUMMARY OF EVALUATIONS

Chemical/exposure	Degree of evidence[a] for		
	Human carcinogenicity	Animal carcinogenicity	Activity in short-term tests
Naturally occurring toxins			
Bracken fern (*Pteridium aquilinum*)	Inadequate	Sufficient	Inadequate
Ptaquiloside	No data	Limited	Inadequate
Shikimic acid	No data	Inadequate	Inadequate
Citrinin	No data	Limited	Inadequate
Patulin	No data	Inadequate	Inadequate
Rugulosin	No data	Inadequate	Limited
Food additives			
Benzyl acetate	No data	Limited	Inadequate
Butylated hydroxyanisole (BHA)	No data	Sufficient	No evidence
Butylated hydroxytoluene (BHT)	No data	Limited	Inadequate
Potassium bromate	No data	Sufficient	Sufficient
Aminoacid pyrolysis products in food			
Glu-P-1 (2-Amino-6-methyldipyrido[1,2-*a*:3′,2′-*d*]-imidazole	No data	Sufficient	Sufficient
Glu-P-2 (2-Aminodipyrido[1,2-*a*:3′,2′-*d*]imidazole)	No data	Sufficient	Sufficient
A-α-C (2-Amino-9*H*-pyrido[2,3-*b*]indole)	No data	Sufficient	Sufficient
MeA-α-C (2-Amino-3-methyl-9*H*-pyrido[2,3-*b*]-indole)	No data	Sufficient	Sufficient
IQ (2-Amino-3-methylimidazo[4,5-*f*]quinoline)	No data	Sufficient	Sufficient
MeIQ (2-Amino-3,4-dimethylimidazo[4,5-*f*]-quinoline)	No data	Inadequate	Sufficient
MeIQx (2-Amino-3,8-dimethylimidazo[4,5-*f*]-quinoxaline)	No data	Inadequate	Limited

Summary of evaluations (contd)

Chemical/exposure	Degree of evidence[a] for		
	Human carcinogenicity	Animal carcinogenicity	Activity in short-term tests
Furocoumarins			
Angelicins			
Angelicin	No data	Inadequate	Inadequate
Angelicin + UVA		Limited	Sufficient
5-Methylangelicin	No data	Inadequate	Inadequate
5-Methylangelicin + UVA		Limited	Sufficient
4,4'-Dimethylangelicin	No data	No data	Inadequate
4,4'-Dimethylangelicin + UVA		No data	Limited
4,5'-Dimethylangelicin	No data	Inadequate	Inadequate
4,5'-Dimethyl angelicin + UVA		Limited	Sufficient
4,4',6-Trimethylangelicin	No data	No data	Inadequate
4,4',6-Trimethylangelicin + UVA		No data	Inadequate
3-Carbethoxypsoralen	No data	Inadequate	Inadequate
3-Carbethoxypsoralen + UVA		No evidence	Sufficient
5-Methoxypsoralen	Inadequate	Inadequate	–
5-Methoxypsoralen + UVA		Sufficient	Sufficient
Pyrido[3,4-c]psoralen	No data	No data	Inadequate
Pyrido[3,4-c]psoralen + UVA		Inadequate	Sufficient
7-Methylpyrido[3,4-c]psoralen	No data	No data	Limited
7-Methylpyrido[3,4-c]psoralen + UVA		Inadequate	Sufficient
4,5',8-Trimethylpsoralen	Inadequate	No data	Inadequate
4,5',8-Trimethylpsoralen + UVA		Inadequate	Sufficient

[a]For definitions of terms see pp. 22, 18 and 20-21 of the Preamble.

APPENDIX

APPENDIX: ULTRAVIOLET RADIATION

1. Nomenclature and Measurement

The nomenclature, measurement and other physical aspects of ultraviolet (UV) radiation have been reviewed (Madden, 1975; WHO, 1979; Diffey, 1980).

The UV region of the electromagnetic radiation spectrum extends from 200-400 nm wavelength. It is adjoined at shorter wavelengths by the vacuum UV region (100-200 nm) and at longer wavelengths by the visible region (400-700 nm).

The UV spectrum has been divided by those studying its biological effects into three segments: UVA, 320-400 nm (also known as long-wave or near UV radiation, or as black light); UVB, 280-320 nm (middle UV or 'sunburn' radiation); and UVC, 200-280 nm (short-wave or far UV radiation, or germicidal radiation). Definitions of the boundaries between the segments vary somewhat, the UVA/UVB boundary ranging from 315-320 nm and the UVB/UVC boundary from 280-290 nm (WHO, 1979; Scotto et al., 1982; Larkö & Diffey, 1983).

Terminology and units commonly used in measuring and describing exposures to UV radiation are given in Table 1.

UV radiation may be measured by a chemical or physical detector, coupled with a monochromator or bandpass filter for wavelength selection. Physical detectors include radiometric devices, which depend for their response on the heating effect of the radiation, and photoelectric devices, in which incident photons are detected by a quantum effect such as the production of electrons (WHO, 1979). Examples of physical detectors of UV radiation have been described (Ruff et al., 1978).

Chemical detectors include photographic emulsions, actinometric solutions and light-sensitive plastic films. Personal dosimeters have been developed based on the change in optical density on exposure to UV light of certain plastic films, such as polysulphone (Challoner et al., 1976; Davis et al., 1976; Challoner et al., 1978; Gibbs et al., 1983; Larkö & Diffey, 1983) and polyvinyl chloride containing nalidixic acid (Tate et al., 1980).

Because the measurement of radiant exposure at individual wavelengths (or within narrow 1-2-nm bands) is time-consuming and expensive, methods for routine monitoring are sometimes designed to measure cumulative exposures over a range of wavelengths. In practice, broad-spectrum detectors are often calibrated against only a narrow waveband. Such devices may incorporate a biological weighting factor. One example is the Robertson-Berger meter, the response of which approximates the sensitivity of human skin to different UV wavelengths — mainly in the UVB region — in producing erythema (Berger, 1976; Scotto et al., 1982).

Table 1. Some basic terminology[a]

Term	International symbol	Definition	SI unit	Comments and synonyms
Wavelength	λ		nm	Nanometer $= 10^{-9}$ m (also called millimicron, mμ)
Radiant energy	Qe		J	1 joule $=$ 1 watt second
Radiant flux	Pe	dQe/dt	W	Rate of radiant energy delivery ('radiant power')
Irradiance	Ee	dPe/dA	W/m²	Radiant flux arriving over a given area ('fluence rate', 'dose-rate', 'intensity'). In photobiology, has also been expressed in W/cm², mW/cm² and μW/cm²
Radiant exposure	He	Ee × t	J/m²	Radiant energy delivered to a given area ('exposure dose', 'dose'); t = time in seconds. Has also been expressed as J/cm², mJ/cm² and μJ/cm²

[a]Adapted from WHO (1979)

2. Sources and Exposures

2.1 Sunlight

The major source of human exposure to UV radiation is sunlight. The wavelengths and relative intensities of solar radiation reaching the earth's surface are affected by a number of factors, including atmospheric absorption, scattering and reflection. Ozone in the stratosphere, with an absorption band centred at 250 nm and extending beyond 350 nm, effectively eliminates all UVC radiation (WHO, 1979). It has been estimated that a 1% decrease in stratospheric ozone results in a 2% increase in erythema-producing UV radiation at the earth's surface (Schulze, 1970; Setlow, 1974).

The effects of molecular scattering by air and aerosols; reflection, scattering and attenuation by clouds, haze and smog; and reflection from the ground have been noted (WHO, 1979). Solar elevation (latitude and season) is a major determining factor, and calculations of irradiance as a function of latitude have been reported (Schulze, 1970). Maps of the calculated world distribution of incident UVB radiation display graphically the interplay of some of these variables. For example, the annual irradiance at 307.5 nm was estimated to range from approximately 50 J/cm² in northern Scandinavia to as high as 450 J/cm² in selected (cloudless) areas near the equator (Schulze, 1978).

Few long-term measurements of actual irradiance in specific locations have been reported. Scotto *et al.* (1976a,b, 1982) monitored ten locations in the USA daily throughout 1974, automatically recording the intensity of erythema-producing radiation at half-hourly intervals with Robertson-Berger meters. On average in these locations, about 60% of the daily dose reached the ground between 10.00 and 14.00 hours and about 85% between 9.00 and 15.00 hours. In general, greater amounts of radiation were found in locations that were closer to the equator (low latitude), that were at higher altitudes and that had less cloud cover. Highest daily doses, as expected, were found in the summer when the days were longest. Robertson (1978) reported similar findings based on earlier measurements at three locations in Australia. Larkö and Diffey (1983), using polysulphone film badges, measured the exposure to UVB of workers in various occupations in Sweden. Monthly exposures in June and August ranged from 0.2-0.4 J/cm² for indoor workers to 1.2-1.5 J/cm² for outdoor workers.

Other compilations have been made of calculated and measured exposures to UV radiation in sunlight (Institute for Defense Analyses, 1975; Kripke & Sass, 1978; National Academy of Sciences, 1979; Scotto *et al.*, 1982; van der Leun & van Weelden, 1983; van der Leun, 1984).

2.2 Artificial sources

The many artificial sources of UV radiation have been reviewed and discussed by a number of authors (e.g., WHO, 1979; Diffey, 1980). These sources range from low-pressure mercury germicidal lamps, emitting principally 254 nm UV radiation (Lill, 1983; Maxwell & Elwood, 1986) to quartz-halogen lamps used for outdoor illumination and emitting primarily >330 nm UV and visible light. Some fluorescent lamps designed for indoor illumination may also emit small amounts of UV radiation (Maxwell & Elwood, 1983). Sunlamps for tanning for cosmetic purposes emitted significant quantities of UVB when first developed, but more recently some sunlamps have been redesigned to emit 'only' UVA. UV radiation, principally UVA, is also used in conjunction with such drugs as the psoralens (see monographs in this volume) in the treatment of various skin disorders. Exposures to a variety of other artificial sources are predominantly occupational. These include certain welding processes and carbon arcs; others have been described in detail (Madden, 1975; WHO, 1979).

3. Biological Data Relevant to the Evaluation of Carcinogenic Risk to Humans

3.1 Carcinogenicity studies in animals

(a) Background

The first animal experiments using UV radiation were performed by Findlay (1928), who showed that daily irradiation of albino mice with UV radiation from a mercury arc induced skin cancer. In a series of studies in the 1930s, Roffo (1934) showed that skin cancer could be induced in rats with natural sunlight, as well as with mercury-arc radiation. Roffo (1939) also performed the first spectral-dependence studies on skin UV radiation carcinogenesis (photocarcinogenesis), in which he demonstrated that clear window-glass [which does not allow the transmission of wavelengths <320 nm] was sufficient to inhibit skin cancer induction by both natural sunlight and mercury-arc radiation.

Between 1940 and 1944, a comprehensive series of experiments on UV carcinogenesis in mice was carried out at the US National Cancer Institute (published in several papers; for review, see Blum, 1959). Repeated exposure of haired albino mice to daily doses of UV radiation led to highly reproducible cancer incidence in the ears of the exposed animals.

The extensive body of literature on photocarcinogenesis has been reviewed by Emmett (1973), Urbach et al. (1974) and Epstein (1978, 1985). The field has also been widely reviewed in the US National Cancer Institute Monograph 50 (Kripke & Sass, 1978) and in the WHO Environmental Health Criteria Document 14 (WHO, 1979). This appendix concentrates on a few representative studies on UVB and describes a few studies on UVA and UVC.

[The Working Group noted that many investigators of photocarcinogenesis, according to standard practice, do not report individual animal survival and/or tumour data as is generally done in long-term chemical carcinogenesis studies. Furthermore, meaningful inter-laboratory comparisons are not always possible because of incomplete descriptions/assessments of UV radiation source, emission spectrum and exposure dose. Some studies do not mention controls not exposed to UV radiation, but it is recognized that the incidence of spontaneous skin tumours in the strains described is rare. The Working Group also noted that UV radiation-induced squamous-cell carcinoma in mouse skin was a model for human skin squamous-cell carcinoma, but that there was no adequate animal model for human skin basal-cell carcinoma or malignant melanoma related to exposure to UV radiation alone.]

(b)   Skin carcinogenesis

Mouse: Of Blum's numerous studies of UV radiation carcinogenesis in mice, those described here (Blum et al., 1941; Grady et al., 1943) involved the ear of the haired A strain mouse. The UV radiation source, an intermediate-pressure mercury arc, emitted mainly UVB but also some UVA and UVC (Blum et al., 1941). The tumours were mostly ear fibrosarcomas, but squamous-cell carcinomas were also observed. Nonexposed mice did not develop skin tumours.

More recently, Kripke (1977) studied the exposure of three differently pigmented strains of mouse to similar dose regimes of UV radiation from Westinghouse FS40T12 sunlamps[a], emitting mainly UVB. Animals were eight weeks old at the start of the experiment; survival

---

[a]Several of the studies described here have involved use of Westinghouse FS40T12 sunlamps. These lamps emit mainly UVB, with <1% below 280 nm, two-thirds at 280-320 nm and one-third at >320 nm.

time was not given. Of a group of 51 BALB/cAnN mice, 46 developed tumours of the ear: ten squamous-cell carcinomas, 28 fibrosarcomas, three mixed tumours, and 17 tumours that were not examined histologically; and/or one squamous-cell carcinoma and five fibrosarcomas of the back; and one fibrosarcoma of the eyelid. Of a group of 19 C57Bl/6N mice, 15 developed tumours of the ear: one squamous-cell carcinoma, four fibrosarcomas and three tumours that were not examined; and of the back: seven fibrosarcomas and three tumours that were not examined histologically. Of a total of 28 irradiated C3H/HeN mice, 24 developed tumours: three squamous-cell carcinomas of the ear; 16 fibrosarcomas, of which one was on the forepaw, two in the eye, ten on the back and three in the ear; two mixed tumours of the ear and two of the back; and five tumours that were not examined histologically: one in the eye, one on the back and three in the ear. Tumours appeared earlier in the albino (BALB/cAnN) strain than in the others.

Dose-response studies to UV radiation were carried out by Forbes *et al.* (1981). Groups of male and female hairless albino Skh:HR mice, seven ($\pm$ one) weeks old at the start of the experiment, were irradiated with Westinghouse FS40T12 sunlamps, emitting mainly UVB. All animals developed skin tumours. A dose-response effect was demonstrated, as assessed by time to tumours in 50% of animals (Table 2). Histological examination showed tumours larger than 4 mm in diameter to be squamous-cell carcinomas, those 1-4 mm to form a continuum from carcinoma *in situ* to squamous-cell carcinoma and those less than 1 mm to show epidermal hyperplasia and evidence of squamous metaplasia tending toward carcinoma *in situ*. Histological similarities to keratoacanthoma were also noted. Less than 1% of tumours were fibrosarcomas.

Extensive dose-response studies have also been carried out by de Gruijl *et al.* (1983), in which six groups of Skh-hr1 hairless albino mice (total, 199) of each sex were exposed to

Table 2. Dose-response to UV radiation of hairless albino Skh:HR mice[a]

Daily dose (J/m²)	Time in weeks to 50% tumour-bearing animals	Terminated at week
420	38.6	45
587	33.3	45
822	29.2	45
1 152	20.0	36
1 613	17.6	36
2 259	12.9	25

[a]From Forbes *et al.* (1981)

daily doses, differing by a factor of 33, of mainly UVB from Westinghouse FS40T12 sunlamps. A clear-cut relationship was shown between daily dose and time required for 50% of animals to develop skin tumours. Two tumours were reported in a total of 24 nonirradiated control mice.

Freeman (1975) studied carcinogenesis induced by chronic exposure to monochromatic UVB produced by a high-intensity diffraction grating monochromator. The wavelengths 300 nm and 310 nm were carcinogenic to the irradiated ears of haired albino mice. In a group of 30 mice exposed to 300 nm, 16 developed 16 squamous-cell carcinomas. In a group of 30 mice exposed to 310 nm, 16 animals survived to 450 days, of which eight had a total of five squamous-cell carcinomas, two fibrosarcomas and one angiosarcoma of the ear.

The recent availability of UVA sources for therapeutic and cosmetic purposes, with and without the use of photosensitizing chemicals such as methoxsalen, has resulted in widespread human exposure to high doses of UVA. There is *sufficient evidence* that the combination of methoxsalen plus UVA is carcinogenic in mouse skin (IARC, 1980, 1982).

A few studies have been designed to study the carcinogenic potential of UVA *per se*. A group of 25 female, lightly pigmented, hairless Oslo/Bom mice, 12 weeks old, was irradiated for five days per week with a Philips TL40W/09 lamp filtered through a 2-mm thick glass plate to eliminate UVB. The daily UVA dose, given for three months only, was 1.08 J/cm³ [10.8×10^3 J/m²]. After 58 weeks of exposure, no tumour was found (Staberg *et al.*, 1983). [The Working Group noted that the dose of UVA and the duration of the irradiation and observation periods were inadequate to assess the carcinogenicity of UVA.]

A group of 200 female A/J mice, six weeks old, was irradiated with Westinghouse 'black light' fluorescent lamps, to give a daily UVA dose of $30\text{-}38 \times 10^4$ J/m². Although glass filters were used, some UVB radiation was emitted (at a daily dose of $8.6\text{-}13 \times 10^3$ J/m²). After 70-90 weeks of exposure, 61 animals examined had six papillomas, six squamous-cell carcinomas and three fibrosarcomas of the ear and tail; 40 animals had hyperplasia of the epidermis; and five showed none of these changes (Zigman *et al.*, 1976). [The Working Group noted that this experiment was inadequate to determine the carcinogenic potential of UVA alone because of the UVB content of the source.]

UVC *per se* has rarely been studied for skin carcinogenicity. A group of 40 female C3H/HeNCr1Br mice were irradiated using a germicidal lamp emitting mainly 254 nm. The weekly dose was 3×10^4 J/m². Three animals died without tumours at nine, 43 and 63 weeks of irradiation, respectively. By 52 weeks, 97% of the animals had developed tumours, the median time of appearance of which was 43 weeks. The mean number of tumours recorded per tumour-bearing mouse was 2.9. Tumour histology was carried out in 29/37 mice. Of a total of 83 suspected tumours, 66 were squamous-cell carcinomas, ten were proliferative squamous lesions, and six were invasive fibrosarcomas (Lill, 1983). [The Working Group noted that the 4% UVB content of the source, representing a weekly dose of 1170 J/m², cannot be excluded as the cause of the tumours.]

Single exposures to UV radiation (Blum *et al.*, 1959; Pound, 1970) were not carcinogenic, possibly due to the low dose. However, a single exposure to an extremely high dose of UVB radiation on mouse skin (Hsu *et al.*, 1975), which caused ulceration and scar formation, resulted in skin tumours. Groups of hairless (HRS/J or Skh-hrl) mice were irradiated with a Westinghouse FS20/40T12 sunlamp at single doses of $3\text{-}24 \times 10^4$ J/m^2. In the group exposed to 12×10^4 J/m^2, a total of 38 (mostly benign) tumours was found in six tumour-bearing animals between 15-28 weeks after irradiation. [The Working Group noted that the dose calculated from the raw data was 8×10^4 J/m^2.]

The results of these and other studies in mice are summarized in Table 3.

Table 3. Skin carcinogenesis induced in mice by ultraviolet radiation

UV source described by author	Strain	Phenotype[a]	No. of animals	No. of TBA[b]	No. of tumours	Reference
UVB/C[c]	A	ah+	605	598	715	Grady *et al.* (1943)
UVB	Albino	ah+	60	24	24	Freeman (1975)
UVB/A	Swiss	ah−	40	20	27	Stenbäck (1975a)
UVB/A	BALB/cAnN	ah+	51	46	48	Kripke (1977)
UVB/A	C57/BL/6N	ph+	19	15	19	Kripke (1977)
UVB/A	C3H/HeN	ph+	28	24	28	Kripke (1977)
UVB/A	C3Hf	ph−	110	88	74[d]	Spikes *et al.* (1977)
UVB/A	C57 (HR)	ph−	11	11	≥11	Winkelmann *et al.* (1963)
UVB/A	Skh/Hr1	ah−	20	20	≥20	Kligman & Kligman
UVB/A	Skh/Hr2	ph−	40	40	≥60	(1981)
UVA	A/J	ah+	61	15[e]	15	Zigman *et al.* (1976)
UVA and UVB	HRA/Skh−1	ah−	22	22	215	Gallagher *et al.* (1984)
UVB; UVA and UVB	Oslo/Bom	ph−[f]	125	49	≥49	Staberg *et al.* (1983)
UVC	C3H	ph+	40	37	107 (mean)	Lill (1983)
UVC	HRS/J	ah−	6	5	24	Forbes & Urbach (1975)

[a]a, albino; p, pigmented; h+, haired; h−, hairless

[b]TBA, tumour-bearing animals

[c]From Blum *et al.* (1941)

[d]Number of tumours examined histologically; total number of tumours not given

[e]Not clear from the paper if TBA or number of tumours

[f]Lightly pigmented

Rat: Early studies by Findlay (1930), Putschar and Holtz (1930) and Hueper (1942) reported malignant skin tumours in rats after exposure to UV radiation.

Groups of six or 12 male CD-1 rats, 28 days of age, were shaved and exposed to varying doses and dose regimes of UV radiation from Westinghouse FS20 sunlamps with a spectral range of 275-375 nm (peak output, 313 nm; UVB), or Westinghouse G36T6L sterilamps emitting only 254 nm (UVC). Survival ranged from 75 to 92% for the separate experimental groups. All groups developed keratoacanthoma-like skin tumours (Strickland *et al.*, 1979).

Skin tumour induction was studied in a group of 40 shaven female NMR albino rats, eight to ten weeks old at the start of the experiment. The animals were irradiated chronically for 60 weeks with Westinghouse FS40T12 sunlamps, emitting mainly UVB (weekly dose, $5.4-10.8 \times 10^4 \, J/m^2$). A total of 25 tumours developed in 16/40 animals, most of which were epidermal ear papillomas (Stenbäck, 1975).

Hamster: Stenbäck (1975) also irradiated 40 shaven female Syrian golden hamsters (a strain sensitive to chemical carcinogenesis), eight to ten weeks of age, with the same irradiation protocol as described above. A total of 30 skin tumours developed in 14/40 animals; 22 were papillomas (14 animals), four were keratoacanthomas (three animals), one was a squamous-cell carcinoma of the skin and three were papillomas of the ear (one animal).

Guinea-pig: Stenbäck (1975) also irradiated 25 shaven female guinea-pigs, eight to ten weeks of age, using the same irradiation protocol. One fibroma and one trichofolliculoma of the skin were observed.

(c)   Eye carcinogenesis

In experimental photocarcinogenesis studies, attention has been focused mainly on skin tumours; however, there have been a few reports of eye tumours. Corneal tumours have been described in mice, rats and hamsters chronically exposed to GE Uviarc UA-3 lamps [dose unspecified] which emit broad-spectrum UVA, UVB and UVC (Freeman & Knox, 1964). Broadband UV radiation also induced a number of eye tumours, such as fibrosarcomas and haemangiosarcomas, in A mice (Lippincott & Blum, 1943), and two fibrosarcomas and another unspecified tumour of the eye were reported in 24 tumour-bearing C3H/HeN mice exposed to UV radiation from Westinghouse FS40T12 sunlamps, emitting mainly UVB radiation (Kripke, 1977).

'Cancer eye', squamous-cell carcinoma of the cornea, in cattle is commonly associated with exposure to solar radiation (Russell *et al.*, 1956).

3.2 Other relevant biological data

(a)   Mutagenesis

Studies with near-visible UV in *Escherichia coli* are unambiguous in demonstrating mutagenic activity (Kubitschek, 1967: UVA, 320-400 nm; Webb & Malina, 1970: UVA, 312-392 nm; Tyrrell, 1982: UVA, 313-405 nm), as are those with UVA (320-400 nm) and UVB

(290-320 nm) in *Saccharomyces cerevisiae* (Hannan *et al.*, 1984) and with 254-313 nm in cultured mammalian cells (for a review, see Kantor, 1985). Broad-spectrum sources that emit in the solar UV region are also mutagenic to cultured mammalian cells, e.g., Chinese hamster ovary and V79 lung cells (Bradley & Sharkey, 1977; Hsie *et al.*, 1977; Burki & Lam, 1978), mouse lymphoma L5178Y cells (Jacobson *et al.*, 1978) and human skin fibroblasts (Patton *et al.*, 1984).

Information is now available to permit some evaluation of the contribution of different wavelength regions.

Exposure to 365 nm (UVA) induced *trp*$^+$ revertants in *E. coli* (Webb, 1977). Using a xenon-mercury lamp and monochromator, mutations were also induced in *E. coli* WP2s (Peak *et al.*, 1984) and in Chinese hamster V79 cells after exposure to 334 and 365 nm (Wells & Han, 1984). In a study by Tyrrell (1984), exposing human TK6 lymphoblastoid cells to the same sources, mutants were not induced.

With UVB radiation, mutation responses have been obtained in *E. coli* (Peak *et al.*, 1984), *S. cerevisiae* (Zölzer & Kiefer, 1983) and in some mammalian cells in culture, such as Chinese hamster ovary and V79 cells (Zelle *et al.*, 1980; Susuki *et al.*, 1981; Wells & Han, 1984; Zölzer & Kiefer, 1984), mouse lymphoma L5178Y cells (Jacobson *et al.*, 1981) and human TK6 lymphoblastoid cells (Tyrrell, 1984).

The studies of Tyrrel and Webb (1973) and Peak *et al.* (1984) in *E. coli*, of Zölzer and Kiefer (1984) in Chinese hamster cells and of Tyrrell (1984) and Tyrrell *et al.* (1984) in human lymphoblastoid cells reveal levels of mutation induction consistent with the known dimer yields (Setlow, 1974).

The inevitable consequence of the absorption spectrum maximum of DNA is that there is a considerable body of positive data on mutagenicity at 254 nm (UVC), which is usually delivered by radiation from germicidal lamps with 90-95% output at 254 nm, for microorganisms (Webb & Malina, 1970; Tyrrell, 1982) and mammalian cells in culture, such as Chinese hamster ovary cells (Zelle *et al.*, 1980), human lymphoblasts (Luca *et al.*, 1983) and human fibroblasts (Maher *et al.*, 1979; Myhr *et al.*, 1979).

(b) Chromosomal damage

No information on chromosomal damage by UVA was available.

Using ICR 2A frog cells, Chao and Rosenstein (1985) demonstrated the induction of sister chromatid exchanges by UV light in the UVB region. The same cells were used to show the induction of chromosomal aberrations by 302 and 313 nm UV radiation from a mercury-arc lamp in conjunction with a monochromator (Rosenstein & Rosenstein, 1985). The photoreactivating sector was greater at 302 than at 313 nm, suggesting that nondimer photoproducts are significant at 313 nm.

UVC has been shown to induce chromosomal aberrations in human fibroblasts (Parrington, 1972), V79 Chinese hamster cells (Griggs & Bender, 1973) and ICR 2A frog cells (Chao & Rosenstein, 1985) and sister chromatid exchanges in V79 Chinese hamster cells (Nishi *et al.*, 1984).

(c)   Cell transformation

Morphological transformation has been demonstrated after exposure of BALB/c 3T3 cells (Withrow *et al.*, 1980) and C3H10T1/2 cells (Kennedy *et al.*, 1980) to broad-spectrum sources. While no information is available on the UVA region, UVB from a sunlamp (emitting 255-400 nm with cut-off at 290 nm) induced malignant transformation of neonatal BALB/c mouse epidermal cells (Ananthaswamy & Kripke, 1981). Suzuki *et al.* (1981) showed by the use of various filters on a sunlamp that transformation of mouse C3H10T1/2 cells was induced by UVB. Doniger *et al.* (1981) showed that monochromatic light in the UVB region induced cell transformation in a Syrian hamster embryo system. The peak of activity in both of these studies correlated with DNA-dimer yields (Setlow, 1974).

Cell transformation by UVC has been demonstrated in the C3H10T1/2 system (Chan & Little, 1976; Suzuki *et al.*, 1981), in the BALB/c 3T3 system (Withrow *et al.*, 1980) and in Syrian hamster embryo cell systems (Doniger *et al.*, 1981).

3.3 Case reports and epidemiological studies of carcinogenicity in humans

Ultraviolet light has been implicated as a possible factor in the etiology of squamous- and basal-cell (non-melanocytic) cancers of the skin, malignant melanoma of the skin, cancer of the lip and malignant melanoma of the eye. The relevant epidemiological studies are discussed here. Few of these assessed the effect of UV light in isolation; the majority were concerned with sunlight, and UV light could not be separated from other components of solar radiation. Latitude of residence and of birth was also sometimes used as an indicator of exposure to UV light. The studies are discussed with respect to the exposures actually measured.

This section does not deal with factors affecting the susceptibility to skin cancer, such as skin colour, genetic defects in repair of UV damage, or other characteristics. While people with sun-sensitive skins are at risk for all skin cancers (see, for example, Vitaliano & Urbach, 1980; Elwood *et al.*, 1984), this is only indirect evidence for a role of sunlight on their etiology. The evidence that the combination of methoxsalen and UVA causes skin cancer in humans (see IARC, 1980, 1982) is also not considered, since it is not possible to distinguish the effects of UV radiation alone from those of methoxsalen or of the combination of the two.

(a)   Non-melanocytic skin cancer

(i)   *Anatomical distribution in relation to solar exposure*

About 80% of non-melanocytic skin cancers arise on the head and neck (Urbach *et al.*, 1966) and these are the parts of the body most exposed to sunlight (Blum, 1948). Urbach *et al.* (1966) illustrated that there is uneven exposure by use of a mannequin head painted with a chemical sensitive to UV light and simulation of the sun's movement in the sky. They showed that maximum exposure occurs to the tops of the ears, the nose, the scalp, the lower lip and the lower portion of the neck. The orbits, nasolabial folds, upper lip and underpart of the chin were relatively protected. These authors then compared the relative distribution of basal-cell and squamous-cell carcinomas on different parts of the head and neck. They found that more than one-third of all basal-cell carcinomas on the head and neck arose in the relatively protected areas (receiving less than 20% of the maximum of UV radiation), while few squamous-cell carcinomas occurred on these sites. Thus, the distribution of squamous-cell carcinomas paralleled the sites found to be maximally exposed to the sun's rays more closely than did the distribution of basal-cell carcinomas.

(ii) *Latitude*

Residence: In what is now known as the US First National Cancer Survey, Dorn (1944a,b,c) showed that the incidence of all skin cancers in ten urban areas of the USA in 1937-1938 was higher in whites in the southern USA than in those in the north of the country. These data were reanalysed according to latitude by Blum (1948), who found that the incidence of skin cancer in males and females was inversely related to latitude. This was not true of any other cancer except buccal cancer (see below). Blum pointed out that UV light intensity was also inversely related to latitude, suggesting that this could explain the relationship between latitude and skin cancer incidence.

Auerbach (1961) analysed data from the US Second National Cancer Survey in ten cities in the USA in 1947-1948 [the same cities for which Dorn (1944) had analysed data for 1937-1938]. He showed that at all ages, and in both males and females, skin cancer incidence increased with decreasing latitude. He estimated that skin cancer incidence rates doubled with every three to four degrees of latitude, or every 265 miles. Similarly, Haenszel (1963) analysed regional cancer incidence in the USA for 1947-1950 and showed that the incidences of squamous-cell and basal-cell skin cancers were inversely related to latitude.

Elwood *et al.* (1974) found a strong inverse relationship between mortality, latitude and estimated UV exposure for non-melanocytic skin cancers in 48 states of the USA and ten provinces of Canada.

Green *et al.* (1976) found a correlation between estimated UV light intensity (estimated principally on the basis of latitude, atmospheric ozone concentration and average cloud cover) and age-specific and age-adjusted incidences of non-melanocytic skin cancer in 30 regions of the USA, UK, Canada and Australia. They also noted that a 1% increase in UV dose was associated with a greater than 1% increase in skin cancer incidence. [No account was taken in the analysis of variations in the completeness of reporting of skin cancer incidence in different parts of the world.]

The studies described above that assessed the relationship of cancer incidence to latitude generally assumed that UV light intensity is directly related to latitude. Rundel and Nachtwey (1978) and Rundel (1983) obtained measurements of the actual UV flux in four regions of the USA (Iowa, Minneapolis-St Paul, San Francisco-Oakland, and Dallas-Fort Worth) and examined their correlation with the incidences of squamous-cell and basal-cell cancers in the Third National Cancer Survey. They found an association between measured UV flux and cancer incidence, noting also that the percentage change in cancer incidence per unit change in UV flux was greater for males than for females and greater for squamous-cell than for basal-cell skin cancer.

Place of birth: Mortality from non-melanocytic cancer of the skin is substantially lower in migrants to Australia (who generally come from higher latitudes and therefore areas of lower sun exposure than Australia) than in native-born Australians. The ratio of the age-standardized mortality rate in males from England and Wales to that in native-born Australians was 0.55, with a 95% confidence interval of 0.43-0.71. There was little evidence of any tendency for relative mortality to increase with increasing duration of residence in Australia (Armstrong *et al.*, 1983).

(iii)   *Exposure to sunlight*

In studies of the relationship between exposure to sunlight and cancer in individuals, exposure has been examined in three main ways: total exposure; exposure to sunlight at work; and exposure during recreation. Each of these is discussed separately.

Total exposure: Lancaster and Nelson (1957) compared a history of 'excessive sun exposure' in 173 patients with non-melanocytic skin cancer and in 173 controls in Sydney, Australia: 21.4% of the patients with cancer and 16.2% of controls with other skin cancers were assessed to have excessive sunlight exposure [$p = 0.13$].

Gellin *et al.* (1965) compared history of outdoor exposure in 861 patients with basal-cell epithelioma and 1938 controls attending a dermatology clinic. Among patients aged 40-79, they found that 75% of cases, but only 35% of controls, spent more than three hours outside each day; and that 29% of cases, but only 10% of controls spent more than six hours outdoors each day ($p < 0.001$ in both cases). [These percentages do not appear to have been adjusted for age. Since the controls were dermatology patients who might stay indoors because of their skin disease, the comparison may be biased.]

Urbach *et al.* (1974) reported on 'cumulative outdoor hour exposure' in patients and controls in Philadelphia, USA, and Galway, Ireland. They reported that, in Philadelphia, 17% of male patients with basal-cell carcinoma and 31% with squamous-cell carcinoma, but only 3% of controls had the highest category of exposure ($p < 0.005$) — more than 50 000 hours of total cumulative outdoor exposure. In Galway, 96% of those with skin cancer and 55% of controls belonged to that category.

Vitaliano (1978) and Vitaliano and Urbach (1980) reported the findings of a case-control study at the Skin and Cancer Hospital, Philadelphia, USA. The 366 patients with basal-cell carcinoma and 58 with squamous-cell carcinoma were compared with 294 controls, of whom 5% had psoriasis. Each subject's cumulative exposure to sunlight was assessed by history of jobs and military service, time spent sunbathing and participation in sports. In a multiple logistic regression analysis, the relative risk associated with maximum outdoor exposure (30 000 hours or more outdoors) compared with minimum exposure group (less than 10 000 hours outdoors) was 3.2 for basal-cell cancers and 7.1 for squamous-cell cancers ($p < 0.001$ in each case). [The age distribution of cases and controls differed markedly and age was treated only as a dichotomous factor in the regression analyses. Since the skin cancer patients were older than the controls, their longer total exposure to sunlight may be at least partly a consequence of their older age. Some of the subjects in this study may also have been included in the study of Urbach *et al.* (1974).]

Occupational exposure: Atkin *et al.* (1949) reported on the occupation of 4378 men in England and Wales who died from non-melanocytic skin cancer between 1911 and 1944. They found that mortality rates were higher in men who had worked outdoors, and were three times higher in those employed in agriculture than in professional men.

Lancaster and Nelson (1957), in a comparison of the work histories of 67 men with non-melanocytic skin cancer and of 67 controls with other cancers in Sydney, Australia, found an association between duration of outdoor work and incidence of skin cancer. Compared to the risk for men who had worked outdoors for less than five years, the estimated relative risk associated with five to ten years' outdoor work was 1.9, and that for ten or more years' outdoor work was 4.2 (p for trend < 0.001).

Silverstone and Gordon (1966) presented data on the association between reported history of skin cancer and outdoor occupation in a survey of 1733 people in two areas of Queensland, Australia. In neither the more northerly, tropical and wet area of Cardwellshire nor the more southerly, subtropical area of Caboolture was a 'significant' association found. Silverstone and Searle (1970), in a survey of 2200 persons in three regions of Queensland, Australia [two of which were included in the report of Silverstone and Gordon (1966)], reported that 12.1% of men and 8.4% of women who worked indoors had a history of skin cancer compared to 15.1% of men and 5.0% of women who worked outdoors. [The diagnosis and reporting of skin cancers in these two studies may have been affected by social class, which in turn may be associated with place of work. It is not clear whether the effects of age on skin cancer occurrence were controlled in the comparison.]

In a survey of 781 cases of squamous-cell carcinoma of the skin reported to the Manchester Regional Cancer Registry, Whitaker *et al.* (1979) found that male farmers had more than twice the expected incidence ($p < 0.001$).

Teppo *et al.* (1980), in a survey of cancer incidence and conditions of life in Finland, found that persons working in areas where farming predominated had lower rates of basal-cell and other non-melanocytic skin cancers than did persons living elsewhere. The authors suggested that registration of skin cancer may not be as complete in farming areas as it is elsewhere.

Beral and Robinson (1981) analysed cancer registration data for England and Wales from 1970 to 1975, classifying the reported occupations of individuals into outdoor and indoor jobs. Those with an outdoor job had a 10% greater incidence of nonmelanocytic skin cancer than did the national population, the small excess being significant ($p < 0.05$). Mortality statistics for England and Wales also showed a significantly higher death rate from nonmelanocytic skin cancer in outdoor workers than indoor workers, the excess being 22% in 1959-1963 and 26% in 1970-1972. In England and Wales, nonmelanocytic skin cancers are more common among people of low social class (Office of Population Censuses and Surveys, 1978) [who are also more likely to work outdoors].

Aubry and MacGibbon (1985) enquired about history of outdoor work from 92 patients with squamous-cell carcinomas of the skin and 174 controls in Montreal, Canada. Using a multiple logistic regression analysis that adjusted for other variables that might affect risk, they found that a 'high index of occupational sunlight exposure' was associated with a relative risk of 1.6 ($p = 0.02$). [The response rate of subjects eligible for the survey was 30%.]

Recreational exposure: Lancaster and Nelson (1957) reported that 55% of patients in Sydney, Australia with nonmelanocytic skin cancer and 49% of controls who had other cancers gave a history of fishing, and that 18% of patients and 22% of controls sunbathed.

In their study in Montreal, Canada, Aubry and MacGibbon (1985) reported that the relative risk for skin cancer in those with a 'high score for non-occupational sunlight exposure' was 1.6 with reference to those with a low score ($p = 0.07$).

Other aspects: In the UK, a seasonal variation was found for nonmelanocytic skin cancer, with a peak in the summer months (Swerdlow, 1985).

(iv) *Exposure to other sources of UV light*

Aubry and MacGibbon (1985) reported use of long-tube sunlamps by four of 92 patients with squamous-cell carcinoma of the skin and by one of 174 controls. Following adjustment for possible confounding effects of colour-complexion, ethnic characteristics and non-occupational and occupational exposure to sunlight, the relative risk associated with use of long-tube sunlamps was estimated to be 13.4, with 95% confidence limits of 1.4-130.5 ($p = 0.008$). [The crude relative risk was 7.9 with $p = 0.05$ by Fisher's exact test. Although data were also collected on exposure to 'round-tube' sunlamps, results for this exposure were not reported. Only 30% of eligible patients were included in the study.]

(b) *Lip cancer*

(i) *Anatomical distribution in relation to sun exposure*

More than 90% of lip cancers are squamous-cell (epidermoid) carcinomas; the remainder are mainly basal-cell carcinomas. The great majority of squamous-cell carcinomas arise on the lower lip (Keller, 1970; Lindqvist, 1979), while basal-cell carcinomas arise with approximately equal frequency on the upper and lower lips (Keller, 1970). The lower lip is more exposed to sunlight than is the upper (Urbach et al., 1966).

(ii) Latitude

Dorn (1944) reported that the incidence of cancer of the buccal cavity (mostly lip cancers) in the USA was higher in the south than in the north of the country. Blum (1948) reanalysed Dorn's data and showed that, as for skin cancer, there was an inverse relation between incidence of buccal cavity cancer and latitude.

Mortality from lip cancer is substantially lower in migrants to Australia than in native-born Australians. The ratio of the age-standardized mortality rate in male migrants to that in native-born Australians was 0.46, with a 95% confidence interval of 0.27-0.78 (Armstrong et al., 1983).

(iii) Exposure to sunlight

Occupational exposure: Atkin et al. (1949) studied the occupations of 1537 men dying from lip cancer in England and Wales between 1911 and 1944. They reported that mortality from cancer of the lip was 13 times higher among men employed in agriculture than in men with professional jobs.

Keller (1970) compared the occupations of 314 men with lip cancer admitted to Veterans' Administration hospitals in the USA with those of two groups of age-matched controls admitted to the same hospitals comprising 304 men with other cancers and 304 men with other diseases. Farming was recorded as the occupation of 27% of men with lip cancer but of only 8% of men with other cancers and 4% of men with other diseases (relative risks in comparison with each control group were 4.0 and 8.4, respectively; $p < 0.001$ in both cases). Any type of outdoor work was recorded for 40% of those with lip cancer, 20% of those with other cancers and 12% of those with other diseases (relative risks of 2.6 and 4.8, respectively; $p < 0.001$). [These relative risk estimates, calculated by the Working Group, were not adjusted for pipe smoking, another risk factor identified in the study.]

Spitzer et al. (1975) obtained information about 366 men with squamous-cell carcinoma of the lip in Newfoundland and 210 male controls chosen from the electoral register and matched by age and geographical location in nine census divisions. An association was found between lip cancer and both reported occupational outdoor exposure (relative risk, 1.52; $p < 0.05$) and fishing (adjusted for outdoor exposure: relative risk, 1.60; $p < 0.05$; adjusted for pipe smoking and for outdoor exposure: relative risk, 1.50; $p < 0.05$).

Lindqvist (1979) compared the reported history of outdoor work of 290 patients with epidermoid carcinoma of the lip in Finland with that of 254 controls with squamous-cell carcinoma of the skin (response rate of 59%). He found that 73% of men with lip cancer had worked outdoors, compared to 49% of those with squamous-cell skin carcinoma ($p < 0.001$). The relative risk estimates ranged from 2.2 to 3.2, according to the calendar period during which the subjects had worked outdoors.

Dardanoni et al. (1984) interviewed 53 men with lip cancer in Ragusa, Sicily, and 106 male controls admitted to the same hospitals. The controls were matched by age and municipality of residence. An association was found between lip cancer and working or spending at least six hours each day outdoors (relative risk, 4.9; $p < 0.001$).

(c) Malignant melanoma of skin

Melanoma of the skin is commonly divided into four histological types, which may bear different relationships to solar exposures. The types are lentigo maligna melanoma (Hutchinson's melanotic freckle), superficial spreading melanoma, nodular melanoma and melanoma of unclassifiable type (Holman & Armstrong, 1984). The epidemiology of malignant melanoma has been reviewed (Gallagher, 1986).

(i) Anatomical distribution in relation to solar exposure

In contrast to non-melanocytic skin cancer, the distribution of melanoma on the skin does not correspond to the distribution of exposure of the body to sunlight (Davis et al., 1966; Lee & Yongchaiyudha, 1971; Crombie, 1981). In Caucasians, only about one-quarter of melanomas arise on the head and neck (Holman et al., 1980). The trunk is the predominant site in males, and the legs the predominant site in females (Lee & Yongchaiyudha, 1971). This site distribution has been offered as a major objection to the solar theory of etiology of melanoma (Anon., 1981). Much of the consideration of site distribution, however, has not taken account of differences in surface area and melanocyte density between different body sites (Elwood et al., 1985a,b; Green et al., 1986), which might be expected to modify the distribution of melanoma.

The majority of melanomas of the face (head or neck), at least in populations with high exposure to the sun, are of the lentigo maligna type, a type which is much less common on other body sites. Lentigo maligna melanomas are more likely than other types to be accompanied by pathological evidence of sun damage in the surrounding skin (McGovern et al., 1980).

(ii) Latitude

Residence: Lancaster (1956) pointed out that the distribution of melanoma, like that of non-melanocytic skin cancer, was inversely related to latitude. He showed that, within Australia, melanoma mortality rates ranged from 23 per million in the most northern state, Queensland, to eight per million in the most southern, Tasmania, and that a gradient existed in intervening states. This pattern still obtains and is seen also in incidence data (Armstrong et al., 1982). Lancaster (1956) reported that mortality from melanoma was higher in the northern than in the southern island of New Zealand; that the rates in Europe were generally lower than those in Australia and New Zealand; and that the death rates from melanoma in Canada were generally below those in the USA. From these data he concluded that, because melanoma rates were generally increased as the equator was approached, sunlight, and UV light in particular, was an important cause of melanoma.

Haenszel (1963) examined cancer incidence in eight to ten cities in the USA for 1947-1950 and showed that the incidence of melanoma was inversely related to latitude, the gradients being stronger for lesions on the face, head, neck and upper extremities than for lesions on the trunk and lower extremities.

Magnus (1973) showed that melanoma incidence in Norway was almost three times as high in the southern as in the northern part of the country.

Elwood *et al.* (1974) examined mortality from melanoma in 48 states of the USA and ten provinces of Canada in relation to latitude and to estimated exposure to UV light. They found a strong relationship between mortality, latitude (inverse) and estimated UV exposure for melanoma. The slope of the regression line for mortality against latitude was steeper for males than for the females.

Teppo *et al.* (1978) found a geographical gradient in cutaneous melanoma incidence in Finland, the highest rates occurring in the south of the country. This gradient largely disappeared, however, once urbanization was considered, the high rates in southern Finland being explained by the high rates of melanoma in urban areas, which are situated in the southern parts of the country.

Eklund and Malec (1978) noted a geographical gradient in cutaneous melanoma incidence in Sweden, the highest rates occurring in the south of the country.

Swerdlow (1979) analysed data on melanoma incidence in 14 health regions of England and Wales, noting a gradient with latitude, the highest rates of the disease occurring in southern England.

Baker-Blocker (1980) compared melanoma mortality in 18 counties of the USA with direct measurements of UV light, and found no significant correlation between the two.

Some additional exceptions to the general finding on latitude and melanoma of the skin have been reported. In Europe, for example, melanoma rates are higher in Scandinavia than in southern Europe (Lancaster, 1956; Crombie, 1979; Jensen & Bolander, 1980). Lancaster (1956) suggested that this may be an artefact due to international differences in recording, but it is now clear that the high rates of melanoma in Scandinavia are real (Crombie, 1979; Jensen & Bolander, 1980). Armstrong (1984) recently reviewed the worldwide variation in the incidence of melanoma and pointed out that the data are best fitted by a U-shaped curve relating melanoma incidence to latitude, with a minimum at about 52° latitude. He discussed several possible explanations for the south-to-north gradient in melanoma risk in Europe: the most plausible was the gradient in the opposite direction in skin pigmentation.

In Israel and Australia, other departures from the general association with latitude suggest that melanoma rates are especially high in coastal areas (Herron, 1969; Anaise *et al.*, 1978; Green & Siskind, 1983). In other populations, there are higher rates of melanoma in urban than in rural areas, and the effect of urbanization may be stronger than any local effect of latitude (Magnus, 1973; Teppo *et al.*, 1978; Holman *et al.*, 1980). A number of explanations have been put forward for these patterns, including the effects of summer cloud on transmission of solar UV, clothing habits and recreation (Armstrong, 1984).

Place of birth: Studies of migrants have demonstrated that persons born further from the equator than their newly adopted home have lower rates of melanoma than does the native-born population (Movshovitz & Modan, 1973; Anaise *et al.*, 1978; Holman *et al.*, 1980; Dobson & Leeder, 1982; Holman & Armstrong, 1984; Green *et al.*, 1986). The younger the age at emigration, or the longer the time since emigration, the more closely the melanoma rates approach those of the population of the newly adopted home (Anaise *et al.*,

1978; Holman *et al.*, 1980; Dobson & Leeder, 1982; Holman & Armstrong, 1984). Age at migration may be the more important of these two highly correlated variables. Moreover, unless people migrate towards the equator in childhood, their risk of melanoma may show little movement towards that of the native-born population of the adopted country (Holman & Armstrong, 1984).

(ii) *Exposure to sunlight*

Total exposure: Lancaster and Nelson (1957) compared 'excessive sun exposure' in 173 melanoma patients with that in 173 controls with cancers other than skin cancer. Of the patients with melanoma, 26.6% were assessed as having 'excessive exposure' as compared with 16.2% of controls [$p = 0.013$].

Gellin *et al.* (1969) interviewed 79 subjects with malignant melanoma and 1037 control patients attending the same dermatology clinic for non-tumour skin conditions. More than three hours were spent outdoors each day on average by 68% of those with melanoma compared to 37% of the control patients ($p < 0.01$). [The average ages of the two groups differed, and no account was taken of this in the analysis. Dermatology patients may not be an ideal comparison group since the amount of time they spend outdoors may be atypical.]

Green (1984) reported on total hours of sunlight exposure in 183 patients with melanoma in Queensland, Australia in 1979-1980, and in an equal number of age- and sex-matched controls chosen from the electoral register. Total hours of exposure to sunlight were estimated by summation of reported occupational and recreational sun hours for the whole of life, taking account of place of residence. Both native-born Australians and migrants to Australia were included in the analysis. She reported that, compared to a total sunlight exposure of 2000 hours, 2000-49 000 hours' exposure was associated with a crude relative risk of 2.0 and 50 000 or more hours exposure with a crude relative risk of 3.3. Neither risk estimate was significantly greater than 1.0.

Holman and Armstrong (1984) reported on a study of 511 patients with melanoma and 511 age- and sex-matched controls in Western Australia. Subjects were asked to give each location in which they had lived for a total of more than six months. Mean annual hours of bright sunshine received in each location were then read from a climatology map. For those who were born in Australia, the relative risks for mean annual hours of bright sunshine, averaged over all places of residence, were: <2600 hours, 1.00; 2600-2799 hours, 1.34; ≥2800 hours, 1.92 (p for trend = 0.003). When each histological type of melanoma was examined separately, the trend was strongest for lentigo maligna melanoma. Similarly, with measurement of chronic solar damage to the skin of the back of the hands by cutaneous microtopography (as an indirect measure of total accumulated UV dose), the relative risk of melanoma increased from 1.00 for damage of grades 1-3, to 1.64 for damage of grade 4, 1.76 for damage of grade 5 and 2.68 for damage of grade 6 ($p = 0.003$). The trend was again steepest for lentigo maligna melanoma.

Elwood *et al.* (1985a) reported on annual sun exposure from all sources assessed in their study in western Canada, described below. No general trend of increasing risk with increasing exposure was found.

Occupational exposure: Occupational groups with characteristically frequent outdoor exposure, such as farmers and fishermen, do not have increased rates of cutaneous melanoma, and, in some populations, the rates are less than for those with indoor occupations (Holman *et al.*, 1980; Lee & Strickland, 1980; Teppo *et al.*, 1980; Beral & Robinson, 1981; Cooke *et al.*, 1984). When melanoma of the head, face and neck was considered separately, an association with outdoor work was noted in England and Wales (Beral & Robinson, 1981). In New Zealand, however, no association was found between head-and-neck melanoma and outdoor occupation (Cooke *et al.*, 1984).

Melanoma is commoner among people of high social class (Holman *et al.*, 1980; Lee & Strickland, 1980; Beral & Robinson, 1981; Cooke *et al.*, 1984). In their analysis of incidence and mortality data in New Zealand, Cooke *et al.* (1984) reclassified occupations in terms of both social class and a three-step scale of outdoor exposure during work. Social-class gradients were observed in both outdoor and indoor workers, whereas there was no evidence of a difference in risk between outdoor and indoor workers of similar social class. [The possible role of factors other than sunlight which are related to social class has not generally been considered in studies of melanoma.]

Lancaster and Nelson (1957) found no clear association between melanoma and outdoor work among 67 men with melanoma and 67 controls with cancers other than skin cancer in Sydney, Australia. Compared to working indoors for less than five years, the estimated relative risk associated with working outdoors for 5-10 years was 0.8, and that with working outdoors for ten or more years was 1.2.

Klepp and Magnus (1979), in a case-control study of 78 patients with melanoma in Norway, reported that 40% of the 35 males and 12% of the 43 females with melanoma had worked outdoors, compared to 32% and 8% of 92 male and 39 female controls, respectively. The controls had either testicular cancer, malignant lymphoma or bone and soft-tissue sarcoma. [Possible confounding effects of age were not considered.]

Paffenbarger *et al.* (1978) found in a prospective study of 50 000 male alumni of US universities that outdoor work in youth was predictive of subsequent development of melanoma (relative risk, 3.9; $p < 0.01$).

Adam *et al.* (1981) found no difference in reported outdoor work history of 169 women aged 15-49 years in southern England with melanoma, compared to 507 age-matched controls chosen from general practioners' registers.

Elwood *et al.* (1985a), in their study of 595 subjects with melanoma other than lentigo maligna melanoma in western Canada and of a similar number of controls drawn at random from the same population, found no association between hours spent working outdoors per year and melanoma risk. Compared to those who spent less than one hour outdoors each summer, the relative risks were 1.8, 1.0, 0.9 and 0.9, respectively, for those spending 1-99, 100-199, 200-399 and 400+ hours outdoors. The 95% confidence intervals included unity in each case, except for the relative risk of 1.8, where the lower bound was 1.2. The response rate among controls was 48% in one centre and 59% in each of the others.

MacKie and Aitchison (1982) interviewed 113 Scottish patients with cutaneous malignant melanoma and 113 age- and sex-matched controls. Men with melanoma were less likely than the controls to have worked outdoors for more than 16 hours each week ($p < 0.05$).

Holman *et al.* (1986a), in their case-control study of 507 patients with melanoma of all types in western Australia, found a decreasing relative risk for melanoma with increasing weekly hours of outdoor work in summer, averaged over the working lifetime ($p = 0.1$). This negative relationship did not appear to apply to lentigo maligna melanoma. In those who had worked outdoors at all in summer, the relative risk for all melanomas was higher in people who usually or sometimes exposed the primary site to the sun (relative risks, 2.1 and 2.5, respectively) than in those who usually covered it ($p = 0.001$). [The possibility of confounding between duration of outdoor work and exposure of the site of melanoma was not considered.]

Green *et al.* (1986), in a case-control study of 236 cases of melanoma in Queensland, Australia, reported no association between melanoma and overall occupational exposure to the sun.

Recreational exposure: Lancaster and Nelson (1957), in the study described above in Sydney, Australia, found that 45% of patients with melanoma gave a history of fishing and 30% gave a history of sunbathing, compared to 49% and 22%, respectively, among the controls.

Klepp and Magnus (1979) found that 19.2% of cases with melanoma in Norway as opposed to 9.2% of controls had gone to southern Europe to sunbathe in the past. The associated relative risk of 2.4 was 'on the border of statistical significance at the 5% level'. [It is not clear whether the data were adjusted for age or sex.]

Adam *et al.* (1981) found that English women with melanoma were only slightly more likely than control women to tan their legs and trunk while abroad (legs: 78% of cases and 73% of controls; trunk: 70% and 67%).

Mackie and Aitchison (1982), in their study of 113 Scottish patients with melanoma and 113 controls, found that those with melanoma were less likely than controls to have spent more than 16 hours each week in outdoor recreational activities ($p < 0.05$). Numbers of continental holidays and total number of days spent in sunny climates were similar in the two groups.

Green *et al.* (1986), in their case-control study of 236 cases of melanoma in Queensland, Australia, found no strong association between recreational hours spent on the beach and risk of melanoma.

Elwood *et al.* (1985a), in their study from western Canada, reported that cases with melanoma spent more hours in outdoor summer recreation than did controls. Compared to those who spent less than one hour outdoors, the relative risks were 1.1, 1.7, 1.8 and 1.7, respectively (p for trend, <0.01), for those spending 1-19, 20-79, 80-159 and 160+ hours in recreation outdoors in the summer. They also reported that those with melanoma took more sunny vacations than controls; compared to those who took no sunny vacations, the relative risks were 1.1, 1.3 and 1.7, respectively, for less than one, one to three and four or more 'sunny vacations' per decade (p for trend, <0.001). These risk estimates were adjusted for hair and skin colour and history of freckling.

In a similar analysis of their 507 case-control pairs, Holman *et al.* (1986a) found no evidence of an effect of total average number of hours spent weekly at outdoor recreation. There were, however, some positive associations between the incidence of melanoma at specific body sites and particular types of outdoor recreation and clothing habits. For example, the relative risk of melanoma of the trunk in women who had usually worn a bikini or bathed nude at 15-24 years of age was 13.0 (95% confidence interval, 2.0-83.9) compared with those who had worn a one-piece bathing-suit with a high back-line. The relative risk associated with wearing a one-piece bathing-suit with a low back-line was intermediate.

The results of several case-control studies have suggested that sunburn may be associated with an increased subsequent risk of melanoma. In their study, MacKie and Aitchison (1982) found a positive association between a history of severe sunburn and risk of melanoma ($p < 0.05$). Green *et al.* (1986) found relative risks of 1.5 (95% confidence interval, 0.7-3.2) for two to five severe sunburns throughout life and 2.4 (95% confidence interval, 1.0-6.1) for six or more sunburns. Elwood *et al.* (1985b) found relative risks of 1.0 for a 'mild' vacation sunburn score, 1.2 for 'moderate', 1.3 for 'severe' and 1.8 for 'very severe' (p for trend, < 0.01) sunburns. They pointed out, however, that when allowance was made for hair colour, skin colour and freckles in adolescence the association disappeared. Similarly, Holman *et al.* (1986a) found no association between sunburn and all melanomas after adjusting for confounding (skin reaction to sunlight, hair colour, ethnic origin, age at arrival in Australia). There was, however, evidence of a residual effect of sunburn on the occurrence of lentigo maligna melanoma ($p = 0.06$).

Recreational exposure to the sun is intermittent. On the basis of the unusual distribution of age, site and occupation of melanoma patients, Fears *et al.* (1977) and McGovern (1977) suggested that intense exposure to sunlight over short periods may be more important than total exposure. Holman *et al.* (1986a), in their case-control study, noted that one measure of the intermittency of solar exposure — the proportion of total outdoor exposure that was recreational — showed no consistent association with risk of melanoma.

Other aspects: The diagnosis of melanoma follows a seasonal pattern, with highest rates occurring during the summer months (Malec & Eklund, 1978; Scotto & Nam, 1980; Hinds *et al.*, 1981; Holman & Armstrong, 1981). It is not clear whether this reflects seasonal changes in diagnosis or a true seasonal change in incidence, although Holman *et al.* (1983) found, on review of the histopathology of 216 melanocytic naevi, that a junctional component was most common in summer months, as was associated inflammation; more naevi diagnosed in the summer months showed mitotic activity (Armstrong *et al.*, 1984).

Houghton *et al.* (1978), in a study of cancer incidence statistics, reported that melanoma incidence fluctuates considerably at certain times, and that there are peaks about every eight to 11 years, lasting for three to five years. They pointed out that these peaks in incidence followed, by zero to two years, periods of sunspot activity. Incidence data from Connecticut and New York followed this general pattern. In Finland, the increased incidence rates were significantly correlated with years of sunspot activity and with the first subsequent year. Wigle (1978) reported a similar finding for Canada.

Swerdlow (1979) reported that fluctuations in melanoma incidence in women in the UK were correlated with the duration of sunny periods two years previously.

(iii)   *Exposure to other sources of UV light*

Beral *et al.* (1982), in a study of 274 women in Sydney aged 18-54 years who had melanoma, reported that working indoors with illumination from fluorescent light was associated with an increased risk of melanoma (RR, 2.1; 95% confidence limits, 1.32-3.32).

Pasternack *et al.* (1983), in a study of 136 patients with melanoma in New York, found that recent exposure to fluorescent light at work was associated with an increased risk of melanoma ($p < 0.01$); Rigel *et al.* (1983) found no such association in 114 patients with melanoma in New York.

A study in Western Australia of 337 cases and 349 controls also found little evidence that exposure to fluorescent light, at home or at work, causes melanoma. There was no overall association, and separate analyses by histological type and body site of melanoma showed, in most instances, no consistent association between incidence rate of melanoma and exposure to fluorescent light without diffusers (English *et al.*, 1985).

Elwood *et al.* (1986), in a case-control study of 83 patients with melanoma in the UK, found a positive trend in the relative risk for malignant melanoma with increasing total exposure to fluorescent light through occupation, which was not, however, statistically significant. In the highest exposure category (more than 50 000 hours), the relative risk was 1.4 for total exposure to fluorescent light and that for exposure to fluorescent lamps without diffusers was 4.0 (trend not statistically significant).

Klepp and Magnus (1979) reported no difference in the use of sunlamps to promote a tan by patients with melanoma compared to controls, but details were not given.

Adam *et al.* (1981) found that women in the UK with melanoma were more likely to have used such lamps in the past (8% *versus* 3%, $p < 0.05$).

In their case-control study of 511 patients with melanoma from Western Australia, Holman *et al.* (1986b) found no association between use of sunlamps and risk of melanoma.

(d)   *Melanoma of the eye*

Individuals with blue eyes and fair hair have a less dense retinal pigment epithelium than other individuals, thus allowing greater light transmission to the uvea. These characteristics have been associated with an increased incidence of ocular melanoma in two case-control studies, one in Canada (Gallagher *et al.*, 1985) and the other in the USA (Tucker *et al.*, 1985). Ocular melanoma is also more common in whites than in blacks or in Asians in the USA (Scotto *et al.*, 1976c; Waterhouse *et al.*, 1982).

(i)   *Latitude*

Melanoma of the eye is not usually distinguished from other cancers of the eye in statistics derived from whole populations (Waterhouse *et al.*, 1982). In the UK, however, it accounts for 80-90% of all eye cancers in adults (Swerdlow, 1983a); for whites, therefore, the incidence and mortality rates of all cancers of the eye may be taken as indicating the incidence and mortality of ocular melanoma (Swerdlow, 1983b). In the USA (Scotto *et al.*, 1976c) and in England and Wales (Swerdlow, 1983b), the incidence of eye cancers does not vary appreciably with latitude, and in Europe the gradient of their mortality in adults with latitude is the opposite of what would be expected from a simple direct relationship with exposure to the sun (Hakulinen *et al.*, 1978).

In a case-control study of 497 white cases and 501 white controls from Philadelphia, USA, Tucker *et al.* (1985) found that those born in the south of the USA had a higher incidence of ocular melanoma than those born in the north (relative risk, 2.7; 95% confidence interval, 1.3-5.9). There was, however, no consistent association between duration of residence in the south and incidence.

(ii)   *Exposure to sunlight*

In 65 case-control pairs from western Canada, Gallagher *et al.* (1985) found no association between ocular melanoma and cumulative lifetime exposure to sun, sun exposure in the decade before diagnosis or occupational, recreational or vacation sun exposure. In contrast, Tucker *et al.* (1985) found that sunbathing, gardening and increased sun exposure during vacations were associated with an increased risk of ocular melanoma, while hunting, camping, fishing and an estimate of total outdoor leisure time were not. Use of eye protection when in the sun (sunglasses, hats or sun visors) appeared to protect against ocular melanoma (relative risk, 1.6; 95% confidence interval, 1.2-2.2 in those who never, rarely or occasionally used protection relative to those who always used it). This effect was particularly strong for melanoma of the iris (relative risks, 3.2, 3.9 and 4.9 for occasional, rare and never use, respectively). Other sun-related effects, however, did not appear to be specific for melanoma of the iris.

(iii)   *Exposure to other sources of UV light*

The study of Tucker *et al.* (1985) found that subjects who had ever worked as welders were at greatly increased risk of ocular melanoma (relative risk, 10.9; 95% confidence interval, 2.1-56.5, relative to those who had never worked as welders).

4. Summary of Data Reported

4.1 Experimental data

Broad-band sources of ultraviolet radiation have been shown to induce skin tumours in at least ten strains of mice of different phenotypes. The most common skin tumour types were squamous-cell carcinoma of the exposed skin in the hairless strains and squamous-cell carcinoma and fibrosarcoma of the ear in the haired strains; other skin tumours occurred. Studies of broad-band ultraviolet radiation cannot identify the carcinogenic potential of different spectral regions. Glass filtration of ultraviolet radiation sources has implicated ultraviolet B radiation as the most potent part of the spectrum. In one study, mono-chromatic ultraviolet B radiation (at 300 nm and 310 nm) was carcinogenic to mouse skin. The few data on the carcinogenicity of ultraviolet A and C radiation *per se* are inconclusive.

Skin tumours were found in two strains of rat and in one strain of hamster after exposure to broad-band ultraviolet B radiation but were not observed in guinea-pigs.

Corneal tumours were observed in rodents after exposure to broad-band ultraviolet radiation.

Ultraviolet radiation in the A, B and C regions induces mutations in microorganisms and cultured mammalian cells. Ultraviolet B and C radiation induce chromosomal aberrations, sister chromatid exchanges (ultraviolet C only) and cell transformation in cultured mammalian cells. No information was available on the effect of ultraviolet A radiation on these endpoints.

4.2 Human data

(a) Non-melanocytic skin cancer

The distribution on the body of non-melanocytic skin cancer parallels closely the parts normally exposed to sunlight. In the USA there is a strong inverse relation between latitude and incidence of non-melanocytic skin cancers, but information from other countries is lacking. One study demonstrated a correlation between incidence of these malignancies in four regions of the USA and measured ultraviolet flux. Outdoor occupations, such as farming, are associated with an increased risk of non-melanocytic skin cancers. Four case-control studies were reviewed. All the findings were consistent in finding that exposure to sunlight is a risk factor, but the studies had major shortcomings. For example, controls for two of the studies were chosen from among dermatology patients, whose outdoor activities may have been affected by their illnesses. Furthermore, cases and controls were of different average ages, and this was not dealt with adequately in the analyses. One study reported a relationship between non-melanocytic skin cancers and the use of sunlamps, but again the study design was weak.

The constitutional, geographical and bodily distribution of non-melanocytic skin cancers is consistent with sunlight being a causal factor. This conclusion receives some support from several methodologically weak case-control studies.

There are no adequate data on which conclusions about the carcinogenic risk of other sources of ultraviolet light could be based.

(b) Lip cancer

The incidence of buccal cancers in the USA, most of which are lip cancers, is inversely related to latitude. Mortality from lip cancer is greater in people in occupational groups involving work out of doors. All five case-control studies reviewed showed consistent and strong associations with outdoor work.

All the evidence — direct and indirect — is consistent with sunlight being a causal factor in lip cancer.

There are no data on the role, if any, of sources of ultraviolet radiation other than sunlight in the etiology of cancer of the lip.

(c) Malignant melanoma of the skin

The distribution of melanomas on the skin does not correspond with the parts of the body most exposed to sunlight.

Mortality and incidence data from many parts of the world show an inverse relationship between melanoma rates and latitude. There are exceptions to this general finding. For example, melanoma rates are higher in the Scandinavian countries than in southern Europe; this could be due to the fact that Scandinavian people have fairer skins.

In one study in which melanoma mortality in 18 counties of the USA was compared with direct measurements of ultraviolet light, no significant correlation was found.

Several studies of migrants have shown that people born further from the equator than their newly adopted home have lower rates of melanoma than do the native-born populations.

Three case-control studies showed a positive association between estimates of total sun exposure and the risk of melanoma. In one of these, chronic solar damage to the skin was also commoner in patients with melanoma. One case-control study showed no general trend of increasing risk of melanoma with increasing annual exposure to the sun.

In five analyses of occupational mortality or incidence, outdoor workers were found to have no increased risk of melanoma. Outdoor work was also assessed in seven case-control studies. Five of these showed no association, while the other two showed a reduced risk in outdoor workers. In one cohort study, outdoor work in youth was associated with an increased risk of melanoma.

Recreational exposure to sunlight was investigated in seven case-control studies. One study showed an increasing risk of melanoma with increasing time spent in outdoor summer recreation and with increasing frequency of sunny vacations. In another study, although there was no evidence of an effect of total average number of hours spent weekly at outdoor recreation, there were some positive associations between melanoma at specific body sites and particular types of outdoor recreation and clothing habits. In one case-control study, patients with melanoma were less likely to have spent more than 16 hours each week in outdoor recreational activities.

Four case-control studies showed an increased risk of melanoma in patients with a history of severe sunburn, although in two instances the association disappeared when allowance was made for confounding by pigmentary characteristics.

Three case-control studies have shown some evidence of an increased risk of melanoma in people exposed to fluorescent light. In two other case-control studies, no such association was found.

In one case-control study, past use of sunlamps was reported by a higher proportion of women with melanoma than by the controls. Two other case-control studies found no association between use of sunlamps and risk of melanoma.

The constitutional risk factors and geographical distribution of malignant melanoma are consistent with exposure to sunlight playing a role in its etiology. This conclusion is supported by some of the results of analytical studies, but the data are not consistent with a simple, direct effect of sunlight.

There are conflicting data concerning the role of ultraviolet sources other than sunlight, and no conclusion can be drawn at present.

(d)   Melanoma of the eye

Cancers of the eye, the majority of which are melanomas in adults, are more common in white than in other populations. Descriptive studies, however, have found no consistent association between latitude of residence and incidence or mortality of these cancers. In two case-control studies, melanoma of the eye was associated with blue eyes and fair hair. In addition, in one of these studies, it was associated with birth near the equator and several indicators of exposure to the sun, and an increased incidence was found in welders.

Both the association of ocular melanoma with indicators of sun sensitivity and the direct link to sun exposure in one study are consistent with a role of sunlight in its etiology. The apparent lack of a consistent inverse relationship with latitude of residence, however, is discordant. On present evidence, therefore, an etiological role for sunlight is not established.

The association of melanoma of the eye with welding, if confirmed in other studies, would suggest an etiological role of ultraviolet light from sources other than the sun.

5. References

Adam, S.A., Sheaves, J.K., Wright, N.H., Mosser, G., Harris, R.W. & Vessey, M.P. (1981) A case-control study of the possible association between oral contraceptives and malignant melanoma. *Br. J. Cancer, 44*, 45-50

Anaise, D., Steinitz, R. & Ben Hur, N. (1978) Solar radiation: a possible etiological factor in malignant melanoma in Israel. A retrospective study (1960-1972). *Cancer, 42*, 299-304

Ananthaswamy, H.N. & Kripke, M.L. (1981) In vitro transformation of primary cultures of neonatal BALB/c mouse epidermal cells with ultraviolet-B radiation. *Cancer Res., 41*, 2882-2890

Anon. (1981) The aetiology of melanoma. *Lancet, i*, 253-255

Armstrong, B.K. (1984) Melanoma of the skin. *Br. med. Bull., 40*, 346-350

Armstrong, B.K., Holman, C.D.J., Ford, J.M. & Woodings, T.L. (1982) *Trends in melanoma incidence and mortality in Australia.* In: Magnus, K., ed., *Trends in Cancer Incidence: Causes and Practical Implications*, Washington DC, Hemisphere, pp. 399-417

Armstrong, B.K., Woodengs, T.L., Stenhouse, N.S. & McCall, M.G. (1983) *Mortality from Cancer in Migrants to Australia. 1962 to 1971*, Perth, University of Western Australia, pp. 21, 81-83

Armstrong, B.K., Heenan, P.J., Caruso, V., Glancy, R.J. & Holman, C.D.J. (1984) Seasonal variation in the junctional component of pigmented naevi. *Int. J. Cancer, 34*, 441-442

Atkin, M., Fenning, J., Heady, J.A., Kennaway, E.L. & Kennaway, N.M. (1949) The mortality from cancer of the skin and lip in certain occupations. *Br. J. Cancer, 3*, 1-15

Aubry, F. & MacGibbon, B. (1985) Risk factors of squamous cell carcinoma of the skin. A case-control study in the Montreal region. *Cancer, 55*, 907-911

Auerbach, H. (1961) Geographic variation in incidence of skin cancer in the United States. *Publ. Health Rep., 76*, 345-348

Baker-Blocker, A. (1980) Ultraviolet radiation and melanoma mortality in the United States. *Environ. Res., 23*, 24-28

Beral, V. & Robinson, N. (1981) The relationship of malignant melanoma, basal and squamous skin cancers to indoor and outdoor work. *Br. J. Cancer, 44*, 886-891

Beral, V., Evans, S., Shaw, H. & Milton, G. (1982) Malignant melanoma and exposure to fluorescent lighting at work. *Lancet, ii*, 290-293

Berger, D.S. (1976) The sunburning ultraviolet meter: design and performance. *Photochem. Photobiol., 24*, 587-593

Blum, H.F. (1948) Sunlight as a causal factor in cancer of the skin of man. *J. natl Cancer Inst., 9*, 247-258

Blum, H.F., Kirby-Smith, J.S. & Grady, H.G. (1941) Quantitative induction of tumors in mice with ultraviolet radiation. *J. natl Cancer Inst, 2*, 259-268

Blum, H.F., Butler, E.G., Dailey, T.H., Daube, J.R., Mawe, R.C. & Soffen, G.A. (1959) Irradiation of mouse skin with single doses of ultraviolet light. *J. natl Cancer Inst., 22*, 979-993

Bradley, M.O. & Sharkey, N.A. (1977) Mutagenicity and toxicity of visible fluorescent light to cultured mammalian cells. *Nature, 266*, 724-726

Burki, H.J. & Lam, C.K. (1978) Comparison of the lethal and mutagenic effects of gold and white fluorescent lights on cultured mammalian cells. *Mutat. Res., 54*, 373-377

Challoner, A.V.J., Corless, D., Davis, A., Deane, G.H.W., Diffey, B.L., Gupta, S.P. & Magnus, I.A. (1976) Personnel monitoring of exposure to ultraviolet radiation. *Clin. exp. Dermatol., 1*, 175-179

Challoner, A.V.J., Corbett, M.F., Davis, A., Diffey, B.L., Leach, J.F. & Magnus, I.A. (1978) Description and application of a personal ultraviolet dosimeter: a review of preliminary studies. *Natl Cancer Inst. Monogr., 50*, 97-100

Chan, G.L. & Little, J.B. (1976) Induction of oncogenic transformation *in vitro* by ultraviolet light. *Nature, 264*, 442-444

Chao, C.C.-K. & Rosenstein, B.S. (1985) Induction of sister-chromatid exchanges in ICR 2A frog cells exposed to 254 NM and solar UV wavelengths. *Photochem. Photobiol.*, *41*, 625-627

Cooke, K.R., Skegg, D.C.G. & Fraser, J. (1984) Socio-economic status, indoor and outdoor work, and malignant melanoma. *Int. J. Cancer*, *34*, 57-62

Crombie, I.K. (1979) Variation of melanoma incidence with latitude in North America and Europe. *Br. J. Cancer*, *40*, 774-781

Crombie, I.K. (1981) Distribution of malignant melanoma on the body surface. *Br. J. Cancer*, *43*, 842-849

Dardoni, L., Gafà, L., Paternò, R. & Parone, G. (1984) A case-control study on lip cancer risk factors in Ragusa (Sicily). *Int. J. Cancer*, *34*, 335-337

Davis, A., Deane, G.H.W. & Diffey, B.L. (1976) Possible dosimeter for ultraviolet radiation. *Nature*, *261*, 169-170

Davis, N.C., Herron, J.J. & McLeod, G.R. (1966) Malignant melanoma in Queensland: analysis of 400 skin lesions. *Lancet*, *ii*, 407-410

DeLuca, J.G., Weinstein, L. & Thilly, W.G. (1983) Ultraviolet light-induced mutation of diploid human lymphoblasts. *Mutat. Res.*, *107*, 347-370

Diffey, B.L. (1980) Ultraviolet radiation physics and the skin. *Phys. med. Biol.*, *25*, 405-426

Dobson, A.J. & Leeder, S.R. (1982) Mortality from malignant melanoma in Australia: effects due to country of birth. *Int. J. Epidemiol.*, *11*, 207-211

Doniger, J., Jacobson, E.D., Krell, K. & DiPaolo, J.A. (1981) Ultraviolet light action spectra for neoplastic transformation and lethality of Syrian hamster embryo cells correlate with spectrum for pyrimidine dimer formation in cellular DNA. *Proc. natl Acad. Sci. USA*, *78*, 2378-2382

Dorn, H.F. (1944a) Illness from cancer in the United States. I. Introduction. *Publ. Health Rep.*, *59*, 33-48

Dorn, H.F. (1944b) Illness from cancer in the United States. IV. Illness from cancer of specific sites classed in broad groups. *Publ. Health Rep.*, *59*, 65-77

Dorn, H.F. (1944c) Illness from cancer in the United States. VI. Regional differences in illness from cancer. *Publ. Health Rep.*, *59*, 97-115

Eklund, G. & Malec, E. (1978) Sunlight and incidence of cutaneous malignant melanoma. Effect of latitude and domicile in Sweden. *Scand. J. plast. reconstr. Surg.*, *12*, 231-241

Elwood, J.M. & Hislop, T.G. (1982) Solar radiation in the etiology of cutaneous malignant melanoma in Caucasians. *Natl Cancer Inst. Monogr.*, *62*, 167-171

Elwood, J.M., Lee, J.A.H., Walter, S.D., Mo, T. & Green, A.E.S. (1974) Relationship of melanoma and other skin cancer mortality to latitude and ultraviolet radiation in the United States and Canada. *Int. J. Epidemiol.*, *3*, 325-332

Elwood, J.M., Gallagher, R.P., Hill, G.B., Spinelli, J.J., Pearson, J.C.G. & Threfall, W. (1984) Pigmentation and skin reaction to sun as risk factors for cutaneous melanoma: Western Canada Melanoma Study. *Br. med. J.*, *288*, 99-102

Elwood, J.M., Gallagher, R.P., Hill, G.B. & Pearson, J.C.G. (1985a) Cutaneous melanoma in relation to intermittent and constant sun exposure — The Western Canada Melanoma Study. *Int. J. Cancer*, *35*, 427-433

Elwood, J.M., Gallagher, R.P., Davison, J. & Hill, G.B. (1985b) Sunburn, suntan and the risk of cutaneous malignant melanoma — The Western Canada Melanoma Study. *Br. J. Cancer*, *51*, 543-549

Elwood, J.M., Williamson, C. & Stapleton, P.J. (1986) Malignant melanoma in relation to moles, pigmentation, and exposure to fluorescent and other lighting sources. *Br. J. Cancer*, *53*, 65-74

Emmett, E.A. (1973) Ultraviolet radiation as a cause of skin tumors. *CRC crit. Rev. Toxicol.*, *2*, 211-255

English, D.R., Rouse, I.L., Xu, Z., Watt, J.D., Holman, C.D.J., Heenan, P.J. & Armstrong, B.K. (1985) Cutaneous malignant melanoma and fluorescent lighting. *J. natl Cancer Inst.*, *74*, 1191-1197

Epstein, J.H. (1978) Photocarcinogenesis: a review. *Natl Cancer Inst. Monogr.*, *50*, 13-25

Epstein, J.H. (1985) *Animal models for studying photocarcinogenesis*. In: Maibach, H.I. & Lowe, N.J., eds, *Models in Dermatology*, Vol. 2, Basel, Karger, pp. 302-312

Fears, T.R., Scotto, J. & Schneiderman, M.A. (1977) Mathematical models of age and ultraviolet effects on the incidence of skin cancer among whites in the United States. *Am. J. Epidemiol.*, *105*, 420-427

Findlay, G.M. (1928) Ultra-violet light and skin cancer. *Lancet*, *ii*, 1070-1075

Findlay, G.M. (1930) Cutaneous papillomata in the rat following exposure to ultraviolet light. *Lancet*, *i*, 1229-1231

Forbes, P.D. & Urbach, F. (1975) Experimental modification of photocarcinogenesis. I. Fluorescent whitening agents and short-wave UVR. *Food Cosmet. Toxicol.*, *13*, 335-337

Forbes, P.D., Blum, H.F. & Davies, R.E. (1981) Photocarcinogenesis in hairless mice: dose-response and the influence of dose-delivery. *Photochem. Photobiol.*, *34*, 361-365

Freeman, R.G. (1975) Data on the action spectrum for ultraviolet carcinogenesis. *J. natl Cancer Inst.*, *55*, 1119-1122

Freeman, R.G. & Knox, J.M. (1964) Ultraviolet-induced corneal tumors in different species and strains of animals. *J. invest. Dermatol.*, *43*, 431-436

Gallagher, C.H., Path, F.R.C., Canfield, P.J., Greenoak, G.E. & Reeve, V.E. (1984) Characterization and histogenesis of tumors in the hairless mouse produced by low-dosage incremental ultraviolet radiation. *J. invest. Dermatol.*, *83*, 169-174

Gallagher, R.P., ed. (1986) *Epidemiology of Malignant Melanoma* (*Recent Results in Cancer Research No. 102*), Berlin (West), Springer-Verlag

Gallagher, R.P., Elwood, J.M., Rootman, J., Spinelli, J.J., Hill, G.B., Threlfall, W.J. & Birdsell, J.M. (1985) Risk factors for ocular melanoma: Western Canada Melanoma Study. *J. natl Cancer Inst.*, *74*, 775-778

Gellin, G.A., Kopf, A.W. & Garfinkel, L. (1965) Basal cell epithelioma. A controlled study of associated factors. *Arch. Dermatol.*, *91*, 38-45

Gellin, G.A., Kopf, A.W. & Garfinkel, L. (1969) Malignant melanoma. A controlled study of possibly associated factors. *Arch. Dermatol.*, *99*, 43-48

Gibbs, N.K., Corbett, M.F. & Young, A.R. (1983) Personnel solar UVR exposure: a method of increasing the reliability of measurements made within film badge dosimeters (Abstract). *Photochem. Photobiol.*, *37*, 102

Grady, H.G., Blum, H.F. & Kirby-Smith, J.S. (1943) Types of tumor induced by ultraviolet radiation and factors influencing their relative incidence. *J. natl Cancer Inst.*, *3*, 371-378

Green, A. (1984) Sun exposure and the risk of melanoma. *Aust. J. Dermatol.*, *25*, 99-102

Green, A. & Siskind, V. (1983) Geographical distribution of cutaneous melanoma in Queensland. *Med. J. Aust.*, *i*, 407-410

Green, A.E.S., Findley, G.B., Jr, Klenk, K.F., Wilson, W.M. & Mo, T. (1976) The ultraviolet dose dependence of non-melanoma skin cancer incidence. *Photochem. Photobiol.*, *24*, 353-362

Green, A., Bain, C., MacLennan, R. & Siskind, B. (1986) Risk factors for cutaneous melanoma in Queensland. *Recent Results Cancer Res.*, *102*, 76-97

Griggs, H.G. & Bender, M.A. (1973) Photoreactivation of ultraviolet-induced chromosomal aberrations. *Science*, *179*, 86-88

de Gruijl, F.R., van der Meer, J.B. & van der Leun, J.C. (1983) Dose-time dependency of tumor formation by chronic UV exposure. *Photochem. Photobiol.*, *37*, 53-62

Haenszel, W. (1963) Variations in skin cancer incidence within the United States. *Natl Cancer Inst. Monogr.*, *10*, 225-243

Hakulinen, T., Teppo, L. & Saxén, E. (1978) Cancer of the eye, a review of trends and differentials. *World Health Stat. Q.*, *31*, 143-158

Hannan, M.A., Paul, M., Amer, M.H. & Al-Watban, F.H. (1984) Study of ultraviolet radiation and genotoxic effects of natural sunlight in relation to skin cancer in Saudi Arabia. *Cancer Res.*, *44*, 2192-2197

Herron, J. (1969) The geographical distribution of malignant melanoma in Queensland. *Med. J. Aust.*, *ii*, 892-894

Hinds, M.W., Lee, J. & Kolonel, L.N. (1981) Seasonal patterns of skin melanoma incidence in Hawaii. *Am. J. publ. Health*, *71*, 496-499

Holman, C.D.J. & Armstrong, B.K. (1984) Cutaneous malignant melanomas and indicators of total accumulated exposure to the sun: an analysis separating histogenetic types. *J. natl Cancer Inst.*, *73*, 75-82

Holman, C.D.J, Mulroney, E.D. & Armstrong, B.K. (1980) Epidemiology of pre-invasive and invasive malignant melanoma in Western Australia. *Int J. Cancer*, *25*, 317-323

Holman, C.D.J., Heenan, P.J., Caruso, V., Glancy, R.J. & Armstrong, B.K. (1983) Seasonal variation in the junctional component of pigmented naevi. *Int. J. Cancer*, *31*, 213-215

Holman, C.D.J., Armstrong, B.K. & Heenan, P.J. (1986a) Relationship of cutaneous malignant melanoma to individual sunlight-exposure habits. *J. natl Cancer Inst.*, *76*, 403-414

Holman, C.D.J., Armstrong, B.K., Heenan, P.J., Blackwell, J.B., Cumming, F.J., English, D.R., Holland, S., Kelsall, G.R.H., Matz, L.R., Rouse, I.L., Singh, A., Ten Seldam, R.E.J., Watt, J.D. & Xu, Z. (1986b) The causes of malignant melanoma: results from the West Australian Lions Melanoma Research Project. *Recent Results Cancer Res.*, *102*, 18-37

Holman, D. & Armstrong, B. (1981) Skin melanoma and seasonal patterns. *Am. J. Epidemiol.*, *113*, 202

Houghton, A., Munster, E.W. & Viola, M.V. (1978) Increased incidence of malignant melanoma after peaks of sunspot activity. *Lancet*, *i*, 759-760

Hsie, A.W., Li, A.P. & Machanoff, R. (1977) A fluence response study of lethality and mutagenicity of white, black, and blue fluorescent light, sunlamp, and sunlight irradiation in Chinese hamster ovary cells. *Mutat. Res.*, *45*, 333-342

Hsu, J., Forbes, P.D., Harber, L.C. & Lakow, E. (1975) Induction of skin tumors in hairless mice by a single exposure to UV radiation. *Photochem. Photobiol.*, *21*, 185-188

Hueper, W.C. (1942) Morphological aspects of experimental actinic and arsenic carcinomas in the skin of rats. *Cancer Res.*, *2*, 551-559

IARC (1980) *IARC Monographs on the Evaluation of the Carcinogenic Risk of Chemicals to Humans*, Vol. 24, *Some Naturally Occurring Substances*, Lyon, pp. 101-124

IARC (1982) *IARC Monographs on the Evaluation of the Carcinogenic Risk of Chemicals to Humans*, Suppl. 4, *Chemicals, Industrial Processes and Industries Associated with Cancer in Humans, IARC Monographs, Volumes 1 to 29*, Lyon, pp. 158-160

Institute for Defense Analyses (1975) *Impacts of Climatic Change on the Biosphere*, Part 1, *Ultraviolet Radiation Effects (CIAP [Climatic Impact Assessment Program] Monogr. No. 5; PB-247724)*, Arlington, VA, Science and Technology Division

Jacobson, E.D., Krell, K. & Dempsey, M.J. (1981) The wavelength dependence of ultraviolet light-induced cell killing and mutagenesis in L5178Y mouse lymphoma cells. *Photochem. Photobiol.*, *33*, 257-260

Jacobson, E.D., Krell, K., Dempsey, M.J., Lugo, M.H., Ellingson, O. & Hench, C.W., II (1978) Toxicity and mutagenicity of radiation from fluorescent lamps and a sunlamp in L5178Y mouse lymphoma cells. *Mutat. Res.*, *51*, 61-75

Jensen, O.M. & Bolander, A.M. (1980) Trends in malignant melanoma of the skin. *World Health Stat. Q.*, *33*, 2-26

Kantor, G.J. (1985) Effects of sunlight on mammalian cells. *Photochem. Photobiol.*, *41*, 741-746

Keller, A.Z. (1970) Cellular types, survival, race, nativity, occupations, habits and associated diseases in the pathogenesis of lip cancers. *Am. J. Epidemiol.*, *91*, 486-499

Kennedy, A.R., Ritter, M.A. & Little, J.B. (1980) Fluorescent light induces malignant transformation in mouse embryo cell cultures. *Science*, *207*, 1209-1211

Klepp, O. & Magnus, K. (1979) Some environmental and bodily characteristics of melanoma patients: a case-control study. *Int. J. Cancer, 23*, 482-486

Kligman, L.H. & Kligman, A.M. (1981) Histogenesis and progression of ultraviolet light-induced tumors in hairless mice. *J. natl Cancer Inst., 67*, 1289-1297

Kripke, M.L. (1977) Latency, histology, and antigenicity of tumors induced by ultraviolet light in three inbred mouse strains. *Cancer Res., 37*, 1395-1400

Kripke, M.L. & Sass, E.R., eds (1978) *Ultraviolet Carcinogenesis (Natl Cancer Inst. Monogr. 50)*, Washington DC, US Department of Health, Education, and Welfare

Kubitschek, H.E. (1967) Mutagenesis by near-visible light. *Science, 155*, 1545-1546

Lancaster, H.O. (1956) Some geographical aspects of the mortality from melanoma in Europeans. *Med. J. Aust., i*, 1082-1087

Lancaster, H.O. & Nelson, J. (1957) Sunlight as a cause of melanoma: a clinical survey. *Med. J. Aust., i*, 452-456

Larkö, O. & Diffey, B.L. (1983) Natural UV-B radiation received by people with outdoor, indoor, and mixed occupations and UV-B treatment of psoriasis. *Clin. exp. Dermatol., 8*, 279-285

Lee, J.A.H. & Strickland, D. (1980) Malignant melanoma: social status and outdoor work. *Br. J. Cancer, 41*, 757-763

Lee, J.A.H. & Yongchaiyudha, S. (1971) Incidence of and mortality from malignant melanoma by anatomical site. *J. natl Cancer Inst, 47*, 253-263

van der Leun, J.C. (1984) UV-carcinogenesis. *Photochem. Photobiol., 39*, 861-868

van der Leun, J.C. & van Weelden, H. (1983) Wavelength interactions in reactions of the skin to light (Abstract No. WAM-F8). *Photochem. Photobiol., 37*, S81

Lill, P.H. (1983) Latent period and antigenicity of murine tumors induced in C3H mice by short-wavelength ultraviolet radiation. *J. invest. Dermatol., 81*, 342-346

Lindqvist, C. (1979) Risk factors in lip cancer: a questionnaire survey. *Am. J. Epidemiol., 109*, 521-530

Lippincott, S.W. & Blum, H.F. (1943) Neoplasms and other lesions of the eye induced by ultraviolet radiation in strain A mice. *J. natl Cancer Inst., 3*, 545-554

Mackie, R.M. & Aitchison, T. (1982) Severe sunburn and subsequent risk of primary cutaneous malignant melanoma in Scotland. *Br. J. Cancer, 46*, 955-960

Madden, R.P. (1975) *Ultraviolet Transfer Standard Detectors and Evaluation and Calibration of NIOSH UV Hazard Monitor (DHEW (NIOSH) Publ. No. 75-131)*, Cincinnati, OH, National Institute for Occupational Safety and Health

Magnus, K. (1973) Incidence of malignant melanoma of the skin in Norway 1955-1970. Variations in time and space and solar radiation. *Cancer, 32*, 1275-1286

Maher, V.M., Dorney, D.J., Mendrala, A.L., Konze-Thomas, B. & McCormick, J.J. (1979) DNA excision-repair processes in human cells can eliminate the cytotoxic and mutagenic consequences of ultraviolet irradiation. *Mutat. Res., 62*, 311-323

Malec, E. & Eklund, G. (1978) The changing incidence of malignant melanoma of the skin in Sweden, 1959-1968. *Scand. J. plast. reconstr. Surg.*, *12*, 19-27

Maxwell, K.J. & Elwood, J.M. (1983) UV radiation from fluorescent lights. *Lancet*, *ii*, 579

Maxwell, K.J. & Elwood, J.M. (1986) Could melanoma be caused by fluorescent light? *Recent Results Cancer Res.*, *102*, 137-143

McGovern, V.J. (1977) Epidemiological aspects of melanoma: a review. *Pathology*, *9*, 233-241

McGovern, V.J., Shaw, H.M., Milton, G.W. & Farago, G.A. (1980) Is malignant melanoma arising in a Hutchinson's melanotic freckle a separate disease entity? *Histopathology*, *4*, 235-242

Movshovitz, M. & Modan, B. (1973) Role of sun exposure in the etiology of malignant melanomas: epidemiologic inference. *J. natl Cancer Inst*, *51*, 777-779

Myhr, B.C., Turnbull, D. & DiPaolo, J.A. (1979) Ultraviolet mutagenesis of normal and xeroderma pigmentosum variant human fibroblasts. *Mutat. Res.*, *62*, 341-353

Nishi, Y., Hasegawa, M.M., Taketomi, M., Ohkawa, Y. & Inui, N. (1984) Comparison of 6-thioguanine-resistant mutation and sister chromatid exchanges in Chinese hamster V79 cells with forty chemical and physical agents. *Cancer Res.*, *44*, 3270-3279

Office of Population Censuses and Surveys (1978) *Occupational Mortality. The Registrar General's Decennial Supplement for England and Wales 1970-72 (Series DS No. 1)*, London, Her Majesty's Stationery Office, p. 48

Paffenbarger, R.S., Jr, Wing, A.L. & Hyde, R.T. (1978) Characteristics in youth predictive of adult onset malignant lymphomas, melanomas, and leukaemias: brief communication. *J. natl Cancer Inst.*, *60*, 89-92

Parrington, J.M. (1972) Ultraviolet-induced chromosome aberrations and mitotic delay in human fibroblast cells. *Cytogenetics*, *11*, 117-131

Pasternack, B.S., Dubin, N. & Moseson, M. (1983) Malignant melanoma and exposure to fluorescent lighting at work. *Lancet*, *i*, 704

Patton, J.D., Rowan, L.A., Mendrala, A.L., Howell, J.N., Maher, V.M. & McCormick, J.J. (1984) Xeroderma pigmentosum fibroblasts including cells from XP variants are abnormally sensitive to the mutagenic and cytotoxic action of broad spectrum sunlight. *Photochem. Photobiol.*, *39*, 37-42

Peak, M.J., Peak, J.G., Moehring, M.P. & Webb, R.B. (1984) Ultraviolet action spectra for DNA dimer induction, lethality and mutagenesis in *Escherichia coli* with emphasis on the UVB region. *Photochem. Photobiol.*, *40*, 613-620

Pound, A.W. (1970) Induced cell proliferation and the initiation of skin tumour formation in mice by ultraviolet light. *Pathology*, *2*, 269-275

Putschar, W. & Holtz, F. (1930) Formation of skin tumour in rats after chronic exposure to ultraviolet radiation (Ger.). *Z. Krebsforsch.*, *33*, 219-260

Rigel, D.S., Friedman, R.J., Levenstein, M. & Greenwald, D.I. (1983) Malignant melanoma and exposure to fluorescent lighting at work. *Lancet*, *i*, 704

Robertson, F. (1978) Measurement of carcinogenic ultraviolet in sunlight. *Natl Cancer Inst. Monogr., 50*, 216-219

Roffo, A.H. (1934) Cancer and sun. Carcinomas and sarcomas produced by the action of sunlight (Fr.). *Bull. Assoc. fr. Etude Cancer, 23*, 590-616

Roffo, A.H. (1939) The physico-chemical etiology of cancer (Ger.). *Strahlentherapie, 66*, 328-350

Rosenstein, B.S. & Rosenstein, R.B. (1985) Induction of chromosome aberrations in ICR 2A frog cells exposed to 265-313 nm monochromatic ultraviolet wavelengths and photoreactivating light. *Photochem. Photobiol., 41*, 57-61

Ruff, R.E., Russell, P.B., Kaplan, S.D., Holt, B.R. & Ryan, J.W. (1978) *Results of Research Related to Stratospheric Ozone Protection (EPA 600/8-78-002; PB-284400)*, Washington DC, US Environmental Protection Agency

Rundel, R.D (1983) Promotional effects of ultraviolet radiation on human basal and squamous cell carcinoma. *Photochem. Photobiol., 38*, 569-575

Rundel, R.D. & Nachtweg, D.S. (1978) Skin cancer and ultraviolet radiation. *Photochem. Photobiol., 28*, 345-356

Russell, W.O., Wynne, E.S., Loquvam, G.S. & Mehl, D.A. (1956) Studies on bovine ocular squamous carcinoma ('cancer eye'). I. Pathological anatomy and historical review. *Cancer, 9*, 1-52

Schulze, R. (1970) *Climate of the Earth: variations in Radiation* (Ger.), Darmstradt, Steinkopf-Verlag, pp. 95-98

Schulze, R. (1978) Measurement of sunlight: the ultraviolet 'B' radiation in sunlight. *Natl Cancer Inst. Monogr., 50*, 213-215

Scotto, J. & Nam, J.-M. (1980) Skin melanoma and seasonal patterns. *Am. J. Epidemiol., 111*, 309-314

Scotto, J., Fears, T.R. & Gori, G.B. (1976a) Ultraviolet exposure patterns. *Environ. Res., 12*, 228-237

Scotto, J., Fears, T.R. & Gori, G.B. (1976b) *Measurements of Ultraviolet Radiation in the United States and Comparisons with Skin Cancer Data (DHEW (NIH) Publ. No. 76-1029)*, Washington DC, US Department of Health, Education, and Welfare

Scotto, J., Fraumeni, J.F., Jr & Lee, J.A.H. (1976c) Melanoma of the eye and other noncutaneous sites. Epidemiologic aspects. *J. natl Cancer Inst., 56*, 489-491

Scotto, J., Fears, T.R. & Fraumeni, J.F., Jr (1982) *Solar radiation*. In: Schottenfeld, D. & Fraumeni, J.F., Jr, eds, *Cancer Epidemiology and Prevention*, Philadelphia, W.B. Saunders Co., pp. 254-276

Setlow, R.B. (1974) The wavelengths in sunlight effective in producing skin cancer: a theoretical analysis. *Proc. natl Acad. Sci. USA, 71*, 3363-3366

Silverstone, H. & Gordon, D. (1966) Regional studies in skin cancer. Second report: wet tropical and subtropical coasts of Queensland. *Med. J. Aust., ii*, 733-740

Silverstone, H. & Searle, J.H.A. (1970) The epidemiology of skin cancer in Queensland: the influence of phenotype and environment. *Br. J. Cancer*, *24*, 235-252

Spikes, J.D., Kripke, M.L., Connor, R.J. & Eichwald, E.J. (1977) Time of appearance and histology of tumors induced in the dorsal skin of C3Hf mice by ultraviolet radiation from a mercury arc lamp. *J. natl Cancer Inst.*, *59*, 1637-1643

Spitzer, W.O., Hill, G.B., Chambers, L.W., Helliwell, B.E. & Murphy, H.B. (1975) The occupation of fishing as a risk factor in cancer of the lip. *New Engl. J. Med.*, *293*, 419-424

Staberg, B., Wulf, H.C., Klemp, P., Poulsen, T. & Brodthagen, H. (1983) The carcinogenic effect of UVA irradiation. *J. invest. Dermatol.*, *81*, 517-519

Stenbäck, F. (1975) Species-specific neoplastic progression by ultraviolet light on the skin of rats, guinea pigs, hamsters and mice. *Oncology*, *31*, 209-225

Strickland, P.T., Burns, F.J. & Albert, R.E. (1979) Induction of skin tumors in the rat by single exposure to ultraviolet radiation. *Photochem. Photobiol.*, *30*, 683-688

Suzuki, F., Han, A., Lankas, G.R., Utsumi, H. & Elkind, M.M. (1981) Spectral dependencies of killing, mutation and transformation in mammalian cells and their relevance to hazards caused by solar ultraviolet radiation. *Cancer Res.*, *41*, 4916-4924

Swerdlow, A.J. (1979) Incidence of malignant melanoma of the skin in England and Wales and its relationship to sunshine. *Br. med. J.*, *ii*, 1324-1327

Swerdlow, A.J. (1983a) Epidemiology of melanoma of the eye in the Oxford region, 1952-78. *Br. J. Cancer*, *47*, 311-313

Swerdlow, A.J. (1983b) Epidemiology of eye cancer in adults in England and Wales, 1962-1977. *Am. J. Epidemiol.*, *118*, 294-300

Swerdlow, A.J. (1985) Seasonality of presentation of cutaneous melanoma, squamous cell cancer and basal cell cancer in the Oxford region. *Br. J. Cancer*, *52*, 893-900

Tate, T.J., Diffey, B.L. & Davis, A. (1980) An ultraviolet radiation dosimeter based on the photosensitizing drug, nalidixic acid. *Photochem. Photobiol.*, *31*, 27-30

Teppo, L., Pakkanen, M. & Hakulinen, T. (1978) Sunlight as a risk factor of malignant melanoma of the skin. *Cancer*, *41*, 2018-2027

Teppo, L., Pukkala, E., Hakama, M., Hakulinen, T., Herva, A. & Saxen, E. (1980) Way of life and cancer incidence in Finland. A municipality-based ecological analysis. *Scand. J. soc. Med.*, *Suppl. 19*, 50-54

Tucker, M.A., Shields, J.A., Hartge, P., Augsburger, J., Hoover, R.N. & Fraumeni, J.F., Jr (1985) Sunlight exposure as risk factor for intraocular malignant melanoma. *New Engl. J. Med.*, *313*, 789-792

Tyrrell, R.M. (1982) *Cell inactivation and mutagenesis by solar ultraviolet radiation*. In: Helène, C., Charlier, M., Montenay-Garestier, T. & Laustriat, G., eds, *Trends in Photobiology*, New York, Plenum Press, pp. 155-172

Tyrrell, R.M. (1984) Mutagenic action of monochromatic UV radiation in the solar range on human cells. *Mutat. Res.*, *129*, 103-110

Tyrrell, R.M. & Webb, R.B. (1973) Reduced dimer excision in bacteria following near ultraviolet (365 nm) radiation. *Mutat. Res., 19*, 361-364

Tyrrell, R.M., Werfelli, P. & Moraes, E.C. (1984) Lethal action of ultraviolet and visible (blue-violet) radiations at defined wavelengths on human lymphoblastoid cells: action spectra and interaction sites. *Photochem. Photobiol., 39*, 183-189

Urbach, F., Davies, R.E. & Forbes, P.D. (1966) Ultraviolet radiation and skin cancer in man. *Adv. Biol. Skin, 7*, 195-214

Urbach, F., Epstein, J.H. & Forbes, P.D. (1974) *Ultraviolet carcinogenesis: experimental, global and genetic aspects.* In: Fitzpatrick, T.B., Pathak, M.A., Harber, L.C., Seiji, M. & Kukita, A., eds, *Sunlight and Man*, Tokyo, Tokyo University Press, pp. 259-283

Vitaliano, P.P. (1978) The use of logistic regression for modelling risk factors: with application to non-melanoma skin cancer. *Am. J. Epidemiol., 108*, 402-414

Vitaliano, P.P. & Urbach, F. (1980) The relative importance of risk factors in nonmelanoma carcinoma. *Arch. Dermatol., 116*, 454-456

Waterhouse, J., Muir, C., Shanmugaratnam, K. & Powell, J., eds (1982) *Cancer Incidence in Five Continents*, Vol. IV (*IARC Scientific Publications No. 42*), Lyon, International Agency for Research on Cancer, pp. 278-351

Webb, R.B. (1977) *Lethal and mutagenic effects of near-ultraviolet radiation.* In: Smith, K.C., ed., *Photochemical and Photobiological Reviews*, Vol. 2, New York, Plenum Press, pp. 169-261

Webb, R.B. & Malina, M.M. (1970) Mutagenic effects of near ultraviolet light and visible radiation energy on continuous culture of *Escherichia coli. Photochem. Photobiol., 12*, 457-468

Wells, R.L. & Han, A. (1984) Action spectra for killing and mutation of Chinese hamster cells exposed to mid- and near-ultraviolet monochromatic light. *Mutat. Res., 129*, 251-258

Whitaker, C.J., Lee, W.R. & Downes, J.E. (1979) Squamous cell skin cancer in the north-west of England, 1967-69, and its relation to occupation. *Br. J. ind. Med., 36*, 43-51

Wigle, D.T. (1978) Malignant melanoma of skin and sunspot activity. *Lancet, ii*, 38

Winkelmann, R.K., Zollman, P.E. & Baldes, E.J. (1965) Squamous cell carcinoma produced by ultraviolet light in hairless mice. *J. invest. Dermatol., 40*, 217-224

Withrow, T.J., Lugo, M.H. & Dempsey, M.J. (1980) Transformation of Balb 3T3 cells exposed to a germicidal UV lamp and a sunlamp. *Photochem. Photobiol., 31*, 135-141

World Health Organization (1979) *Ultraviolet Radiation* (*Environmental Health Criteria 14*), Geneva

Zelle, B., Reynolds, R.J., Kottenhagen, M.J., Schuite, A. & Lohman, P.H.M. (1980) The influence of the wavelength of ultraviolet radiation on survival, mutation induction and DNA repair in irradiated Chinese hamster cells. *Mutat. Res., 72*, 491-509

Zigman, S., Fowler, E. & Kraus, A.L. (1976) Black light induction of skin tumors in mice. *J. invest. Dermatol.*, *67*, 723-725

Zölzer, F. & Kiefer, J. (1983) Wavelength dependence of inactivation and mutagenesis in haploid yeast cells of different sensitivities. *Photochem. Photobiol.*, *37*, 39-48

Zölzer, F. & Kiefer, J. (1984) Wavelength dependence of inactivation and mutation induction to 6-thioguanine-resistance in V79 Chinese hamster fibroblasts. *Photochem. Photobiol.*, *40*, 49-53

SUPPLEMENTARY CORRIGENDA TO VOLUMES 1-39

Corrigenda covering volumes 1-6 appeared in volume 7; others appeared in volumes 8, 10-13 and 15-38.

Volume 18

p. 47   *Delete footnote*

Supplement 4

p. 149   paragraph 1, 2nd line from   *replace* extended [3-5] *by*
                       bottom   extended [3,4]

Volume 36

p.120   *Replace table by*

	Genetic activity			Cell transformation
	DNA damage	Mutation	Chromosomal effects	
Prokaryotes	+	+		
Fungi/Green plants		+	+	
Insects				
Mammalian cells (*in vitro*)			+	
Mammals (*in vivo*)			+	
Humans (*in vivo*)				
Degree of evidence in short-term tests for genetic activity: **Sufficient**				Cell transformation: No data

p. 208   Column 1, entry 3   *replace* Hogstedt *by* Högstedt

Volume 37

p. 73   Table 25, heading   *replace* μg/g *by* μg/kg

Volume 38

p. 40	Table 1	*delete the line* Osteoporosis... <0.1 *from section* Γ *and add to section* C
p. 41	section D, lines 6-7	*replace* osteoporosis, with its attendant risk of fractured neck of the femur *by* cancer of the endometrium

Volume 39

p. 169	section 3.3, paragraph 2, line 2	*replace* 1656 *by* 1662
p. 170	line 13	*delete* statistically significant
	line 13, after 278	*add* These SMRs were not statistically significant.
p. 248		*replace structure of caprolactam by*

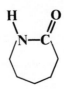

p. 322	Ulrich reference	*replace* Vol. 13 *by* Vol. 23

CUMULATIVE INDEX TO IARC MONOGRAPHS
ON THE EVALUATION OF THE CARCINOGENIC RISK
OF CHEMICALS TO HUMANS

Numbers in italics indicate volume, and other numbers indicate page. References to corrigenda are given in parentheses. Compounds marked with an asterisk(*) were considered by the working groups in the year indicated, but monographs were not prepared because adequate data on carcinogenicity were not available.

A

A-α-C (2-Amino-9*H*-pyrido[2,3-*b*]indole)	*40*, 245
Acetaldehyde	*36*, 101 (corr. *40*, 419)
Acetaldehyde formylmethylhydrazone	*31*, 163
Acetamide	*7*, 197
Acetylsalicylic acid (1976)*	
Acridine orange	*16*, 145
Acriflavinium chloride	*13*, 31
Acrolein	*19*, 479
	36, 133
Acrylamide	*39*, 41
Acrylic acid	*19*, 47
Acrylic fibres	*19*, 86
Acrylonitrile	*19*, 73
	Suppl. 4, 25
Acrylonitrile-butadiene-styrene copolymers	*19*, 9
Actinomycins	*10*, 29 (corr. *29*, 399; *34*, 197)
	Suppl. 4, 27
Adipic acid (1978)*	
Adriamycin	*10*, 43
	Suppl. 4, 29
AF-2	*31*, 47
Aflatoxins	*1*, 145 (corr. *7*, 319; *8*, 349)
	10, 51
	Suppl. 4, 31
Agaritine	*31*, 63
Aldrin	*5*, 25
	Suppl. 4, 35
Allyl chloride	*36*, 39

Benzene	7, 203 (corr. 11, 295)
	29, 93, 391
	Suppl. 4, 56 (corr. 35, 249)
Benzidine and its salts	1, 80
	29, 149, 391
	Suppl. 4, 57
Benzo[b]fluoranthene	3, 69
	32, 147
Benzo[j]fluoranthene	3, 82
	32, 155
Benzo[k]fluoranthene	32, 163
Benzo[ghi]fluoranthene	32, 171
Benzo[a]fluorene	32, 177
Benzo[b]fluorene	32, 183
Benzo[c]fluorene	32, 189
Benzo[ghi]perylene	32, 195
Benzo[c]phenanthrene	32, 205
Benzo[a]pyrene	3, 91
	Suppl. 4, 227
	32, 211
Benzo[e]pyrene	3, 137
	32, 225
para-Benzoquinone dioxime	29, 185
Benzotrichloride	29, 73
	Suppl. 4, 84
Benzoyl chloride	29, 83
	Suppl. 4, 84
Benzoyl peroxide	36, 267
Benzyl acetate	40, 109
Benzyl chloride	11, 217 (corr. 13, 243)
	29, 49 (corr. 30, 407)
	Suppl. 4, 84
Benzyl violet 4B	16, 153
Beryllium and beryllium compounds	1, 17
Bertrandite	23, 143 (corr. 25, 392)
Beryllium acetate	Suppl. 4, 60
Beryllium acetate, basic	
Beryllium-aluminium alloy	
Beryllium carbonate	
Beryllium chloride	
Beryllium-copper alloy	
Beryllium-copper-cobalt alloy	
Beryllium fluoride	
Beryllium hydroxide	
Beryllium-nickel alloy	
Beryllium oxide	
Beryllium phosphate	

Calcium saccharin	*22*, 120 (corr. *25*, 391)
	Suppl. 4, 225
Cantharidin	*10*, 79
Caprolactam	*19*, 115 (corr. *31*, 293)
	39, 247 (corr. *40*, 418)
Captan	*30*, 295
Carbaryl	*12*, 37
Carbazole	*32*, 239
3-Carbethoxypsoralen	*40*, 317
Carbon blacks	*3*, 22
	33, 35
Carbon tetrachloride	*1*, 53
	20, 371
	Suppl. 4, 74
Carmoisine	*8*, 83
Carpentry and joinery	*25*, 139
	Suppl. 4, 139
Carrageenan	*10*, 181 (corr. *11*, 295)
	31, 79
Catechol	*15*, 155
Chloramben (1982)*	
Chlorambucil	*9*, 125
	26, 115
	Suppl. 4, 77
Chloramphenicol	*10*, 85
	Suppl. 4, 79
Chlordane	*20*, 45 (corr. *25*, 391)
	Suppl. 4, 80
Chlordecone (Kepone)	*20*, 67
Chlordimeform	*30*, 61
Chlorinated dibenzodioxins	*15*, 41
	Suppl. 4, 211, 238
Chlorinated toluenes (production of)	*Suppl. 4*, 84
Chlormadinone acetate	*6*, 149
	21, 365
	Suppl. 4, 192
Chlorobenzilate	*5*, 75
	30, 73
1-(2-Chloroethyl)-3-cyclohexyl-1-nitrosourea (CCNU)	*26*, 173 (corr. *35*, 249)
	Suppl. 4, 83

Oestradiol-17β   6, 99
                                                  21, 279
                                                  Suppl. 4, 190
Oestradiol 3-benzoate   21, 281
Oestradiol dipropionate   21, 283
Oestradiol mustard   9, 217
Oestradiol-17β-valerate   21, 284
Oestriol   6, 117
                                                  21, 327
Oestrone   6, 123
                                                  21, 343 (corr. 25, 391)
                                                  Suppl. 4, 191
Oestrone benzoate   21, 345
                                                  Suppl. 4, 191
Oil Orange SS   8, 165
Oral contraceptives
  Combined   21, 103,133
                                                  Suppl. 4, 173
  Sequential   21, 111
                                                  Suppl. 4, 177
Orange I   8, 173
Orange G   8, 181
Oxazepam   13, 58
Oxymetholone   13, 131
                                                  Suppl. 4, 203
Oxyphenbutazone   13, 185

P

Panfuran S (Dihydroxymethylfuratrizine)   24, 77
Parasorbic acid   10, 199 (corr. 12, 271)
Parathion   30, 153
Patulin   10, 205
                                                  40, 83
Penicillic acid   10, 211
Pentachlorophenol   20, 203
                                                  Suppl. 4, 88, 205
Pentobarbital sodium (1976)*
Perylene   32, 411
Petasitenine   31, 207
Phenacetin   3, 141
                                                  24,135
                                                  Suppl. 4, 47

Polyvinyl chloride

7, 306
19, 402

Polyvinylidene fluoride (1978)*
Polyvinyl pyrrolidone

19, 463

Ponceau MX

8, 189

Ponceau 3R

8, 199

Ponceau SX

8, 207

Potassium bis(2-hydroxyethyl)dithiocarbamate

12, 183

Potassium bromate

40, 207

Prednisone

26, 293
Suppl. 4, 219

Procarbazine hydrochloride

26, 311
Suppl. 4, 220

Proflavine and its salts

24, 195

Progesterone

6, 135
21, 491 (corr. 25, 391)
Suppl. 4, 202

Pronetalol hydrochloride

13, 227 (corr. 16, 387)

1,3-Propane sultone

4, 253 (corr. 13, 243; 20, 591)

Propham

12, 189

β-Propiolactone

4, 259 (corr. 15, 341)

n-Propyl carbamate

12, 201

Propylene

19, 213

Propylene oxide

11, 191
36, 227 (corr. 38, 397)

Propylthiouracil

7, 67
Suppl. 4, 222

The pulp and paper industry

25, 157
Suppl. 4, 144

Pyrazinamide (1976)*
Pyrene

32, 431

Pyrido[3,4-c]psoralen

40, 349

Pyrimethamine

13, 233

Pyrrolizidine alkaloids

10, 333

Q

Quercetin

31, 213

Quinoestradol (1978)*
Quinoestrol (1978)*
para-Quinone

15, 255

Quintozene (Pentachloronitrobenzene)

5, 211

R

Reserpine

10, 217
24, 211 (corr. 26, 387; 30, 407)
Suppl. 4, 222

Urethane   *7*, 111

V

Vinblastine sulphate   *26*, 349 (corr. *34*, 197)
                                                Suppl. 4, 257
Vincristine sulphate   *26, 365*
                                                Suppl. 4, 259
Vinyl acetate   *19*, 341
                                                39, 113
Vinyl bromide   *19*, 367
                                                39, 133
Vinyl chloride   *7*, 291
                                                19, 377
                                                Suppl. 4, 260
Vinyl chloride-vinyl acetate copolymers   *7*, 311
                                                19, 412
4-Vinylcyclohexene   *11*, 277
                                                39, 181
Vinyl fluoride   *39*, 147
Vinylidene chloride   *19*, 439
                                                Suppl. 4, 262 (corr. *31*, 293)
                                                39, 195
Vinylidene chloride-vinyl chloride copolymers   *19*, 448

Vinylidene fluoride   *39*, 227
N-Vinyl-2-pyrrolidine   *19*, 461

X

2,4-Xylidine and its hydrochloride   *16*, 367
2,5-Xylidine and its hydrochloride   *16*, 377
2,6-Xylidine (1977)*

Y

Yellow AB   *8*, 279
Yellow OB   *8*, 287

Z

Zearalenone   *31*, 279
Zectran   *12*, 237
Zineb   *12*, 245
Ziram   *12*, 259

PUBLICATIONS OF THE INTERNATIONAL AGENCY FOR RESEARCH ON CANCER

SCIENTIFIC PUBLICATIONS SERIES

(Available from Oxford University Press)

SCIENTIFIC PUBLICATIONS SERIES

SCIENTIFIC PUBLICATIONS SERIES

No. 36 CANCER MORTALITY BY
OCCUPATION AND SOCIAL CLASS
1851-1971 (1982)
By W.P.D. Logan
253 pages

No. 37 LABORATORY DECONTAMI-
NATION AND DESTRUCTION OF
AFLATOXINS B_1, B_2, G_1, G_2 IN
LABORATORY WASTES (1980)
Edited by M. Castegnaro, D.C. Hunt,
E.B. Sansone, P.L. Schuller,
M.G. Siriwardana, G.M. Telling,
H.P. Van Egmond & E.A. Walker,
59 pages

No. 38 DIRECTORY OF ON-GOING
RESEARCH IN CANCER EPI-
DEMIOLOGY 1981 (1981)
Edited by C.S. Muir & G. Wagner,
696 pages; out of print

No. 39 HOST FACTORS IN HUMAN
CARCINOGENESIS (1982)
Edited by H. Bartsch & B. Armstrong
583 pages

No. 40 ENVIRONMENTAL CARCINOGENS
SELECTED METHODS OF ANALYSIS
Editor-in-Chief H. Egan
Vol. 4. SOME AROMATIC AMINES AND
AZO DYES IN THE GENERAL AND
INDUSTRIAL ENVIRONMENT (1981)
Edited by L. Fishbein, M. Castegnaro,
I.K. O'Neill & H. Bartsch
347 pages

No. 41 N-NITROSO COMPOUNDS:
OCCURRENCE AND BIOLOGICAL
EFFECTS (1982)
Edited by H. Bartsch, I.K. O'Neill,
M. Castegnaro & M. Okada,
755 pages

No. 42 CANCER INCIDENCE IN FIVE
CONTINENTS. VOLUME IV (1982)
Edited by J. Waterhouse, C. Muir,
K. Shanmugaratnam & J. Powell,
811 pages

No. 43 LABORATORY DECONTAMI-
NATION AND DESTRUCTION OF
CARCINOGENS IN LABORATORY
WASTES: SOME N-NITROSAMINES
(1982) Edited by M. Castegnaro,
G. Eisenbrand, G. Ellen, L. Keefer,
D. Klein, E.B. Sansone, D. Spincer,
G. Telling & K. Webb
73 pages

No. 44 ENVIRONMENTAL CARCINOGENS.
SELECTED METHODS OF ANALYSIS
Editor-in-Chief H. Egan
Vol. 5. SOME MYCOTOXINS (1983)
Edited by L. Stoloff, M. Castegnaro,
P. Scott, I.K. O'Neill & H. Bartsch,
455 pages

No. 45 ENVIRONMENTAL CARCINOGENS.
SELECTED METHODS OF ANALYSIS
Editor-in-Chief H. Egan
Vol. 6: N-NITROSO COMPOUNDS
(1983)
Edited by R. Preussmann, I.K. O'Neill,
G. Eisenbrand, B. Spiegelhalder &
H. Bartsch
508 pages

No. 46 DIRECTORY OF ON-GOING
RESEARCH IN CANCER EPI-
DEMIOLOGY 1982 (1982)
Edited by C.S. Muir & G. Wagner,
722 pages; out of print

No. 47 CANCER INCIDENCE IN
SINGAPORE (1982)
Edited by K. Shanmugaratnam, H.P. Lee
& N.E. Day
174 pages; out of print

No. 48 CANCER INCIDENCE IN
THE USSR Second Revised
Edition (1983)
Edited by N.P. Napalkov,
G.F. Tserkovny, V.M. Merabishvili,
D.M. Parkin, M. Smans & C.S. Muir,
75 pages

No. 49 LABORATORY DECONTAMI-
NATION AND DESTRUCTION OF
CARCINOGENS IN LABORATORY
WASTES: SOME POLYCYCLIC
AROMATIC HYDROCARBONS (1983)
Edited by M. Castegnaro, G. Grimmer,
O. Hutzinger, W. Karcher, H. Kunte,
M. Lafontaine, E.B. Sansone, G. Telling
& S.P. Tucker
81 pages

No. 50 DIRECTORY OF ON-GOING
RESEARCH IN CANCER EPI-
DEMIOLOGY 1983 (1983)
Edited by C.S. Muir & G. Wagner,
740 pages; out of print

No. 51 MODULATORS OF EXPERI-
MENTAL CARCINOGENESIS (1983)
Edited by V. Turusov & R. Montesano
307 pages

No. 52 SECOND CANCER IN
RELATION TO RADIATION
TREATMENT FOR CERVICAL
CANCER: RESULTS OF A CANCER
REGISTRY COLLABORATION (1984)
Edited by N.E. Day & J.C. Boice, Jr,
207 pages

No. 53 NICKEL IN THE HUMAN
ENVIRONMENT (1984)
Editor-in-Chief, F.W. Sunderman, Jr,
529 pages

No. 54 LABORATORY DECONTAMI-
NATION AND DESTRUCTION OF
CARCINOGENS IN LABORATORY WASTES:
SOME HYDRAZINES (1983)
Edited by M. Castegnaro, G. Ellen,
M. Lafontaine, H.C. van der Plas,
E.B. Sansone & S.P. Tucker,
87 pages

No. 55 LABORATORY DECONTAMI-
NATION AND DESTRUCTION OF
CARCINOGENS IN LABORATORY WASTES:
SOME N-NITROSAMIDES (1984)
Edited by M. Castegnaro,
M. Benard, L.W. van Broekhoven,
D. Fine, R. Massey, E.B. Sansone,
P.L.R. Smith, B. Spiegelhalder,
A. Stacchini, G. Telling & J.J. Vallon,
65 pages

No. 56 MODELS, MECHANISMS AND
ETIOLOGY OF TUMOUR PROMOTION
(1984)
Edited by M. Börszönyi, N.E. Day,
K. Lapis & H. Yamasaki
532 pages

No. 57 N-NITROSO COMPOUNDS:
OCCURRENCE, BIOLOGICAL EFFECTS
AND RELEVANCE TO HUMAN
CANCER (1984)
Edited by I.K. O'Neill, R.C. von Borstel,
C.T. Miller, J. Long & H. Bartsch,
1013 pages

No. 58 AGE-RELATED FACTORS
IN CARCINOGENESIS (1985)
Edited by A. Likhachev, V. Anisimov
& R. Montesano
288 pages

No. 59 MONITORING HUMAN
EXPOSURE TO CARCINOGENIC AND
MUTAGENIC AGENTS (1984)
Edited by A. Berlin, M. Draper,
K. Hemminki & H. Vainio
457 pages

No. 60 BURKITT'S LYMPHOMA: A
HUMAN CANCER MODEL (1985)
Edited by G. Lenoir, G. O'Conor
& C.L.M. Olweny
484 pages

No. 61 LABORATORY DECONTAMI-
NATION AND DESTRUCTION OF
CARCINOGENS IN LABORATORY
WASTES: SOME HALOETHERS (1984)
Edited by M. Castegnaro,
M. Alvarez, M. Iovu, E.B. Sansone,
G.M. Telling & D.T. Williams
55 pages

No. 62 DIRECTORY OF ON-GOING
RESEARCH IN CANCER EPI-
DEMIOLOGY 1984 (1984)
Edited by C.S. Muir & G.Wagner 728 pages

No. 63 VIRUS-ASSOCIATED CANCERS
IN AFRICA (1984)
Edited by A.O. Williams, G.T. O'Conor,
G.B. de-Thé & C.A. Johnson,
773 pages

No. 64 LABORATORY DECONTAMI-
NATION AND DESTRUCTION OF
CARCINOGENS IN LABORATORY
WASTES: SOME AROMATIC AMINES
AND 4-NITROBIPHENYL (1985)
Edited by M. Castegnaro, J. Barek,
J. Dennis, G. Ellen, M. Klibanov,
M. Lafontaine, R. Mitchum,
P. Van Roosmalen, E.B. Sansone,
L.A. Sternson & M. Vahl
85 pages

No. 65 INTERPRETATION OF NEGATIVE
EPIDEMIOLOGICAL EVIDENCE FOR
CARCINOGENICITY (1985)
Edited by N.J. Wald & R. Doll
232 pages

No. 66 THE ROLE OF THE REGISTRY
IN CANCER CONTROL (1985)
Edited by D.M. Parkin, G. Wagner
& C.S. Muir
155 pages

SCIENTIFIC PUBLICATIONS SERIES

NON-SERIAL PUBLICATIONS

(Available from IARC)

ALCOOL ET CANCER (1978)
By A.J. Tuyns (in French only)
42 pages

CANCER MORBIDITY AND CAUSES OF
DEATH AMONG DANISH BREWERY
WORKERS (1980)
By O.M. Jensen
145 pages

DIRECTORY OF COMPUTER SYSTEMS
USED IN CANCER REGISTRIES (1986)
By H.R. Menck & D.M. Parkin
236 pages

IARC MONOGRAPHS ON THE EVALUATION OF THE CARCINOGENIC RISK OF CHEMICALS TO HUMANS

(English editions only)

(Available from WHO Sales Agents)

IARC MONOGRAPHS SERIES

Volume 23
Some metals and metallic compounds (1980)
438 pp.

Volume 24
Some pharmaceutical drugs (1980)
337 pp.

Volume 25
Wood, leather and some associated industries (1981)
412 pp.

Volume 26
Some antineoplastic and immuno-suppressive agents
(1981)
411 pp.

Volume 27
Some aromatic amines, anthraquinones and nitroso
compounds, and inorganic
fluorides used in drinking-water and
dental preparations (1982)
341 pp.

Volume 28
The rubber industry (1982)
486 pp.

Volume 29
Some industrial chemicals and dyestuffs (1982)
416 pp.

Volume 30
Miscellaneous pesticides (1983)
424 pp.

Volume 31
Some food additives, feed additives and
naturally occurring substances (1983)
314 pp.

Volume 32
Polynuclear aromatic compounds,
Part 1, Environmental and experimental data (1984)
477 pp.

Volume 33
Polynuclear aromatic compounds, Part 2, Carbon
blacks, mineral oils and some nitroarene compounds
(1984)
245 pp.

Volume 34
Polynuclear aromatic compounds,
Part 3, Industrial exposures
in aluminium production, coal gasification, coke
production, and iron and steel founding (1984)
219 pp.

Volume 35
Polynuclear aromatic compounds,
Part 4, Bitumens, coal-tar and
derived products, shale-oils and soots
(1985)
271 pp.

Volume 36
Allyl Compounds, aldehydes,
epoxides and peroxides (1985)
369 pp.

Volume 37
Tobacco habits other than smoking; betel-quid and
areca-nut chewing;
and some related nitrosamines (1985)
291 pp.

Volume 38
Tobacco smoking (1986)
421 pp.

Volume 39
Some chemicals used in plastics and elastomers
(1986)
403 pp.

Volume 40
Some naturally occurring and synthetic food
components, furocoumarins and ultra-violet
radiation (1986)
444 pp.

Volume 41
Some halogenated hydrocarbons and pesticide
exposures (1986)
434 pp.

Supplement No. 1
Chemicals and industrial processes associated with
cancer in humans (IARC Monographs,
Volumes 1 to 20) (1979)
71 pp.; out of print

Supplement No. 2
Long-term and short-term screening assays
for carcinogens: a critical appraisal (1980)
426 pp.; US$25.00; Sw.fr. 40.-

Supplement No. 3
Cross index of synonyms and trade
names in Volumes 1 to 26 (1982)
199 pp.

Supplement No. 4
Chemicals, industrial processes and
industries associated with cancer in humans
(IARC Monographs, Volumes 1 to 29) (1982)
292 pp.

Supplement No. 5
*Cross index of synonyms and trade
names in Volumes 1 to 36* (1985)
259 pp.

INFORMATION BULLETINS ON THE
SURVEY OF CHEMICALS BEING
TESTED FOR CARCINOGENICITY

(Available from IARC)

No. 8 (1979)
Edited by M.-J. Ghess, H. Bartsch
& L. Tomatis
604 pp.; US$20.00; Sw.fr. 40.-

No. 9 (1981)
Edited by M.-J. Ghess, J.D. Wilbourn,
H. Bartsch & L. Tomatis
294 pp.; US$20.00; Sw.fr. 41.-

No. 10 (1982)
Edited by M.-J. Ghess, J.D. Wilbourn
H. Bartsch
326 pp.; US$20.00; Sw.fr. 42.-

No. 11 (1984)
Edited by M.-J. Ghess, J.D. Wilbourn,
H. Vainio & H. Bartsch
336 pp.; US$20.00; Sw.fr. 48.-

No. 12 (1986)
Edited by M.-J. Ghess, J.D. Wilbourn,
A. Tossavainen & H. Vainio
389 pp.